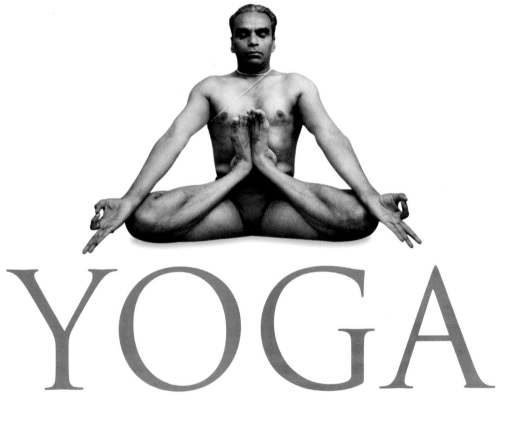

YOGA

THE PATH TO HOLISTIC HEALTH

Dorling **DK** Kindersley

LONDON, NEW YORK, SYDNEY, DELHI, PARIS,
MUNICH, and JOHANNESBURG

PROJECT EDITOR: Ranjana Sengupta
PROJECT DESIGNER: Aparna Sharma
EDITORS: Dipali Singh, Sheema Mookherjee
DESIGNERS: Ankita Saha, Nikki Duggal
DTP SUPPORT: Sunil Sharma
MANAGING EDITOR: Prita Maitra
MANAGING ART EDITOR: Shuka Jain

US EDITORIAL DIRECTOR: LaVonne Carlson
US PROJECT EDITOR: Barbara Minton
US CONSULTANT: Joan Budilovsky
US EDITOR: Jennifer Quasha

◆

First published in Great Britain in 2001
by Dorling Kindersley Limited
80 Strand, London, WC2R ORL

A Library of Congress catalog card number is available upon request

ISBN 0–7894–7165–5

◆

Reproduced by Colorscan, Singapore
Printed in China by Toppan

◆

see our complete product line at
www.dk.com

YOGA

THE PATH TO HOLISTIC HEALTH

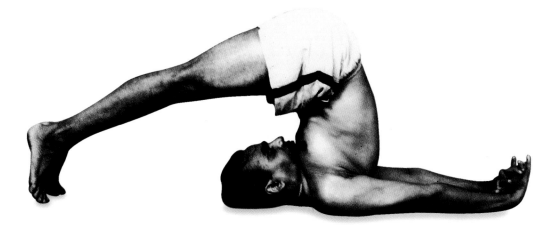

B.K.S. IYENGAR

A DORLING KINDERSLEY BOOK

Contents

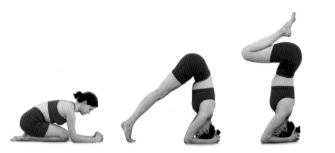

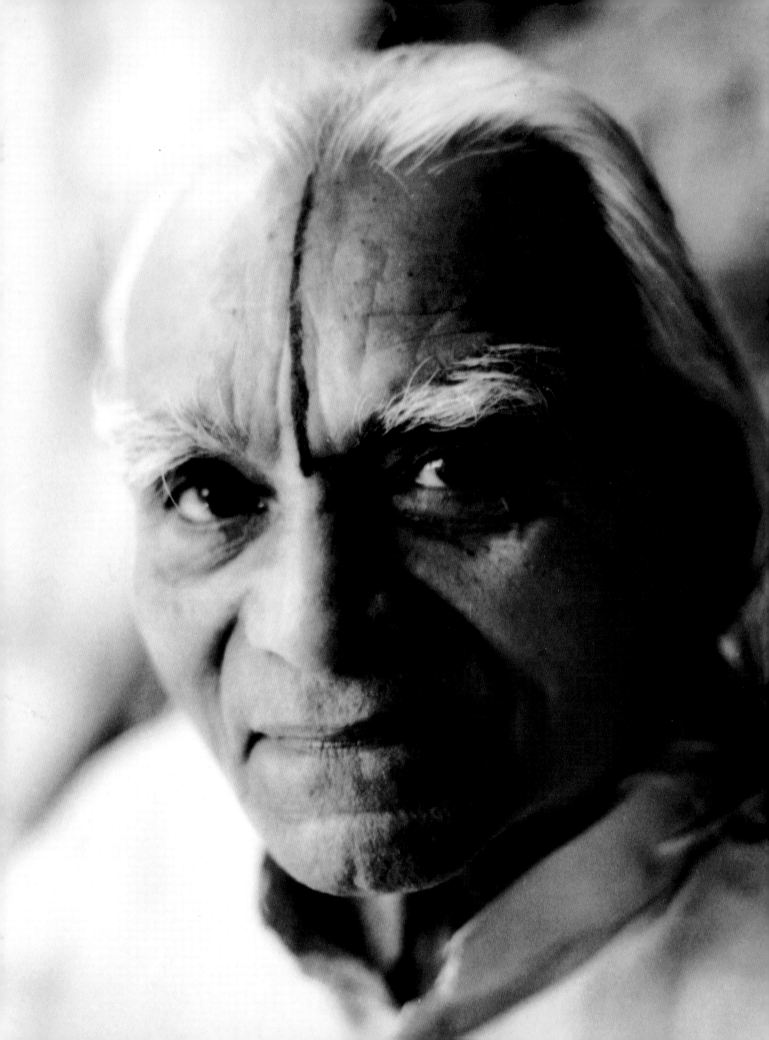

FOREWORD

by Yogacharya B.K.S. Iyengar

Yoga is for everyone. You do not need to be an expert or at the peak of physical fitness to practice the asanas described in this book. The strain of modern life can lead to physical pain and illness, as our bodies' well being is neglected in the race for material success. The stress of modern life can also lead to mental suffering like feelings of inadequacy, isolation, or powerlessness. Yoga helps integrate the mental and the physical plane, and it offers a sense of inner and outer balance, or *alignment*. True alignment means that the inner mind reaches every cell and fiber of the body.

During my sixty years of teaching and practicing yoga, I have observed that some students only pay attention to the physical aspect of yoga. Their practice is like a fast-flowing stream, tumbling and falling, which lacks depth and direction. By attending to the mental and spiritual side of yoga, a sincere student becomes like a smoothly flowing river, irrigating and fertilizing the land around it. Just as one cannot dip into the same river twice, so each and every asana refreshes your life force with new energy each time you practice it.

This book focuses on techniques, so that even a beginner will have a thorough understanding of how to practice the asanas in order to obtain the maximum benefit. By using a few simple props, students with different capabilities can gradually build up strength, confidence, and flexibility without the threat of strain or injury. The yoga techniques described and illustrated in this book can also help those with specific ailments. Regular practice builds up the body's inner strength and natural resistance, helps alleviate pain, and tackles the root, rather than the symptoms, of the problem. Across the world, there is now a growing awareness that alternative therapies are more conducive to health than conventional ones. It is my hope that this book will help all those who want to change their lives through yoga. May yoga's blessing be on all of you.

CHAPTER 1

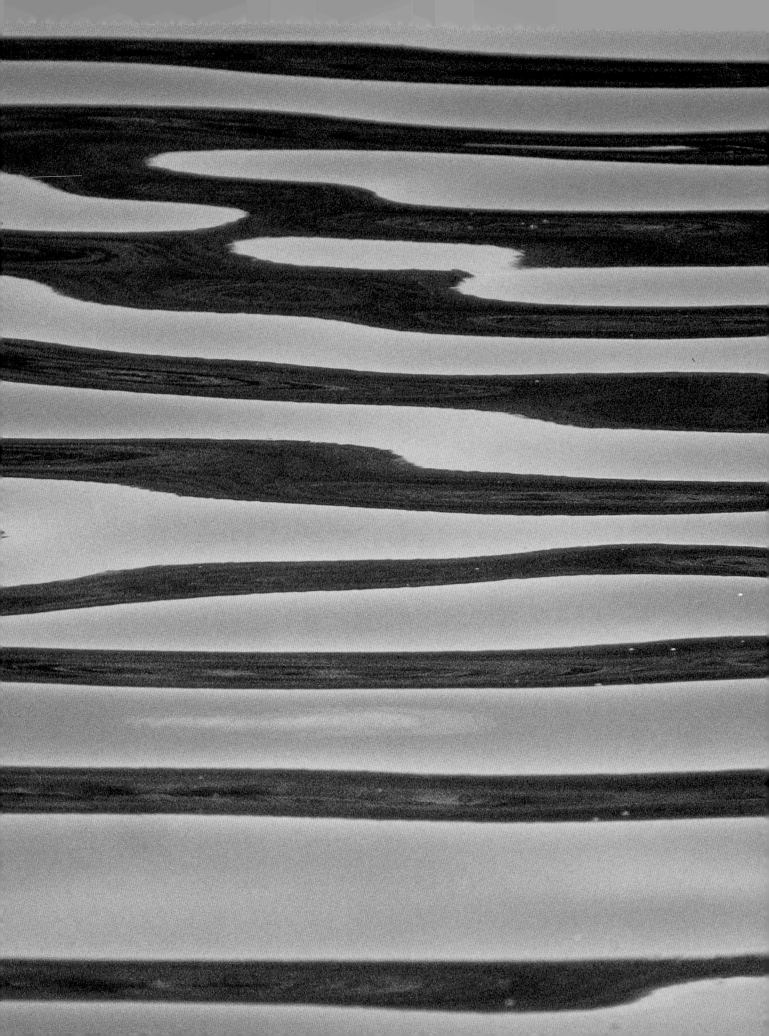

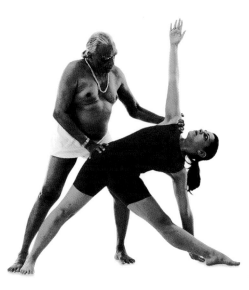

"Yoga is a light which, once lit, will never dim. The better your practice, the brighter the flame."

Yoga for You

The primary aim of yoga is to restore the mind to simplicity and peace, and free it from confusion and distress. This sense of calm comes from the practice of yogic asanas and pranayama. Unlike other forms of exercise which strain muscles and bones, yoga gently rejuvenates the body. By restoring the body, yoga frees the mind from the negative feelings caused by the fast pace of modern life. The practice of yoga fills up the reservoirs of hope and optimism within you. It helps you overcome all obstacles on the path to perfect health and spiritual contentment. It is a rebirth.

Aims of Yoga

*The practice of yoga aims to overcome the limitations of the body.
Yoga teaches us that the goal of every individual's life is to take the inner journey
to the soul. Yoga offers both the goal and the means to reach it.*

When there is perfect harmony between body and mind, we achieve self-realization. Yoga teaches us that the obstacles in the path of our self-realization show themselves in a physical or mental indisposition. When our physical state is not perfect it causes an imbalance in our mental state, which is known in Sanskrit as *chittavritti*. The practice of yoga helps us overcome that imbalance. Yogic asanas, or postures, can cure *vyadhi*, or physical ailments, and redress *angamejaytatva*, or unsteadiness, in the body. *Shvasa-prashvasa*, which translates as "uneven respiration," an indication of stress, is alleviated by the practice of yoga. Asanas tone the whole body. They strengthen bones and muscles, correct posture, improve breathing, and increase energy. This physical well-being strengthens and calms the mind.

ASANAS AND PRANAYAMA

Practicing asanas cleanses the body. Just as a goldsmith heats gold in a fire to burn out its impurities, similarly, asanas, by increasing the circulation of fresh blood through the body, purge it of the diseases and toxins which are the consequences of an irregular lifestyle, unhealthy habits, and poor posture. Regular practice of the stretches, twists, bends, and inversions, which are the basic movements of asanas, restores strength and stamina to the body. Asanas, together with pranayama, or the control of breath, rectify physical, physiological, and psychological disorders. They have a positive impact on the effects of stress and disease. Among the many ailments that benefit from the practice of asanas are osteoarthritis, high and low blood pressure, diabetes, asthma, and anorexia.

HARMONY BETWEEN BODY AND SOUL
This 10th-century figure, the Yoga Narayan, from Khajuraho, India, depicts the god Vishnu in a state of yogic calm

MIND AND BODY

The body and the mind are in a state of constant interaction. Yogic science does not demarcate where the body ends and the mind begins, but approaches both as a single, integrated entity. The turmoil of daily life brings stress to the body and the mind. This creates anxiety, depression, restlessness, and rage. Yoga asanas, while appearing to deal with the physical body alone, actually influence the chemical balance of the brain, which in turn improves one's mental state of being.

The obstacles to this perfect balance were outlined by the sage, Patanjali, 2,000 years ago in the *Yoga Sutras*. Historians disagree on the exact dates, but it is known that the *sutras*, or aphorisms on the philosophy and practice of yoga, were compiled sometime between 300 BC and AD 300, and the entire corpus was called the *Patanjali Yoga Darshana*. In the final chapter of the *Yoga Sutras*, the *Samadhi Pada*, Patanjali discusses the disorders that are the root cause of suffering. According to the sage, *vyadhi*, or physical ailments, create emotional upheaval. The task of yoga is to tackle both.

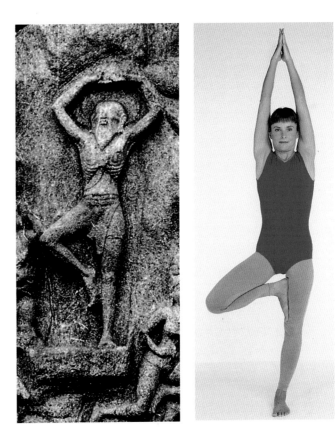

TIMELESS TRADITION
The 4th-century figure from Mahabalipuram, India (left), and this modern woman show that certain classic movements are eternal

"After a session of yoga, the mind becomes tranquil and passive."

Even today, the alleviation of pain is one of the main reasons most people journey into yoga. Yoga asanas also work specific parts of the body to soothe and relax the mind as well. Inverted asanas, for instance, simultaneously calm and stimulate the brain. These asanas activate glands and vital organs by supplying fresh blood to the brain, making it alert but relaxed.

Yoga possesses the unique ability to calm nerves. The nerves function as the medium between the physiological body and the psychological body (*see page* 42). Practicing yoga has the holistic impact of relaxing the body and calming the mind.

USTRASANA OR CAMEL POSTURE
Yoga activates all the muscles, bones, and organs of the body

STAGES OF YOGA

The primary aim of yoga is to restore the mind to simplicity, peace, and poise, and free it from confusion and distress. This simplicity, this sense of order and calm, comes from the practice of asanas and pranayama. Yoga asanas integrate the body, the mind, the intelligence, and, finally, the self, in four stages. The first stage, *arambhavastha*, is when we practice at the level of the physical body. The second stage is *ghatavastha*, when the mind learns to move in unison with the body. The third level, *parichayavastha*, occurs when the intelligence and the body become one. The final stage is *nispattyavastha*, the state of perfection (*see page 42*).

Spiritual awareness flows into the student of yoga through these stages. *Dukha*, which is misery or pain, vanishes, and the art of living in simplicity and peace is realized.

YOGA FILLS THE SPIRITUAL VOID

The world today is overwhelmingly materialistic, and this has created a great spiritual void in our lives. Our lifestyles are unduly complex and we become stressed primarily as a result of our own actions. Our existence feels barren and devoid of meaning. There is a lack of spiritual dimension in our lives and in our relationships. This has led many reflective people to realize that solace, inspiration, peace, and happiness cannot come from the external environment, but must come from within.

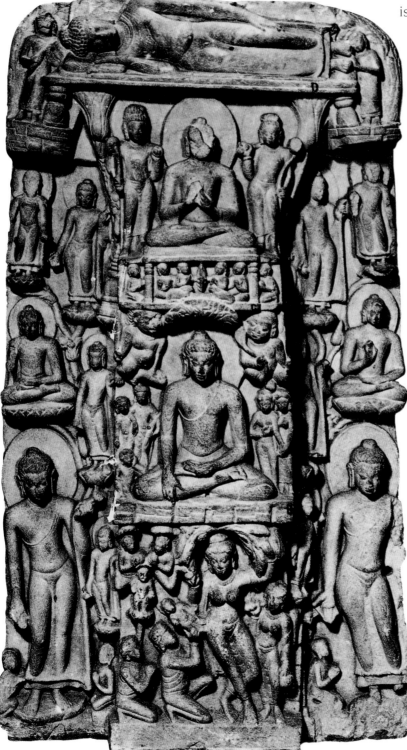

THE FOUR STAGES OF THE BUDDHA'S JOURNEY TO SELF-REALIZATION
This 5th-century frieze from Sarnath, India, shows the four defining events of the Buddha's life. (From the bottom) Buddha's birth from his mother's hip; attaining enlightenment in Bodhgaya; preaching to his disciples; the ascent to the celestial realms

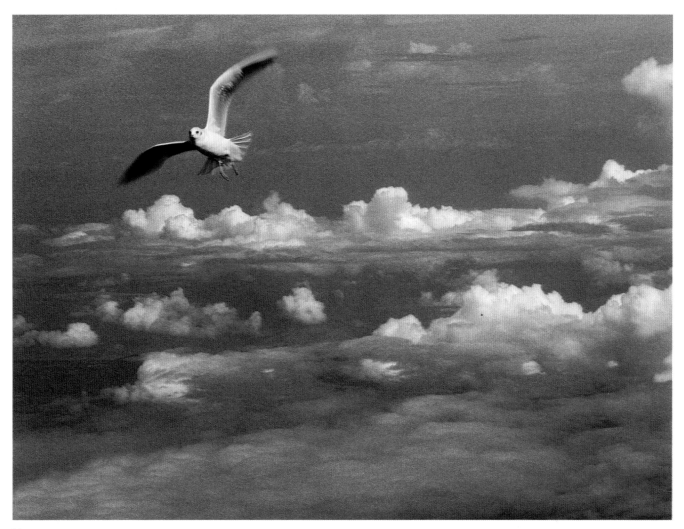

YOGA LIBERATES YOU
When you practice yoga, your mind becomes unfettered and free

THE FREEDOM OF YOGA

The impact of yoga is never purely physical. Asanas, if correctly practiced, bridge the divide between the physical and the mental spheres. Yoga stems the feelings of pain, fatigue, doubt, confusion, indifference, laziness, self-delusion, and despair that assail us from time to time. The yogic mind simply refuses to accept such negative emotions and seeks to overcome these turbulent currents on the voyage to the total liberation of the self. Once we become sincere practitioners of yoga, we cease to be tormented by these unhappy and discouraging states of mind.

Yoga illuminates your life. If you practice sincerely, with seriousness and honesty, its light will spread to all aspects of your life. Regular practice will bring you to look at yourself and your goals in a new light. It will help remove the obstacles to good health and stable emotions. In this way, yoga will help you achieve emancipation and self-realization, which is the ultimate goal of every person's life.

UNWAVERING FLAME
Yoga illuminates your life, helping you see yourself in a new light

Meaning of Yoga

Yoga is an ancient art based on an extremely subtle science, one of the body, mind, and soul. The prolonged practice of yoga will, in time, lead the student to a sense of peace and a feeling of being at one with his or her environment.

Most people know that the practice of yoga makes the body strong and flexible. It is also well known that yoga improves the functioning of the respiratory, circulatory, digestive, and hormonal systems. Yoga also brings emotional stability and clarity of mind, but that is only the beginning of the journey to *samadhi*, or self-realization, which is the ultimate aim of yoga.

The ancient sages, who meditated on the human condition 2,000 years ago, outlined four ways to self-realization: *jnana marg*, or the path to knowledge when the seeker learns to discriminate between the real and the unreal, *karma marg*, the path of selfless service without thought of reward, *bhakti marg*, the path of love and devotion, and finally, *yoga marg*, the path by which the mind and its actions are brought under control. All these paths lead to the same goal: *samadhi*.

The word "yoga" is derived from the Sanskrit root *yuj* which means "tó join" or "to yoke;" the related meaning is "to focus attention on" or "to use." In philosophical terms, the union of the individual self, *jivatma*, with the universal self, *paramatma*, is yoga. The union results in a pure and perfect state of consciousness in which the feeling of "I" simply does not exist. Prior to this union is the union of the body with the mind, and the mind with the self. Yoga is therefore a dynamic, internal experience which integrates the body, the senses, the mind, and the intelligence with the self. The sage Patanjali was a master of yoga and a fully evolved soul. However, this great thinker had the ability to empathize with the joys and sorrows of ordinary people. His reflections and those of other ancient sages on the ways through which every person could realize his full potential were outlined in the 196 *Yoga Sutras*.

YOGACHARYA IYENGAR IN
URDHVA DHANURASANA
*Asanas improve the working of all
the systems of the body*

WHERE YOGA CAN TAKE YOU

According to Patanjali, the aim of yoga is to calm the chaos of conflicting impulses and thoughts. The mind, which is responsible for our thoughts and impulses, is naturally inclined to *asmita* or egoism. From this spring the prejudice and biases which lead to pain and distress in our daily lives. Yogic science centers the intelligence in two areas, the heart and the head. The intelligence of the heart, sometimes also called the "root mind," is the actual agent of *ahankara*, or false pride, which disturbs the intelligence of the head, and causes fluctuations in the body and mind.

Patanjali describes these afflictions as: *vyadhi*, or physical ailments, *styana*, or the reluctance to work, *samshaya*, or doubt, *pramadha*, or indifference, *alasya*, or laziness, *avirati*, or the desire for sensual satisfaction, *bharanti darshana*, or false knowledge, *alabdha bhumikatva*, or indisposition, *angamejaytatva*, or unsteadiness in the body, and, lastly, *shvasa-prashvasa*, or unsteady respiration. Only yoga eradicates these afflictions, and disciplines the mind, emotions, intellect, and reason.

ASTANGA YOGA

Yoga is also known as Astanga yoga. A*stanga* means "8 limbs" or "steps" (*see page* 29) and is divided into 3 disciplines. The discipline, *bahiranga-sadhana*, comprises ethical practices in the form of *yama*, or general ethical principles, *niyama*, or self-restraint, and physical practices in the form of asanas and pranayama.

The second discipline, *antaranga-sadhana*, is emotional or mental discipline brought to maturity by pranayama and *pratyahara*, or mental detachment. Lastly, *antaratma-sadhana* is the successful quest of the soul through *dharana*, *dhyana*, and *samadhi* (*see page* 29).

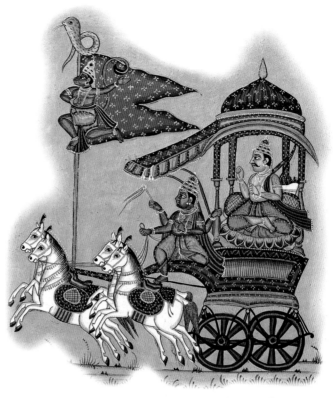

KRISHNA DRIVING THE CHARIOT OF THE WARRIOR, ARJUN
Their discourses are narrated in the Bhagvad Gita, *the main source of yogic philosophy*

In this spiritual quest, it is important to remember the role of the body. The *Kathopanishad*, an ancient text compiled between 300-400 BC, compares the body to a chariot, the senses to the horses, and the mind to the reins. The intellect is the charioteer and the soul is the master of the chariot. If anything were to go wrong with the chariot, the horses, the reins, or the charioteer, the chariot and the charioteer would come to grief, and so would the master of the chariot.

However, writes Patanjali in *Yoga Sutra* 11.28, "The practice of yoga destroys the impurities of the body and mind, after which maturity in intelligence and wisdom radiate from the core of the being to function in unison with the body, senses, mind, intelligence, and the consciousness."

"*The aim of yoga is to calm the chaos of conflicting impulses.*"

The Way to Health

Good health results from perfect communication between each part of the body and mind, and when each cell communes with every other. Although yoga is essentially a spiritual science, it leads to a sense of physical and emotional well-being.

Health is not just freedom from disease. For good health, the joints, tissues, muscles, cells, nerves, glands, and each system of the body must all be in a state of perfect balance and harmony. Health is the perfect equilibrium of the body and mind, intellect, and soul.

Health is like the flowing water of a river, always fresh and pure, in a constant state of flux. Humans are a combination of the senses of perception, the organs of action, the mind, the intelligence, the inner consciousness, and the conscience. Each of these is worked on by the practice of yoga. Yoga asanas help ensure an even distribution of bioenergy, or life force, which brings the mind to a state of calm. A practitioner of yoga faces life not as a victim, but as a master, in control of his or her life situations, circumstances, and environment. Asanas balance the respiratory, circulatory, nervous, hormonal, digestive, excretory, and reproductive systems perfectly. The equilibrium in the body then brings mental peace and enhances intellectual clarity.

GOOD HEALTH
A healthy body is like the flowing water of a river, always fresh and pure

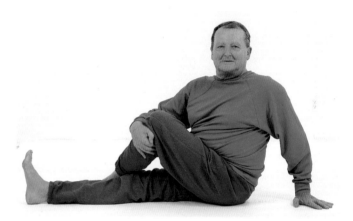

YOGA IS FOR EVERYONE
There are asanas to suit every constitution, irrespective of age or physical condition

HARMONY OF BODY AND MIND

Asanas cater to the needs of each individual according to his or her specific constitution and physical condition. They involve vertical, horizontal, and cyclical movements, which provide energy to the system by directing the blood supply to the areas of the body which need it most. In yoga, each cell is observed, attended to, and provided with a fresh supply of blood, allowing it to function smoothly.

The mind is naturally active and dynamic, while the soul is luminous. However, unhealthy bodies tend to house inert, dull, and sluggish minds. It is the practice of yoga which removes this sluggishness from the body and brings it to the level of the active mind. Ultimately, both the body and mind rise to the level of the illuminated self.

The practice of yoga stimulates and changes emotional attitudes, and convert apprehensiveness into courage, indecision and poor judgement into positive decision-making skills, and emotional instability into confidence and mental equilibrium.

Benefits of Postures

Asanas are based on the three basic human postures of standing, sitting, or lying down. But they are not a series of movements to be followed mechanically. They have a logic which must be internalized if the posture is to be practiced correctly.

The Sanskrit term, *asana*, is sometimes translated as "pose" and sometimes as "posture." Neither translation is wholly accurate, since they do not convey the element of thought or consciousness that must inform each movement of the asana. The final posture of an asana is achieved when all the parts of the body are positioned correctly, with full awareness and intelligence.

To achieve this, you must think through the structure of the asana. Realize the fundamental points by imagining how you will adjust and arrange each part of your anatomical body, especially the limbs, in the given movements.

Then, mold the body to fit the structure of the asana, making sure that the balance between both sides of the body is perfect, until there is no undue stress on any one organ, muscle, bone, or joint.

IMPORTANCE OF PRACTICING ASANAS
The practice of asanas has a beneficial impact on the whole body. Asanas not only tone the muscles, tissues, ligaments, joints, and nerves, but also maintain the smooth functioning and health of all the body's systems. They relax the body and mind, allowing both to recover from fatigue or weakness and the stress of daily life. Asanas also boost metabolism, lymphatic circulation, and hormonal secretions, and bring about a chemical balance in the body.

It is important to keep practicing until you are absolutely comfortable in the final posture. It is only then that you experience the full benefits of the asana. The sage Patanjali observes in *Yoga Sutra* 11.47, "Perfection in an asana is achieved when the effort to perform it becomes effortless, and the infinite being within is reached."

PERFECT BALANCE
Yogacharya Iyengar supports a student in Salamba Sarvangasana

Yoga & Fitness

Most types of exercise are competitive. Yoga, although noncompetitive, is nevertheless challenging. The challenge is to one's own will power. It is a competition between one's self and one's body.

Exercise usually involves quick and forceful body movements. It has repeated actions which often lead to exertion, tension, and fatigue. Yoga asanas, on the other hand, involve movements which bring stability to the body, the senses, the mind, the intellect, the consciousness, and finally, to the conscience. The very essence of an asana is steady movement, a process that does not simply end, but finds fulfilment in tranquillity.

Most diseases are caused by the fluctuations in the brain and in the behavioral pattern of the body. In yogic practice, the brain is quiet, the senses are stilled, and perceptions are altered, which all generates a calm feeling of detachment. With practice, the student of yoga learns to treat the brain as an object and the body as a subject. Energy is diffused from the brain to the other parts of the body. The brain and body then work together and energy is evenly balanced between the two. Yoga is therefore termed *sarvaanga sadhana* or "holistic practice." No other form of exercise so completely involves the mind and self with the body, and results in all-around development and harmony. Other forms of exercise address only particular parts of the body. Such forms are termed *angabhaga sadhana* or "physical exercise."

STIMULATIVE EXERCISE

Yoga asanas are stimulative exercises, while other endurance exercises are irritative. For instance, medical experts claim that jogging stimulates the heart. In fact, though the heartbeat of the jogger increases, the heart is not stimulated in the yogic sense of being energized and invigorated. For example, in yoga, back bends are more physically demanding than jogging, but the heart beats at a steady, rhythmic pace.

Asanas do not lead to breathlessness. When practicing yoga, strength and power play separate roles to achieve a perfect balance in every part of the body, as well as the mind. After such stimulating exercise, a sense of rejuvenation and a fresh surge of energy follow.

Exercise can also be exhausting. Many forms of exercise require physical strength and endurance and can lead to a feeling of fatigue after 15 minutes of practice. Many exercises improve energy levels by boosting nerve function, but ultimately, this exhausts the cellular reserves and endocrine glands. Cellular toxins increase, and though circulation is enhanced, it is at the cost of irritating the other body systems and increasing the pulse rate and blood pressure. Ultimately, the heart is overworked.

JOGGING
This form of exercise raises the heartbeat, but can tire you out

An athlete's strong lung capacity is achieved by hard and forceful usage, which is not conducive to preserving the health of the lungs. Furthermore, ordinary physical exercise, such as in jogging, tennis, or football, lends itself to repetitive injuries of the bones, joints, and ligaments.

STRENGTHENING IMMUNITIES
Children benefit from yoga as much as adults do

Such forms of exercise work with, and for, the skeletal and muscular systems. They cannot penetrate beyond these limits. However, asanas penetrate each layer of the body and, ultimately, the consciousness itself. Only in yoga can you keep both the body and the mind relaxed, even as you stretch, extend, rotate, and flex your body.

Yoga, unlike other forms of exercise, keeps the nervous system elastic and capable of bearing stress. Although all forms of exercise bring about a feeling of well-being, they also stress the body. Yoga refreshes the body, while other systems exhaust it. Yoga involves the equal exertion of all parts of the body and does not overstrain any one part.

In other forms of exercise, the movements are restricted to a part or parts. They are reflex actions, which do not involve the intelligence in their execution. There is little space for precision and perfection, without extra expenditure of energy.

YOGA CAN BE PRACTICED AT ANY AGE

With advancing age, physically vigorous exercises cannot be performed easily because of stiffening joints and muscles that have lost tone. Isometric exercises, for example, cannot be practiced with increasing age, since they lead to sprained muscles, painful joints, strained body systems, and the degeneration of organs. The great advantage of yoga is that it can be practiced by anyone, irrespective of age, sex, and physical condition.

In fact, yoga is particularly beneficial in middle age and after. Yoga is a gift to older people when the recuperative power of the body is declining and resistance to illness is weakened. Yoga generates energy and does not dissipate it. With yoga one can look forward to a satisfying, healthier future, rather than reflecting on one's youthful past.

Unlike other exercises, yoga results in the concentration of immunity cells in areas affected by disease, and therefore improves immunity. That is why the ancient sages called yoga a therapeutic as well as a preventive science.

CALM AND REJUVENATED
Expectant mother in Baddhakonasana

Yoga & Stress

Yoga minimizes the impact of stress on the individual. Yogic science believes that the regular practice of asanas and pranayama strengthens the nervous system and helps people face stressful situations positively.

We have all experienced the way unrelieved tension results in both mental disorders and physical ill health. This is not a modern phenomenon. In the centuries-old *Yoga Sutras*, the sage Patanjali attributed the causes of mental affliction to the ego, spiritual ignorance, desire, hatred of others, and attachment to life. He called these *kleshas* or "sorrows."

ORIGINS OF STRESS

Through advances in science and technology, modern civilization has been able to conquer ignorance in many fields, but its pride in

grasp at in their desperate search for consolation. However, while these measures may provide temporary distraction or oblivion, the root of unhappiness, stress, remains unresolved.

Yoga is not a miracle cure that can free a person from all stress, but it can help minimize it. The worries of modern life deplete our reserves of bioenergy, because we draw on our vital energy from our storehouse, the nerve cells. This can, ultimately, exhaust our energy reserves and lead to the collapse of mental and physical equilibrium.

Yogic science believes that the nerves control the unconscious mind, and that when the nervous

"Regular practice of yoga can help you face the turmoil of life with steadiness and stability."

technological achievement is excessive and misplaced. It has triggered widespread feelings of competitiveness and envy. Financial tensions, emotional upheavals, environmental pollution, and, above all, a sense of being overtaken by the speed of events, have all increased the stress of daily life.

All these factors strain the body, cause nervous tension, and adversely affect the mind. This is when feelings of isolation and loneliness take over.

To deal with this, people turn to artificial solutions to cope with the pressures of daily life. Substance abuse, eating disorders, and destructive relationships are some of the substitutes people

system is strong, a person faces stressful situations more positively. Asanas improve blood flow to all the cells of the body, and revitalize the nerve cells. This flow strengthens the nervous system and its capacity for enduring stress.

RELIEVING STRESS

The diaphragm, according to yogic science, is the seat of the intelligence of the heart and the window to the soul. During stressful situations, however, when you inhale and exhale, the diaphragm becomes too taut to alter its shape. Yogic exercises address this problem by developing elasticity in the diaphragm, so that, when stretched, it can handle any amount of stress, whether intellectual, emotional, or physical.

The practice of asanas and pranayama helps integrate the body, breath, mind, and intellect. Slow, effortless exhalation during practice of an asana brings serenity to the body cells, relaxes the facial muscles, and releases all tension from the organs of perception, the eyes, ears, nose, tongue, and skin.

When this happens, the brain, which is in constant communication with the organs of action, becomes *shunya*, or void, and all thoughts are stilled. Then, invading fears and anxieties cannot penetrate to the brain. When you develop this ability, you perform your daily activities with efficiency and economy. You do not dissipate your valuable bioenergy. You enter the state of true clarity of intellect. Your mind is free of stress and is filled with calm and tranquillity.

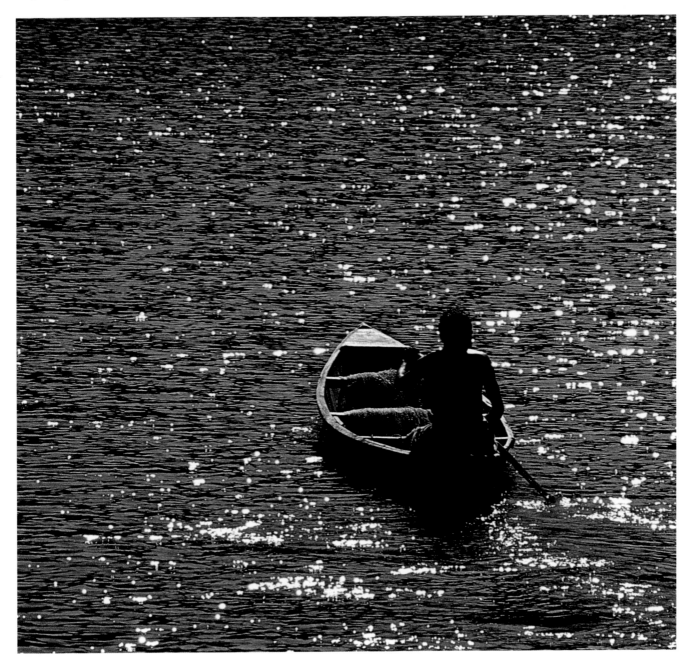

A VIEW OF THE SOUL
Yoga can minimize the worries of modern life

CHAPTER 2

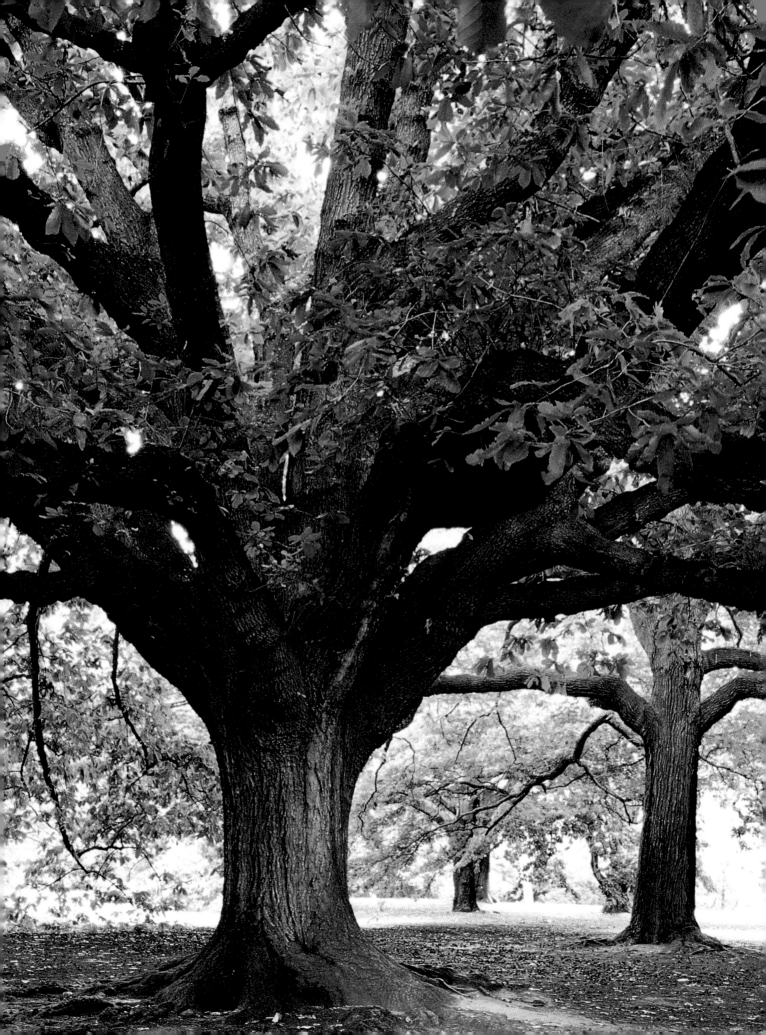

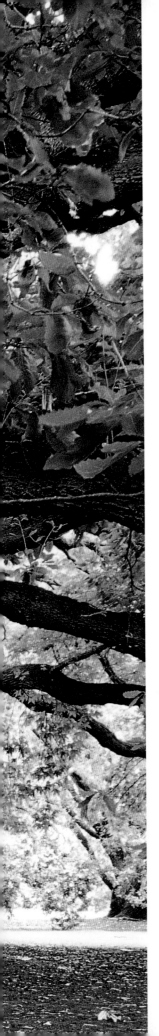

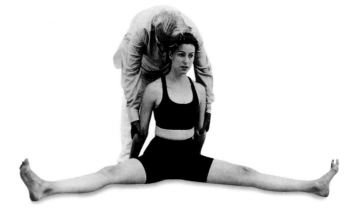

"Yoga is the union of the individual self with the universal self."

Philosophy of Yoga

Yoga is a fine art and seeks to express the artist's abilities to the fullest possible extent. While most artists need an instrument, such as a paint brush or a violin, to express their art, the only instruments a yogi needs are his body and his mind. The ancient sages compared yoga to a fruit tree. From a single seed grow the roots, trunk, branches, and leaves. The leaves bring life-giving energy to the entire tree, which then blossoms into flowers and sweet, luscious fruit. Just as the fruit is the natural culmination of the tree, yoga, too, transforms darkness into light, ignorance into knowledge, knowledge into wisdom, and wisdom into unalloyed peace and spiritual bliss.

Philosophy of Asanas

Asanas, one of yoga's most significant "tools," help the sincere student develop physically and spiritually. The ancient sages believed that if you put your whole heart into your practice, you become a master of your circumstances and time.

Asanas are one of the major "tools" of yoga. Their benefits range from the physical level to the spiritual. That is why yoga is called *sarvaanga sadhana*, or holistic practice. "Asana" is the positioning of the body in various postures, with the total involvement of the mind and self, in order to establish communication between our external and internal selves.

Yogic philosophy looks at the body as being made up of three layers and five sheaths. The three layers are the causal body, or *karana sharira*, the subtle body, or *suksma sharira*, and the gross body, or *karya sharira*. Every individual functions in mind, matter, energy, and pure consciousness through five sheaths. These are the anatomical sheath, or *annamaya kosha*, which is dealt with by asanas, the life-force sheath or *pranamaya kosha*, which is treated by pranayama, the psychological sheath, or *manomaya kosha*, is worked on by meditation, and the intellectual sheath, or *vijnamaya kosha*, is transformed by studying the scriptures with sincerity and discrimination. Once these goals are addressed, you reach the *anandamaya kosha*, or the sheath of bliss.

Yoga integrates the three layers of the body with the five sheaths, enabling the individual to develop as a total being. The separation between the body and the mind and the mind and the soul, then vanishes, as all planes fuse into one. In this way, asanas help transform an individual by bringing him or her away from the awareness of the body toward the consciousness of the soul.

THE JOURNEY OF YOGA

The *Hathayoga Pradipika* is a practical treatise on yoga, and is thought to have been compiled in the 15th century. The author, the sage Svatmarama, gives practical guidelines to beginners on the journey that they must make from the culture of the body toward the vision of the soul. Unlike Patanjali, who discusses the sighting of the soul through the restraint of consciousness or *chitta*, Svatmarama begins his treatise with the restraint of energy, or *prana*. Sighting the soul through the restraint of energy is called Hatha yoga, whereas sighting the soul through the restraint of consciousness is known as Raja yoga.

SAMADHI
The Buddha attaining enlightenment at Bodhgaya. The 3rd-century sculpture is from Sarnath, India

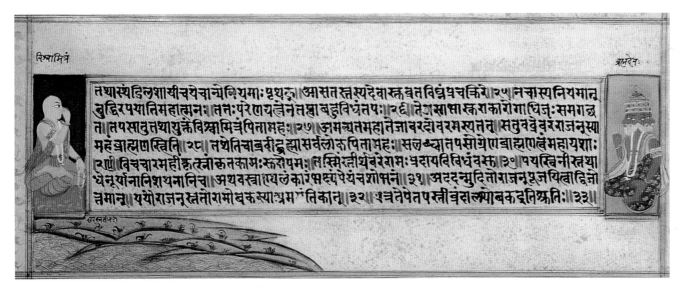

A FOLIO FROM THE ANCIENT INDIAN EPIC, THE MAHABHARATA.
The essentials of yoga philosophy are found in the Bhagvad Gita, which forms a part of the epic

In *Hathayoga Pradipika* 4.29, the author stresses the importance of the breath by saying that if the mind is the king of the senses, the master of the mind is breath. If breath is made to move rhythmically, with a controlled, sustained sound, the mind becomes calm. In that calmness, the king of the mind, or soul, becomes the supreme commander of the senses, mind, breath, and consciousness. When you learn to focus on the inhaled breath and the exhaled breath, you experience a neutralizing effect on the mind. This reaction led Svatmarama to conclude that the control of *prana* is the key to super-awareness or *samadhi*.

In the chapter *Samadhi Prakarana* of the *Hathayoga Pradipika*, Svatmarama gives glimpses of his experiences of *samadhi*. He says, "If one learns not to think of external things and simultaneously keeps away inner thoughts, one experiences *samadhi*. When the mind is dissolved in the sea of the soul, an absolute state of existence is reached. This is *kaivalya*, the freedom of emancipation."

The goal of yoga is a state of equilibrium and peace. Patanjali warns the student of yoga not to be deceived by this quietness, for it could lead to a state of *yogabhrastha* or "falling from the grace of yoga." He also says, "The practice of yoga must

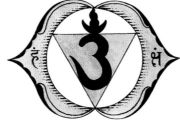

AJNA CHAKRA
This symbol represents the potential for spirituality in every individual

continue, as it has to culminate in the sight of the soul," he says. This stage, when the individual becomes one with the core of his or her being, is known as *nirbija* (seedless) *samadhi*.

IMPACT OF YOGA

In his third chapter of the *Yoga Sutras*, *Vibhuti Pada*, Patanjali speaks of the effects of yoga. Although they seem exotic to our modern conciousness, they indicate the potential of the powers of human nature. These spiritual powers and gifts have to be conquered in their turn. Otherwise, they become a trap, diverting the seeker from the true aim of yoga. When the soul is free from the bondage of body, mind, power, and pride of success, it reaches the state of *kaivalya* or freedom. This aspect is covered in the fourth chapter of the *Yoga Sutras*, *Kaivalya Padha*, the chapter on absolute liberation.

The person who practices yoga regularly will not become a victim but a master of his or her circumstances and time. The yoga practitioner lives to love and serve the world. This is the essence of life. Peace within, peace without, and peace in the individual, in the family unit, in society, and in the world at large.

States of Mind

The mind is the vital link between the body and the consciousness. The individual can live with awareness, discrimination, and confidence only once the mind is calm and focused. Yoga is the alchemy that generates this equilibrium.

In yogic terminology, consciousness, or *chitta*, encompasses the mind, or *manas*, intelligence, or *buddhi*, and ego, or *ahankara*. The Sanskrit word for man, *manusya* or *manava*, means "one who is endowed with this special consciousness." The mind does not have an actual location in the body. It is latent, elusive, and exists everywhere. The mind desires, wills, remembers, perceives, and experiences. Sensations of pain and pleasure, heat and cold, and honor and dishonor, are experienced and interpreted by the mind. The mind reflects both the external and the internal worlds, but though it has the capacity to perceive things within and without, its natural tendency is to be preoccupied with the outside world.

NATURE OF THE MIND

When the mind is fully absorbed by objects seen, heard, smelled, felt, or tasted, this leads to stress, fatigue, and unhappiness. The mind can be a secret enemy and a treacherous friend. It influences our behavior before we have the time to consider causes and consequences. Yoga trains the mind and inculcates a sense of discrimination, so that objects and events are seen for what they are and are not allowed to gain mastery over us.

FIVE MENTAL FACULTIES

We have five mental faculties which can be used in a positive or a negative way. These are correct observation and knowledge, perception, imagination, dreamless sleep, and memory. Sometimes the mind loses its stability and clarity, and is either incapable of using its various faculties properly, or uses them in a negative way. The practice of yoga leads us to use these mental faculties in a positive way, thereby bringing the mind to a discriminative and attentive state. Awareness, together with discrimination and memory, target bad habits, which are essentially repetitive actions based on mistaken perception. These are then replaced by good habits. In this way, an individual becomes stronger, honest, and gains maturity. He or she is able to perceive and understand people, situations, and events with clarity. This seasoned, mature mind gradually transcends its frontiers to reach beyond mundane observation and experience, making the journey from confusion to clarity, one of the greatest benefits of yoga.

CLARITY OF MIND
Practicing yoga gives you the ability to recognize situations for what they are, and to deal with them.

"The seasoned, mature mind transcends frontiers to reach beyond mundane observation."

DIFFERENT STATES OF MIND

Yogic science distinguishes between five basic states of mind. These are not grouped in stages, nor are they, except the last, unchangeable. According to Patanjali, these states of mind are dull and lethargic, distracted, scattered, focused, and controlled. Patanjali described the lowest level of the mind as dull, or *mudha*. A person in this state of mind is disinclined to observe, act, or react. This state is rarely inherent or permanent. It is usually caused by a traumatic experience, for instance, bereavement, or when a desired goal presents so many obstacles that the goal seems impossible to attain. After successive failures to take control of their lives, many people withdraw into dullness and lethargy. Often, this is exacerbated by either insomnia or oversleeping, comfort eating, or the ingestion of tranquillizers and other substances which make the original problem worse. Yoga gradually transforms this feeling of defeat and helplessness into optimism and energy. The distracted state of mind is one where thoughts, feelings, and perceptions churn around in the consciousness, but leave no lasting impressions and hence serve no purpose. Patanjali calls this state, *ksipta*. Someone in a state of *ksipta* is unstable, and unable to prioritize or focus on goals, usually because of flawed signals from the senses of perception he or she accepts and follows unthinkingly. This clouds the intellect and disturbs mental equilibrium. Such a state has to be calmed and brought to confront the factual knowledge of reality through the regular practice of yoga asanas and pranayama.

The most common state of mind is the scattered mind. In such a state, though the brain is active, it lacks purpose and direction. This state of mind is known as *viksipta*. Constantly plagued by doubt and fear, it alternates between decisiveness and lack of confidence. The regular practice of yoga gradually encourages the seeds of awareness and discrimination to take root, giving rise to a positive attitude and mental equilibrium.

THE DISTURBED MIND
Unable to concentrate, resisting realities, and lurching between priorities, this state of mind responds to the practice of yoga

The ancient sages characterized the focused state of mind, or *ekagra*, as one that indicated a higher state of being. This is a liberated mind which has confronted afflictions and obstacles and conquered them. Such a mind has direction, concentration, and awareness. A person in this category of mental intelligence lives in the present without being caught in the past or future, undisturbed by external circumstances.

The fifth and highest state of mind is *niruddha*, or the controlled, restrained mind. According to Patanjali, *niruddha* is attained through the persistent practice of yoga, which allows an individual to conquer the lower levels of the mind.

At this level, the mind is linked exclusively with the object of its attention. It has the power to become totally absorbed in an activity, allowing nothing to disturb its absorption. When the brain is quiet, the intellect is at peace, the individual is serene and balanced, neither free nor bound, but poised in pure consciousness.

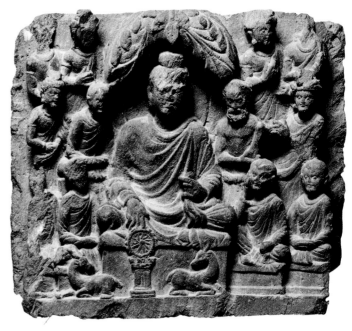

AN ENLIGHTENED MIND
The Buddha teaching his disciples the value of truth and contentment, from a frieze found at Sarnath, India

THE FINAL STAGE
The persistent practice of yoga allows you to conquer the lower levels of the mind and reach the peaks of self-realization

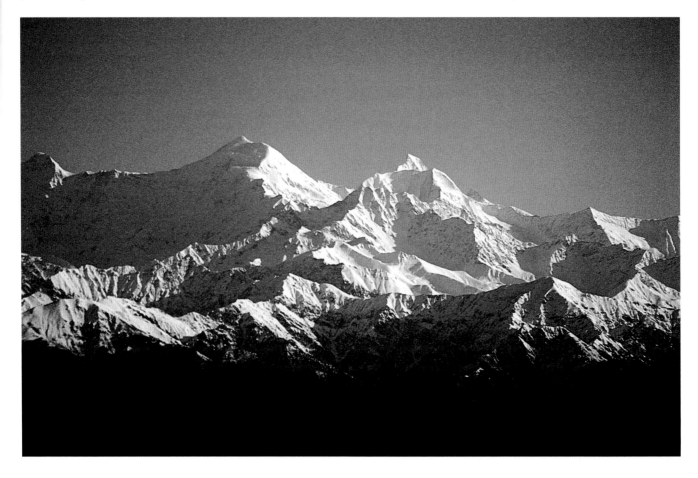

Eight Limbs

The basic tenets of yoga are described in the form of eight limbs, or steps, described by the sage, Patanjali. These are aphorisms, explaining the codes of ethical behavior which will ultimately lead to self-realization.

The sage Patanjali reflected on the nature of man and the norms of society during his time. Then, very systematically, he expressed his observations in the form of aphorisms which deal with the entire span of life, beginning with a code of correct conduct and ending with the ultimate goal, emancipation and freedom. These aphorisms outline the fundamental tenets of yoga, known as the eight limbs, or *astanga.*

ASTANGA YOGA

The eight limbs or steps are *yama, niyama, asana, pranayama, pratyahara, dharana, dhyana,* and *samadhi.* These are sequential stages in an individual's life journey through yoga. Each step must be understood and followed to attain the ultimate goal of Astanga Yoga, that of emancipation of the self. *Yama,* or general ethical principles, and *niyama,* or self-restraint, prescribe a code of conduct that molds individual morality and behavior.

Asanas, or yogic postures, and pranayama, or breath control, discipline the body and the mind by basic practices conducive to physical, physiological, psychological, and mental health. Pranayama controls the mind, taming base instincts, while

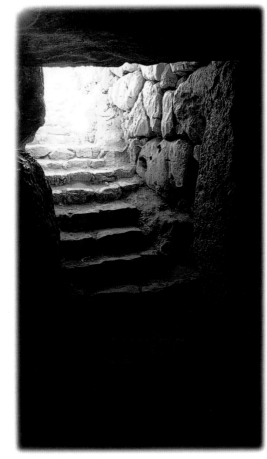

STEPS TO SELF-REALIZATION
Understand and absorb each stage to reach the ultimate goal

pratyahara, or detachment from the external world, stems the outgoing flow of the senses, withdrawing those of perception and the organs of action from worldly pleasures. D*harana,* or concentration, guides the consciousness to focus attention rigorously on one point. D*hyana,* or prolonged concentration, saturates the mind until it permeates to the source of existence, and the intellectual and conscious energy dissolves in the seat of the soul. It is then that *samadhi,* when you lose the sense of your separate existence, is attained. Nothing else remains except the core of one's being: the soul.

YAMA

Yama and *niyama* require tremendous inner discipline. *Yama* explains the codes of ethical behavior to be observed and followed in everyday life, reminding us of our responsibilities as social beings. *Yama* has 5 principles. These are: *ahimsa* or nonviolence, *asteya,* or freedom from avarice, *satya,* or truthfulness, *brahmacharya,* or chastity, and *aparigraha,* or freedom from desire. A*himsa* needs introspection to replace negative, destructive thoughts and actions by positive, constructive ones. Anger, cruelty, or harassment of others are facets of the violence latent in all of us.

These contradict the principles of *ahimsa*, while lying, cheating, dishonesty, and deception break the principles of *satya*. *Brahmacharya* does not mean total abstinence, but denotes a disciplined sexual life, promoting contentment and moral strength from within. *Parigraha* means "possession" or "covetousness," the instinct within all of us that traps us in the *karmic* cycle of reincarnation after death. However, while you may be able to give up material possessiveness, what about emotional or intellectual possessiveness? This is where Astanga yoga helps to discipline the mind, freeing it from the desire to possess, bringing it into a state of *aparigraha*, or freedom from desire, as well as *asteya*, or freedom from greed.

NIYAMA

Niyama is the positive current that brings discipline, removes inertia, and gives shape to the inner desire to follow the yogic path. The principles of *niyama* are *saucha*, or cleanliness, *santosa*, or contentment, *tapas*, or austerity, *svadhyaya*, or the study of one's own self, which includes the body, mind, intellect, and ego. The final principle of *niyama* is *isvara pranidhana* or devotion to God. Contentment or *santosa* helps curb desire, anger, ambition, and greed, while *tapas*, or austerity, involves self-discipline and the desire to purify the body, senses, and mind. The study and practice of yoga with devotional attention to the self and God is *tapas*.

ASANAS, PRANAYAMA, AND PRATYAHARA

According to the *Gheranda Samhita*, a text dating to the 15th century, written by the yogic sage, Gheranda says, "The body soon decays like unbaked earthen pots thrown in water. Strengthen and purify

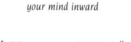

POSITIVE CURRENTS
Focus on your inner body and draw your mind inward

the body by baking it in the fire of yoga." Performing an asana helps create and generate energy. Staying in an asana organizes and distributes this energy, while coming out of the posture protects the energy, preventing it from dissipating. In *Yoga Sutra* 111.47, Patanjali explains the effects of an asana as *"Rupa lavanya bala vaira samhananatvani kayasampat."* This means that a perfected body has beauty, grace, and strength which is comparable to the hardness and brilliance of a diamond. While practicing an asana, one must focus attention on the inner body, drawing the mind inward to sharpen the intelligence.

Then, the asana becomes effortless as the blemishes on both the gross and the subtle body are washed off. This is the turning point in the practice of asanas, when the body, mind, and self unite. From this state begins the *isvara pranidhana*, or devotion to God. Asanas and pranayama are interrelated and interwoven. Patanjali clearly specifies that pranayama should be attempted only after the asanas are mastered. *Prana* is "vital energy", which includes will power and ambition, while *ayama* means "stretch, expansion, and extension." Pranayama can be described as the "expansion and extension of energy or life force." Patanjali begins pranayama with the simple movement of breathing, and leads us deeper and deeper into ourselves by teaching us to observe the very act of respiration. Pranayama has three movements, prolonged inhalation, deep exhalation, and prolonged, stable retention, all of which have to be performed with precision. Pranayama is the actual process of directing energy inward, making the mind fit for *pratyahara*, or the detachment of the senses, which evolves from pranayama. When the senses withdraw from objects of desire, the mind is released from the power of the senses, which in turn become passive. Then the mind turns inward and is set free from the tyranny of the senses. This is *pratyahara*.

SAMAYAMA – TOWARD THE LIBERATION OF THE SELF

Patanjali groups *dharana*, *dhyana*, and *samadhi* under the term *samayama*, or the integration of the body, breath, mind, intellect, and self. It is not easy to explain the last three aspects of yoga as separate entities. The controlled mind that is gained in *pratyahara* is made to intensify its attention on a single thought in *dharana*. When this concentration is prolonged, it becomes *dhyana*. In *dhyana*, release,

expansion, quietness, and peace are experienced. This prolonged state of quietness frees an individual from attachment and results in indifference to the joys of pleasure or the sorrows of pain. The experience of *samadhi* is achieved when the knower, the knowable, and the known become one. When the object of meditation engulfs the meditator and becomes the subject, self-awareness is lost. This is *samadhi*, or a state of total absorption. *Sama* means "level" or "alike", while *adhi* means "over" and "above." Though *samadhi* can be explained at the intellectual level, it can only be experienced at the level of the heart. It is the maintenance of the intelligence in a balanced state. Ultimately, it is *samadhi* that is the fruit of the discipline of Astanga Yoga.

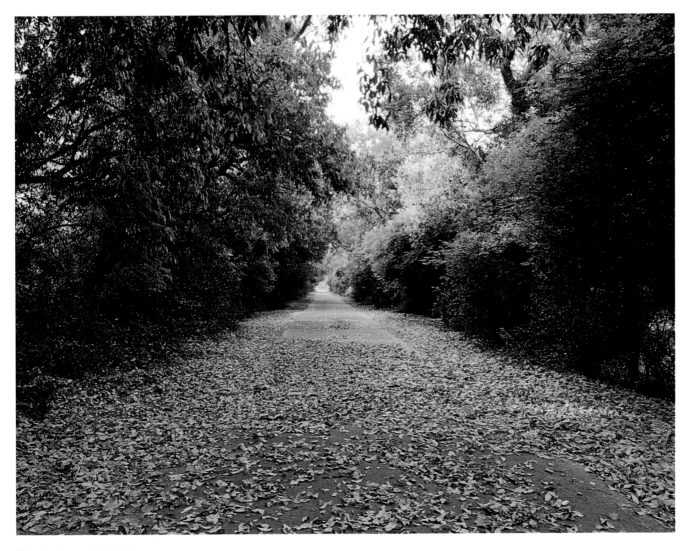

THE ROAD TO SAMADHI
The practice of yoga requires discipline and intense concentration, but the fruits of the journey are truth and tranquillity

Pranayama

Prana *is the life force which permeates both the individual as well as the universe at all levels. It is at once physical, sexual, mental, intellectual, spiritual, and cosmic.* Prana, *the breath, and the mind are inextricably linked to each other.*

The ancient yogis advocated the practice of pranayama to unite the breath with the mind, and therefore with the *prana* or life force. *Prana* is energy, and *ayama* is the storing and distribution of that energy. *Ayama* has three aspects or movements: vertical extension, horizontal extension, and cyclical extension. By practicing pranayama, we learn to move energy vertically, horizontally, and cyclically to the frontiers of the body.

BREATH IN PRANAYAMA

Pranayama is not deep breathing. Deep breathing tenses the facial muscles, makes the skull and scalp rigid, tightens the chest, and applies external force to the intake or release of breath. This creates hardness in the fibers of the lungs and chest, and prevents the percolation of breath through the body.

In pranayama, the cells of the brain and the facial muscles remain soft and receptive, and the breath is drawn in or released gently. During inhalation, each molecule,

fiber, and cell of the body is independently felt by the mind, and is allowed to receive and absorb the *prana*. There are no sudden movements and one becomes aware of the gradual expansion of the respiratory organs, and feels the breath reaching the most remote parts of the lungs.

In exhalation, the release of breath is gradual, and this gives the air cells sufficient time to reabsorb the residual *prana* to the maximum possible extent. This allows for the full utilization of energy, therefore building emotional stability and calming the mind.

The practice of asanas removes the obstructions which impede the flow of *prana*. During pranayama, one should be totally absorbed in the fineness of inhalation, exhalation, and in the naturalness of retention. One should not disturb or jerk the vital organs and nerves, or stress the brain cells. The brain is the instrument which observes the smooth flow of inhalation and exhalation. One must be aware of the interruptions which occur during a single inhalation and exhalation.

YOGACHARYA IYENGAR
IN PRANAYAMA
Practicing pranayama while sitting up is very difficult and should not be attempted by beginners

Check these, and a smooth flow will set in. Similarly, during retention of breath, learn to retain the first indrawn breath with stability. If this stability is lost, it is better to release the breath, rather than strain to hold it. While inhaling or retaining the breath in a pranayamic cycle, remember to ensure that the abdomen does not swell.

THE FINAL GOAL

Attempt pranayama only when the yoga asanas have been mastered. Patanjali reiterates this several times, most emphatically in *Yoga Sutra* II, 49. The next *sutra*, *Yoga Sutra* II, 50, explains that inhalation, exhalation, and retention must be precise. The *sutra* begins with control over the movement of exhalation, or *bahya*, and inhalation, or *abhyantara*. Each inhalation activates the central nervous system into stimulating the peripheral nerves, and each exhalation triggers the reverse process. During the retention of breath, both processes take place. The *Hathayoga Pradipika* speaks of *antara-kumbhaka* and *bahya-kumbhaka*, or the suspension of breath with empty or full lungs, as well as inhalation, and exhalation. Pranayama is a complex process composed of all of these. It has to be practiced with the greatest sincerity and precision. You cannot achieve pranayama just because you want to. You have to be ready for it.

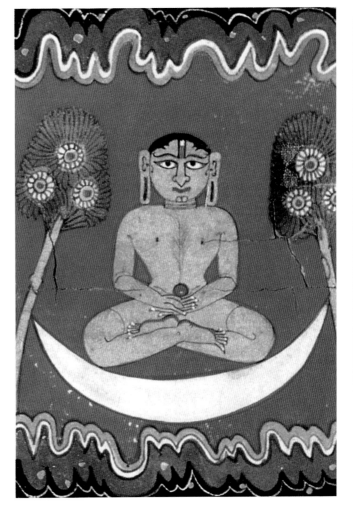

A YOGI IN PRANAYAMA
For more than a thousand years, sages have practiced pranayama, controlling their breath and with it, their mind

ANCIENT TRADITIONS
An illustrated folio from the Kalpasutra, 15th-century texts describing the path to health and spirituality

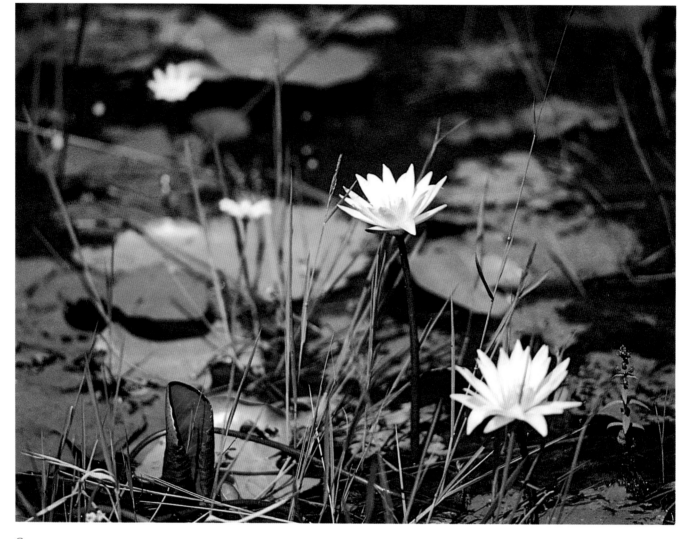

SPIRITUAL PRANAYAMA
The pranayamic mind blossoms, becomes completely free, and dissolves in the self

In pranayamic breathing, the brain is quiet, and this allows the nervous system to function more effectively. Inhalation is the art of receiving primeval energy into the body in the form of breath, and bringing the spiritual cosmic breath into contact with the individual breath. Exhalation is the removal of toxins from the system.

BETWEEN THE MATERIAL AND SPIRITUAL WORLD
Pranayama is also the link between the physiological and spiritual organisms of man. At first, pranayama is difficult and requires great effort. Mastery is achieved when pranayama becomes effortless. Just as the diaphragm is the meeting point of the physiological and spiritual body, the retention of

energy, or *kumbhaka*, is realizing the very core of your body. Once the external movements are controlled, there is internal silence. In such a silence there is no thought as the mind has then dissolved in the self.

In the *Hathayoga Pradipika*, the sage Svatmarama gives a detailed description of the ways in which an individual comes to experience the elevated state of oneness with the self through the practice of pranayama. Hence, practicing it is not only very difficult, but also highly absorbing. If you fail after a few cycles, be content with the knowledge that you have practiced three or four cycles with awareness and attention. Do not turn away from failures. Accept them and learn from them. Gradually, you will learn to master pranayama.

Chakras

Yogic science recognizes that spiritual health is activated by a system of chakras, or "nerve" centers, said to be located within the spinal column. Cosmic energy lies coiled within these chakras and has to be awakened for self-realization.

Modern technology has provided us with the means to examine the state of our bodies. However, nothing has helped us discern character, personality, or the potential for goodness yet. The most important aspect of a human being is the part which lies between the outer skin and the innermost soul, the *shakti*, which includes the mind, intellect, emotions, vital energy, the sense of "I," the powers of will and discrimination, and the conscience. These are different in every human being, and that makes us individually both mysterious and unique. In yogic terminology, the soul is called *purusha shakti*, while *prakriti shakti*, or the energy of nature, came to be called *kundalini* by the ancient yogis.

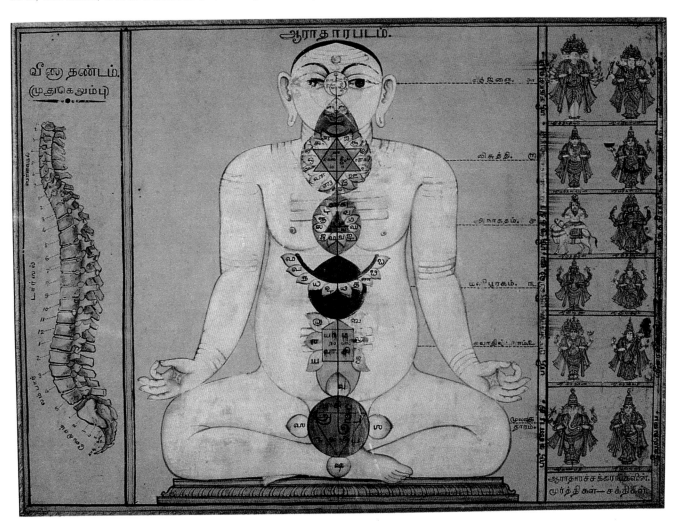

THE 7 MAIN CHAKRAS OF THE BODY
Yogic sages believed chakras were located along the spinal column

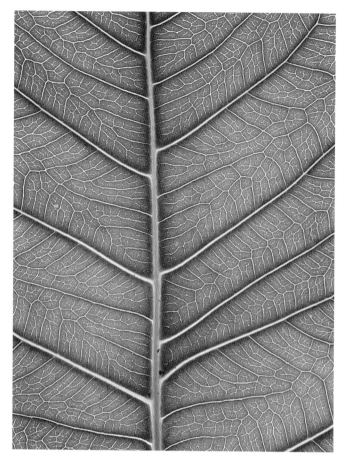

EACH CELL IS AN ENTITY
Energy spreads through a leaf, from each tiny cell connected to the other, permeating from the stalks to the entire plant

We have always known that health is important, but it is time to realize, as proponents of yoga have known for generations, that our physical condition is inextricably linked to our state of mind.

Yogic science recognized this connection from the very beginning. In order to achieve perfect physical health, the ancient sages concluded that you must activate the body's *chakras*. *Chakras* are located along the spine, from the brain to the tailbone. However, while the spine is a physical entity, *chakras* are not composed of matter. Although they possess no physicality, they govern all the elements of the body.

THE MEANING OF CHAKRAS

Chakra means "wheel" or "ring" in Sanskrit and our personal *chakras* have energy coiled within them. They are the critical junctions which determine the state of the body and mind. Just as the brain controls physical, mental, and intellectual functions through the nerve cells or neurons, similarly *chakras* tap the *prana*, or cosmic energy which is within all living beings and transform it into spiritual energy. This is spread through the body by the *nadis*, or channels.

Being invisible, *chakras* are tangible only through their effects. They can be accessed once the student of yoga has achieved all the eight aspects of yoga (*see page* 29), when the human self merges with the divine self.

Kundalini is the divine, cosmic energy which exists as a latent force in everyone. When the *prakriti shakti* is awakened, it gravitates toward the very core of the soul or *purusha shakti*.

AWAKENING COSMIC ENERGY

This fire of divine, cosmic energy is ignited by *yoga-agni*, the fire of yoga. When a fire is covered with ashes, it goes out. In the same way, if our senses are inert, or if we are motivated by pride, self-indulgence, and envy, the *kundalini* is kept in a dormant state. If we allow such negative qualities to dominate our thinking over long periods, our spiritual evolution is not merely hampered, but actually halted.

A SYMBOLIC REPRESENTATION OF THE MULADHARA CHAKRA
Chakras transform cosmic energy into spiritual energy

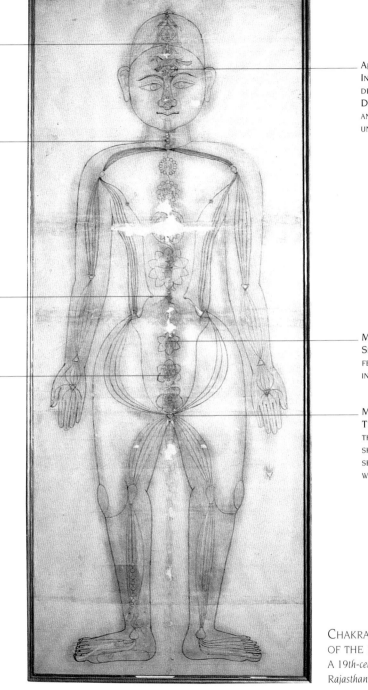

Sahasrara Chakra
Uncoiled through
intuitive knowledge, it
allows the seeker to
achieve freedom

Vishuddhi Chakra
Seat of intellectual
awareness

Anahata chakra
When uncoiled,
it develops compassion,
spirituality, and
knowledge

Swadhishtana chakra
Influences worldly
desires when coiled

Ajna Chakra
Influences pride and
desire when coiled.
Develops humanity
and spirituality when
uncoiled

Manipuraka chakra
Site of the sense of
fear; when uncoiled,
induces calm

Muladhara chakra
The foundation of
the anatomical
sheath controls
sexual energy
when coiled.

CHAKRAS AND NADIS
OF THE HUMAN BODY
*A 19th-century painting from
Rajasthan, India*

There are 11 *chakras* of which 7 are crucial (*see diagram above*), and the others dependent. The most important is the Sahasrara *chakra*, where *prakriti shakti* or energy, unites with *purusha shakti*, or soul.

The practice of yoga is directed at awakening the divine energy within every human being. Asanas and pranayama uncoil and alert the *chakras*. In the process, the *nadis* are activated. This causes the *chakras* to vibrate and generate energy, which is then circulated all over the body through the *nadis*. The emotions rooted in the *chakras* are transformed as divine energy is awakened and circulated.

To achieve self-realization the sincere student of yoga will, with persistent, rigorous practice, conquer the 6 main obstacles to happiness, desire, anger, greed, infatuation, pride, and envy.

The Guru & the Yogi

The tradition of the guru, or master, and the yogi, or disciple, is an ancient one. All learning from generation to generation has been handed down this way. The guru must be compassionate, yet exacting. The yogi must be sincere and dedicated.

How do we distinguish between the true guru and the false one? The cult of the guru, or master, is an Asian concept. To other societies, the concept might seem exotic, mysterious, or even abhorrent, a brake on individual freedom or judgment. Some thinkers have declared that a guru is not needed at all, while others believe that you cannot reach your goal without one. Perhaps the importance of the guru can be explained by examining its Sanskrit root. *Gu* means "darkness" and *ru* means "light." Therefore, a guru is one who leads you from darkness to light. Although the *sadhaka*, or seeker, has to tread the spiritual path to self-realization alone, the guru's guidance is essential to show the right path and to safeguard the yogi, the student of yoga, who decides to follow it.

AN ANCIENT TRADITION

The guru is the voice of consciousness during the process of spiritual awakening. In India, the relationship between a guru and a disciple is an ancient tradition, and has been the foundation of all learning. The *guru-sishya parampara* (*sishya* means "disciple" and *parampara* means "tradition") has been the system through which knowledge has been handed down, generation to generation and age to age. The energy that the guru has imbibed from *his* teacher is passed on to his disciple, and keep the process of communication alive from one epoch to the next. The guru opens the disciple's eyes to awareness. Knowledge exists, but ignorance veils it,

YOGACHARYA IYENGAR WITH A STUDENT
The guru does not only teach asanas, he teaches you how to live

and it is the guru who removes this veil from the intellect of the *sishya*. The guru is the guide who opens the gate of the student's dormant faculties and awakens the latent power and energy within. Being with the guru is like being in the sunlight, and the glow lasts for eternity.

The relationship between the teacher and the disciple is a unique one. It is similar, but not identical, to a mother and child. Just as a mother loves, nourishes, guides, cajoles into obedience, rebukes, educates, and protects her child, the guru takes the disciple into his care, making it his life's work to mold his student into perfect shape, physically, mentally, and spiritually.

THE GURU

Yoga is a discipline and the yogic texts aptly begin with the emphasis on discipline, or *anusasanami*, and say, "Without discipline, nothing can be achieved." The guru does not enforce discipline with strictness, but builds an awareness of it in his student, allowing the latter to develop inner discipline. A wise guru does not lay down codes of conduct, but motivates the disciple by precept and example.

The guru does not demand attention, he commands it. In the process of teaching, he creates total confidence in the disciple, and helps him or her develop the will power to face all circumstances with equanimity. The guru constantly improves on his teaching techniques, opening the disciple's eyes, improvising where necessary to create new dimensions in his teaching. The guru is compassionate, but does not expect emotional attachment from his disciple, nor does he become emotionally attached himself.

The guru should be confident, challenging, caring, cautious, constructive, and courageous. The clarity and creativity of his teaching should reflect his devotion and dedication to his subject, in this case, the complexities and subtleties of yoga.

THE DISCIPLE

An ideal disciple is obedient, earnest, serious, and always ready to follow the teachings of his or her guru. This is not unthinking obedience, but one based on respect and a sincere desire to learn. Disciples can be dull, average, or superior. The dull student has little enthusiasm, is unstable, timorous, and self-indulgent. He or she is unwilling to put in the hard work required which is needed to attain self-realization.

The average student is indecisive, attracted equally to worldly pleasures as to spiritual matters.

While conscious of the highest good, this student lacks the determination to persevere, and is unable to hold on steadfastly to the yogic path. He or she needs firmness and discipline from his or her guru, a fact the guru recognizes at once.

The superior or intense student, on the other hand, has vision, enthusiasm, and courage. He or she resists temptations and does not hesitate to cast off qualities that distract him or her from the goal. This student becomes steady, stable, and skillful. The guru guides this kind of student to the ultimate goal of self-realization.

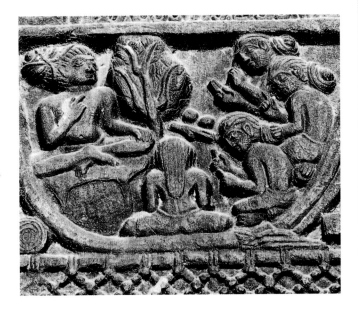

A SAGE TEACHING HIS PUPILS
This 2nd-century BC frieze from Bharhut, India, points to the antiquity of the guru-yogi tradition

While practicing yoga, the disciple must recall and deliberate on each word and action of the guru and consolidate each learning experience. Today's disciple may become the guru of tomorrow. Clarity of mind and firmness of resolve to tread the path to self-realization is essential. The yogi must have *riti* and *niti*, or method and morality, to impart to the disciple the learning, the experience, and wisdom gleaned over the years. The tradition of the guru and the yogi is carried on for yet another generation.

This book is my attempt to disseminate my knowledge of yoga to people all over the world who wish to become true followers of yoga.

CHAPTER 3

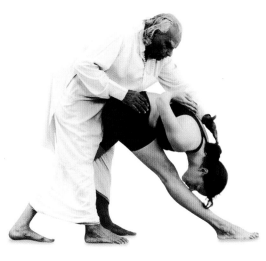

"The body is your temple. Keep it pure and clean for the soul to reside in."

Asanas for You

The science of yoga is like the art of music. There is a rhythm within the body, and that can only be maintained by paying attention to each step of the asana, and to the progression between asanas. In your practice of yoga, there has to be a physical, physiological, psychological, and spiritual rhythm. Unless there is harmony and melody, the music will not be worth listening to. The body is a truly sensitive and receptive instrument, and its vibrations, like sound, express the harmony or dissonance within it. Each of these vibrations must synchronize in the movement, which is the asana.

Classic Postures

Yoga asanas cover the basic positions of standing, sitting, forward bends, twists, inversions, back bends, and lying down. The 23 classic postures must be practiced with physical coordination, as well as intelligence and sincerity.

There is more to practicing asanas correctly than merely the physical aligning of the body. The classic postures, when practiced with discrimination and awareness, bring the body, mind, intelligence, nerves, consciousness, and the self together into a single, harmonious whole. Asanas may appear to deal with the physical body alone but, in fact, different asanas can affect the chemical messages sent to and from the brain and improve and stabilize your mental state. Yoga's unique ability to soothe the nerves, the medium between the physiological body and the psychological body, calms the brain, makes the mind fresh and tranquil, and relaxes the entire body.

I have selected these 23 asanas because they cover all the basic positions of yoga: standing, sitting, forward bends, twists, inversions, back bends, and lying down. The regular practice of these asanas, stimulates and activates all the organs, tissues, and cells of the body. The mind becomes alert and strong, the body healthy and active.

The anatomical body comprises the limbs and the actual parts of the body. The physical body is made up of bones, muscles, skin, and tissue. The physiological body is composed of the heart, lungs, liver, spleen, pancreas, intestines, and the other organs. The nerves, brain, and intellect make up the psychological body. To practice asanas correctly, you have to learn to bring all these levels together.

STAGES OF LEARNING YOGA

Newcomers to yoga approach asanas with "uncultured" minds. They have to learn that at first asanas are practiced at the level of the anatomical body alone, the stage called *arambhavastha*. This beginner's stage is important and should not be hurried through. In order to learn the asanas, beginners should be primarily concerned with getting their movements right. In the step-by-step instructions to the asanas in this chapter, I have highlighted the points you should concentrate on, the important motions and movements in the posture you need to take note of. Beginners have to grasp the whole asana, and not lose themselves in the finer details. It is more important for you to start by striving for stability within a posture. This provides a strong foundation. You will then enter the intermediate stage, or *ghatavastha*, in which the mind is affected by changes in the body. When you reach this stage, you are practicing the movements correctly, and your body is

INTEGRATING BODY AND SPIRIT
Yogacharya Iyengar in Adhomukha Svanasana

"Asanas keep your body, as well as your mind, healthy and active."

under your control, but you must now push your mind to touch every part of your body. In my instructions to the asanas in this chapter, I have pointed out that students of yoga at this stage must practice the asanas with reflective and meditative attention. You must become aware of your tissues, organs, skin, and even individual cells. Your mind must flow along with all these parts.

Parichayavastha, or the advanced stage, comes next. This is the stage of intimate knowledge, when your mind brings your body in touch with your intelligence. Once this happens, the mind ceases to be a separate entity, and the intelligence and the body become one. I have included the concepts that the advanced practitioner of yoga should focus on. Your adjustments are more subtle and discriminating now, and are in the realm of the mental and physiological body, rather than merely in your muscles, bones, and joints. The final stage, nispattyavastha, is the state of perfection. Once the intelligence feels the oneness between the flesh and the skin, it introduces the atman, the self or soul. This frees the body and integrates it with the soul in the journey from the finite to the infinite. Then the body, mind, and self become one. At this stage, asanas become meditative and spiritual. This may be termed "dynamic meditation."

WHAT IS AN ASANA?

An asana is not a posture that you assume mechanically. It involves a thoughtful process at the end of which a balance is achieved between movement and resistance. Your weight has to be evenly distributed over muscles, bones, and

joints, just as your intelligence must be engaged at every level. You have to create space in your muscles and your skin, fitting the fine network of your entire body into the asana. This helps the organs of perception (the eyes, ears, nose, tongue, and skin) discern the subtlety of each movement. This conjunction between the organs of action and organs of perception occurs when the student reaches a subjective understanding of an asana, and begins, through instinct as well as knowledge, to adjust his or her movements correctly. Practice with dedication. Be completely absorbed by the asana.

Once both sides of the body become symmetrical, undue stress is removed from the circulatory, respiratory, digestive, reproductive, and excretory systems. In each asana, different organs are placed in different anatomical positions, and are squeezed and spread, dampened and dried, heated and cooled. The organs are supplied with fresh blood, and are gently massaged, relaxed, and toned into a state of optimum health.

MOVEMENT AND RESISTANCE
The final posture of Utthita Parsvakonasana

RELIEVING TENSION
AND STRESS
*The torso is stretched
in Bharadvajasana*

SITTING ASANAS

All sitting asanas bring elasticity to the hips, knees, ankles, and muscles of the groin. These postures remove tension and hardness in the diaphragm and throat, making breathing smoother and easier. They keep the spine steady, pacifying the mind and stretching the muscles of the heart. Blood circulation increases to all parts of the body.

STANDING ASANAS

Standing asanas strengthen the leg muscles and joints, and increase the suppleness and strength of the spine. Owing to their rotational and flexing movements, the spinal muscles and intervertebral joints are kept mobile and well aligned. The arteries of the legs are stretched, increasing the blood supply to the lower limbs, and preventing thrombosis in the calf muscles. These asanas also tone the cardiovascular system. The lateral wall of the heart is fully stretched, increasing the supply of fresh blood to the heart.

FORWARD BENDS

In forward bends, the abdominal organs are compressed. This has a unique effect on the nervous system. As these organs relax, the frontal brain is cooled, and the flow of blood to the entire brain is regulated. The sympathetic nervous system is rested, bringing down the pulse and blood pressure. Stress is removed from the organs of perception and the senses relax. The adrenal glands are also soothed and function more efficiently. Since the body is in a horizontal position in forward bends, the heart is relieved of the strain of pumping blood against gravity, and blood circulates through all parts of the body easily. Forward bends also strengthen the paraspinal muscles, intervertebral joints, and ligaments.

TWISTS

These asanas teach us the importance of a healthy spine and inner body. In twists, the pelvic and abdominal organs are squeezed and flushed with blood. They improve the suppleness of the diaphragm, and relieve spinal, hip, and groin disorders. The spine also becomes more supple, and this improves the flow of blood to the spinal nerves and increases energy levels.

INVERSIONS

Some people fear that if they practice inverted postures, their blood pressure will rise or their blood vessels will burst. These are misconceptions. After all, standing for long periods can lead to thrombosis and varicose veins, but no one is going to stop standing up! Standing upright is a result of evolution. Just as the human body has adjusted to an upright position, it can also learn to perform inversions without any risk or harm. In contrast to the twisting asanas, inverted asanas have a drying effect on the pelvic and abdominal organs, while vital organs like the brain, heart, and lungs are flushed with blood. According to the third chapter of the sage Svatmarama's *Hathayoga Pradipika,*

Salamba Sirsasana (headstand, *see page* 118) is the king of asanas, and Salamba Sarvangasana (shoulderstand, *see page* 124) the queen of asanas. The health of your body and mind is greatly enhanced by the practice of these two asanas.

BACK BENDS

All back bends stimulate the central nervous system and increase its ability to bear stress. They help relieve and prevent headaches, hypertension, and nervous exhaustion. These asanas stimulate and energize the body, and are invaluable to people suffering from depression. In Urdhva Dhanurasana (*see page* 140) and Viparita Dandasana (*see page* 220), the liver and spleen are fully stretched, and can therefore function more effectively.

RECLINING ASANAS

Reclining asanas are restful postures which soothe the body and refresh the mind. While reclining asanas are often sequenced at the end of a yoga session, they are also preparatory asanas, since they help relax the body and strengthen the joints. They give the body the required energy for the more strenuous asanas. Savasana (*see page* 150), for instance, helps recover the breath and cool the body and the mind. Reclining asanas prepare you for pranayama.

PRACTICING CLASSIC POSTURES

Read the instructions for practice (*see page* 386). Practice classic postures when you feel confident of the suppleness of your body and the stability of your mind. In the 20-Week Yoga Course (*see page* 388), I recommend that beginners and those with stiff muscles or joints, or people with specific ailments, might prefer to practice with props for the first 6 to 8 months. If you normally practice classic postures without props, you may, however, wish to use them on

STRETCHING OUT
Paschimottanasana extends the spine

days when you are feeling tired, or if a particular part of your body feels stiff. Always sequence your asanas with care. Beginners should follow the order given in the 20-Week Yoga Course. Whenever you practice, take care not to "harden" your brain. This occurs when you hold your breath, and your head becomes tense and heavy, particularly common when practicing standing asanas and forward bends. This can also happen in a standing asana when you use force to descend without fully extending your spine. Since the action is achieved by force, rather than by utilizing the intelligence of the spine, this results in tension in the spine. I call this situation "hardening the brain," because it means you are not allowing your brain to be sufficiently sensitive to your body's actions. Similarly, in back bends, if force, not intelligence is applied while extending the back, the cervical region remains hard. This, too, "hardens the brain."

"BRAIN" OF THE POSTURE

In each asana, a specific part of your body is the "brain" of the posture. The outstretched arm, for instance, is the "brain" of Utthita Parsvakonasana (*see page* 60), the center of balance in the posture. When you practice, observe this specific part carefully and focus on it. Bring a

PRACTICE WITHOUT FEAR
Inversions, like Salamba Sarvangasana, are good for your body and mind

firmness and steadiness to it. This will spread to the rest of your body and bring it under your control. You will then be able to experience the posture at the physiological level, and not merely the physical level.

Standing Asanas

"An asana is not a posture which you assume mechanically. It involves thought, at the end of which a balance is achieved between movement and resistance."

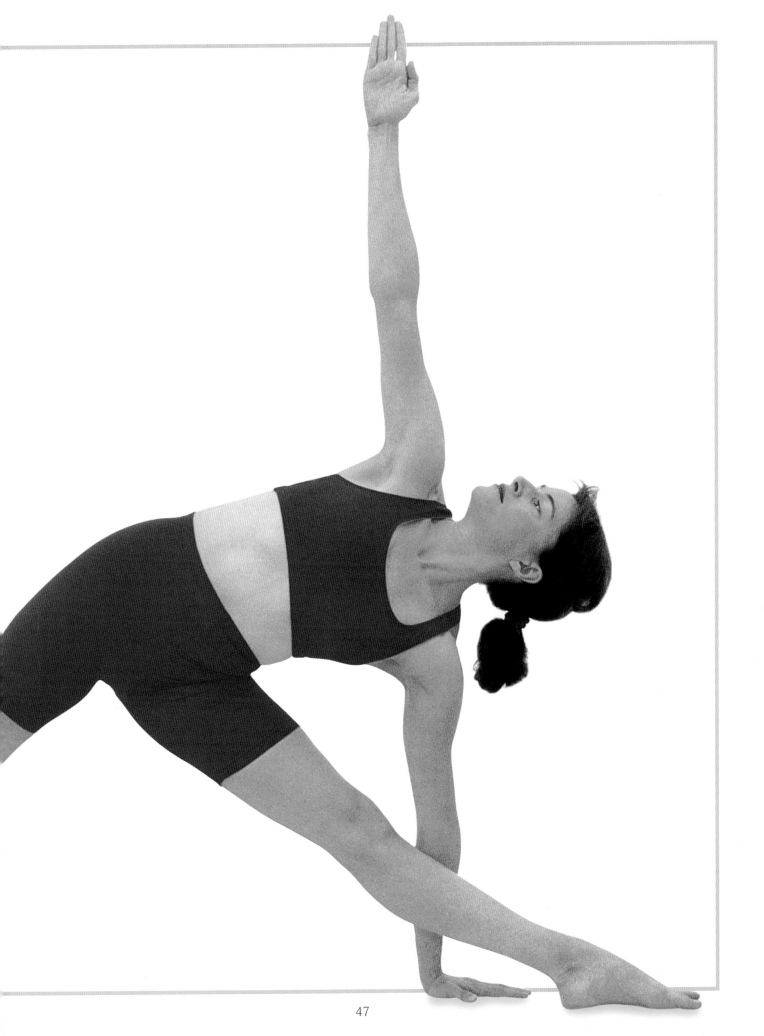

ताडासन
Tadasana

- Mountain posture -

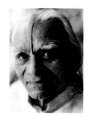

I N THIS POSTURE you learn to stand as firm and erect as a mountain. The word *tada* in Sanskrit means "mountain." Most people do not balance perfectly on both legs, leading to ailments which can be avoided. Tadasana teaches you the art of standing correctly and increases your awareness of your body. It is the foundation stone for other asanas. Practicing it gives rise to a sense of firmness, strength, stillness, and steadiness.

CAUTIONS
◆

If you have Parkinson's disease or a spinal disc disorder, you may find it helpful to stand facing a wall with your palms placed on it. People with scoliosis should rest the spine against the protruding edge of two adjoining walls.

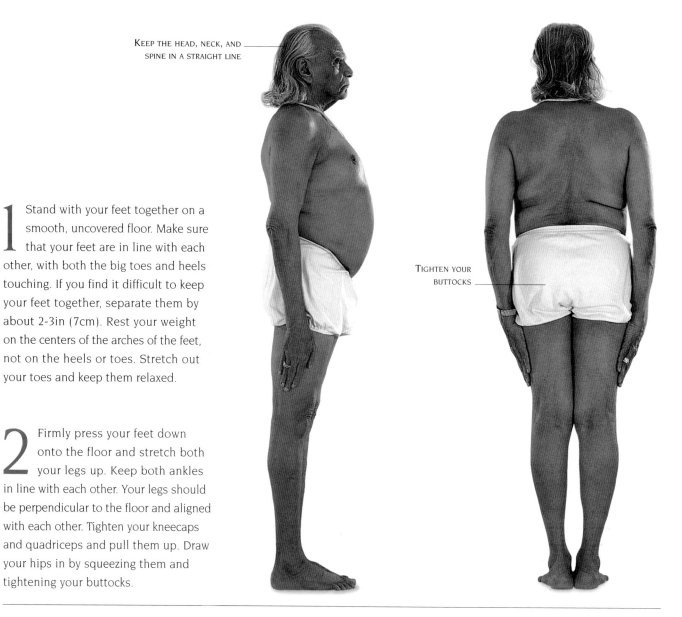

KEEP THE HEAD, NECK, AND SPINE IN A STRAIGHT LINE

TIGHTEN YOUR BUTTOCKS

1 Stand with your feet together on a smooth, uncovered floor. Make sure that your feet are in line with each other, with both the big toes and heels touching. If you find it difficult to keep your feet together, separate them by about 2-3in (7cm). Rest your weight on the centers of the arches of the feet, not on the heels or toes. Stretch out your toes and keep them relaxed.

2 Firmly press your feet down onto the floor and stretch both your legs up. Keep both ankles in line with each other. Your legs should be perpendicular to the floor and aligned with each other. Tighten your kneecaps and quadriceps and pull them up. Draw your hips in by squeezing them and tightening your buttocks.

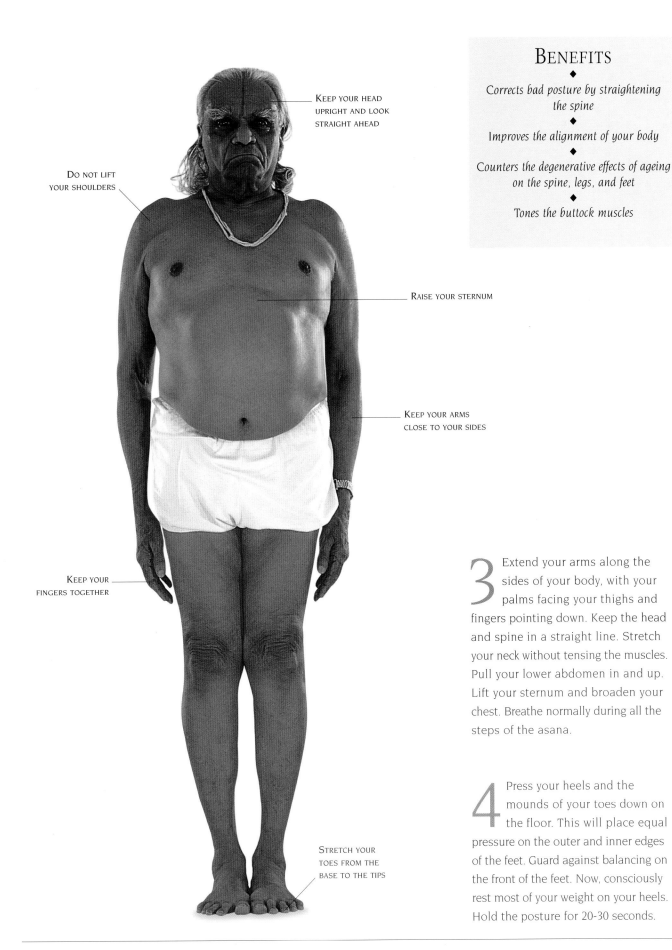

KEEP YOUR HEAD
UPRIGHT AND LOOK
STRAIGHT AHEAD

DO NOT LIFT
YOUR SHOULDERS

KEEP YOUR
FINGERS TOGETHER

RAISE YOUR STERNUM

KEEP YOUR ARMS
CLOSE TO YOUR SIDES

STRETCH YOUR
TOES FROM THE
BASE TO THE TIPS

BENEFITS

◆

*Corrects bad posture by straightening
the spine*

◆

Improves the alignment of your body

◆

*Counters the degenerative effects of ageing
on the spine, legs, and feet*

◆

Tones the buttock muscles

3 Extend your arms along the
sides of your body, with your
palms facing your thighs and
fingers pointing down. Keep the head
and spine in a straight line. Stretch
your neck without tensing the muscles.
Pull your lower abdomen in and up.
Lift your sternum and broaden your
chest. Breathe normally during all the
steps of the asana.

4 Press your heels and the
mounds of your toes down on
the floor. This will place equal
pressure on the outer and inner edges
of the feet. Guard against balancing on
the front of the feet. Now, consciously
rest most of your weight on your heels.
Hold the posture for 20-30 seconds.

उत्थित त्रिकोणासन

Utthita Trikonasana

- Extended triangle posture -

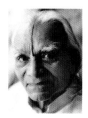

IN THIS ASANA, your body takes the shape of an extended triangle, giving an intense stretch to your trunk and legs. *Utthita* means "extended" in Sanskrit, *tri* means "three," and *kona* indicates an angle. With practice, you will learn to move from your physical body into your physiological body (*see page* 42). You will learn to activate the organs, glands, and nerves, which form the physiological body, by controlling the movements of your limbs. This posture tones the ligaments and improves flexibility.

CAUTIONS

◆

If you are prone to dizzy spells, vertigo, or high blood pressure, look down at the floor in the final posture. Do not turn your head up. If you have a cardiac condition, practice against a wall. Do not raise the arm, but rest it along your hip.

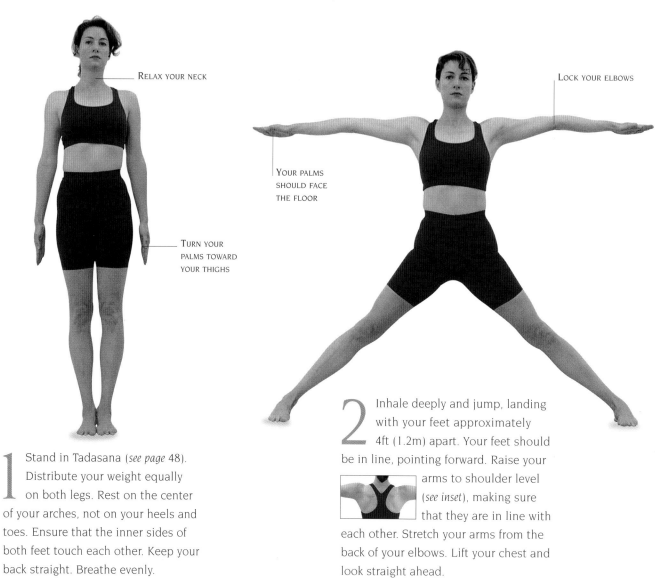

RELAX YOUR NECK

TURN YOUR PALMS TOWARD YOUR THIGHS

YOUR PALMS SHOULD FACE THE FLOOR

LOCK YOUR ELBOWS

1 Stand in Tadasana (*see page* 48). Distribute your weight equally on both legs. Rest on the center of your arches, not on your heels and toes. Ensure that the inner sides of both feet touch each other. Keep your back straight. Breathe evenly.

2 Inhale deeply and jump, landing with your feet approximately 4ft (1.2m) apart. Your feet should be in line, pointing forward. Raise your arms to shoulder level (*see inset*), making sure that they are in line with each other. Stretch your arms from the back of your elbows. Lift your chest and look straight ahead.

3 Turn in your right foot, slightly to the left, maintaining the stretch of your other leg. Then, turn your left foot 90° to the left, keeping the right leg stretched and tightened at the knee. Make sure that your arms do not waver. Keep them fully stretched.

BEGINNERS To maintain your balance during this step, always keep to the sequence of turning in your right foot first. Once you have done this, turn out your left foot.

INTERMEDIATES For a better stretch in the final posture, press your left heel down on the floor and raise your toes toward the ceiling (*see inset*). Then tighten the left knee and flatten your foot to the floor again.

CORRECTING YOURSELF

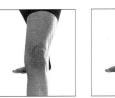

THE RIGHT KNEE

WRONG *If your right knee rotates to the right, this will impair your stretch in the final posture.*

RIGHT *Keep your right kneecap facing front. Ensure that your right thigh does not turn in.*

THE LEFT KNEE

WRONG *If the left knee rotates too far to the left, your balance in the asana will be affected.*

RIGHT *Keep your left knee tightened, and in line with the center of your left foot, shin, and thigh.*

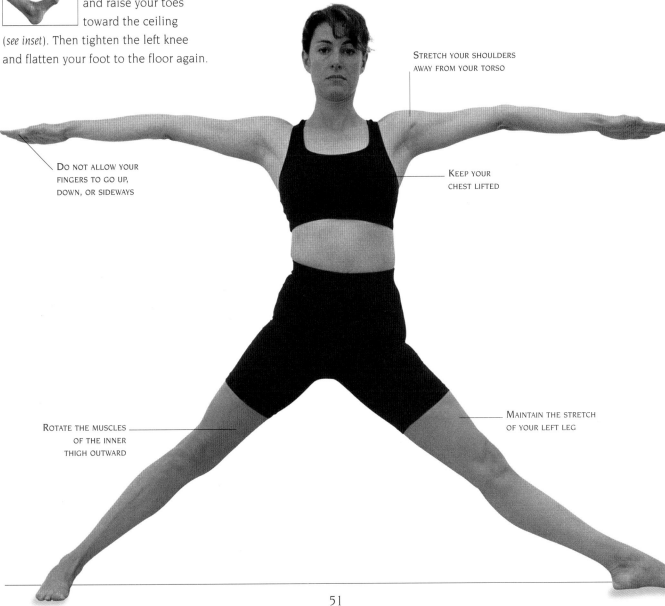

STRETCH YOUR SHOULDERS AWAY FROM YOUR TORSO

KEEP YOUR CHEST LIFTED

DO NOT ALLOW YOUR FINGERS TO GO UP, DOWN, OR SIDEWAYS

MAINTAIN THE STRETCH OF YOUR LEFT LEG

ROTATE THE MUSCLES OF THE INNER THIGH OUTWARD

UTTHITA TRIKONASANA – EXTENDED TRIANGLE POSTURE

उत्थित त्रिकोणासन

Utthita Trikonasana

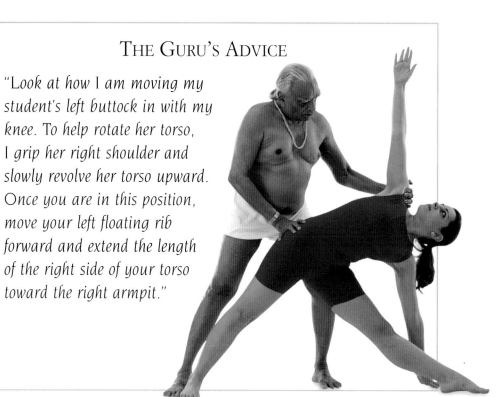

THE GURU'S ADVICE

"Look at how I am moving my student's left buttock in with my knee. To help rotate her torso, I grip her right shoulder and slowly revolve her torso upward. Once you are in this position, move your left floating rib forward and extend the length of the right side of your torso toward the right armpit."

CORRECTING YOURSELF

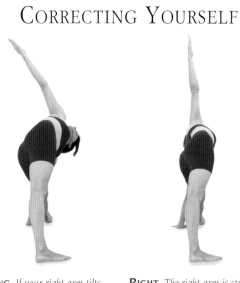

WRONG *If your right arm tilts back, you will lose the correct alignment of the hips and buttocks. Your neck and head will jut forward and your weight will fall on your left palm, and not on your left heel.*

RIGHT *The right arm is stretched straight up from the armpit and kept steady. Keep the back of your head aligned with your spine, and keep your shoulder blades in line with each other.*

KEEP YOUR KNEECAP
FACING FRONT

MAKE SURE
YOUR RIGHT LEG IS
FULLY STRETCHED

4 Exhale and bend your torso sideways to the left. Place your left palm flat on the floor and press your left heel down on the floor. Adjust your posture until your weight rests on your left heel and not on your left palm. Raise your right arm up toward the ceiling in line with your shoulders and left arm. Turn your head keeping your neck passive and fix your eyes on your right thumb. Stay in the posture for 20-30 seconds. Do not take deep breaths, but breathe evenly.

BEGINNERS When you bend, first grip your left ankle with your left hand. Bring the left buttock slightly forward. Place your right hand on your right hip. Once you feel steady in this posture, follow the instructions above.

KEEP YOUR RIGHT PALM OPEN AND FULLY STRETCHED

BENEFITS

Relieves gastritis, indigestion, acidity, and flatulence

Improves the flexibility of the spine

Alleviates backache

Corrects alignment of the shoulders

Helps to treat neck sprains

Massages and tones the pelvic area

Strengthens the ankles

Reduces discomfort during menstruation

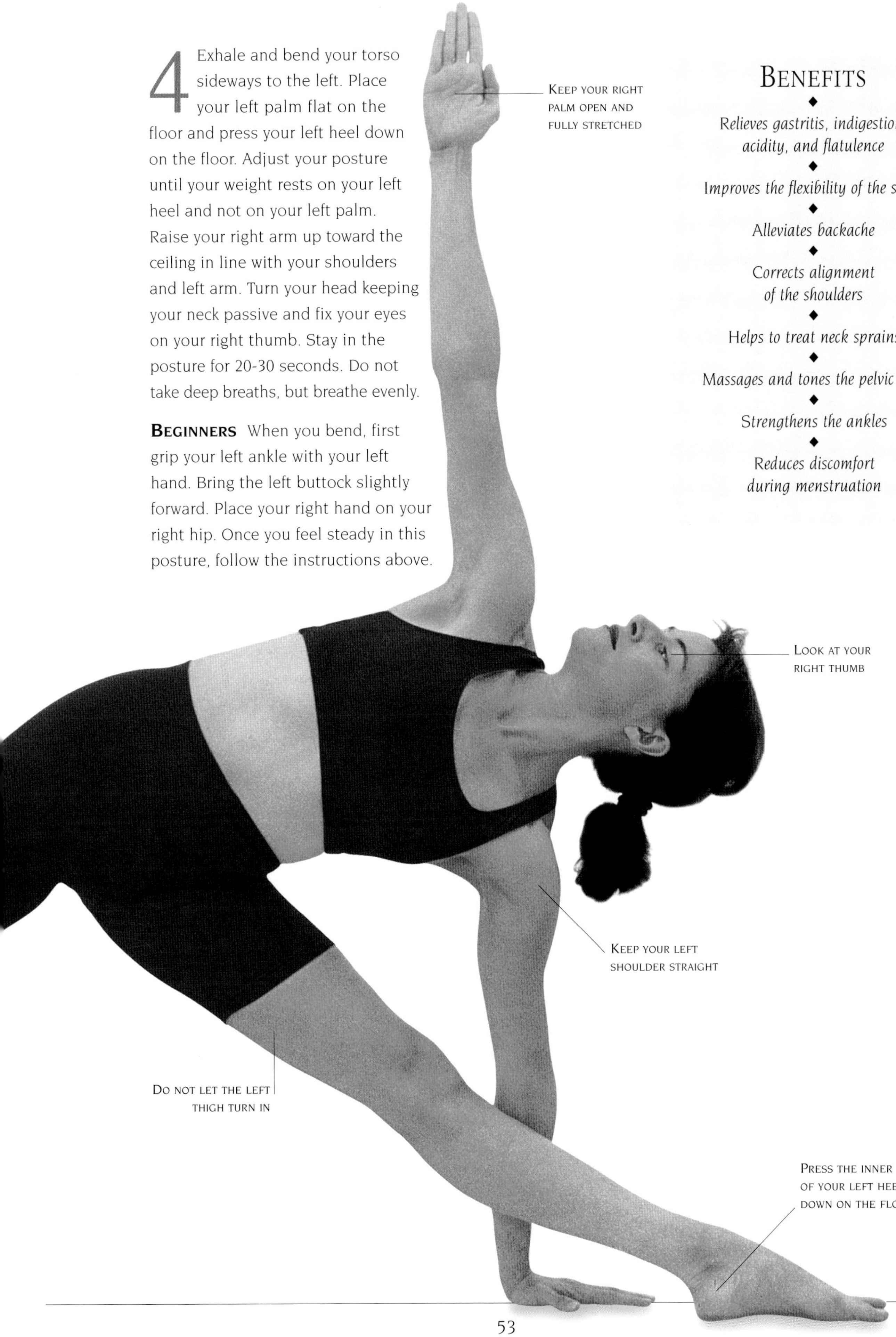

LOOK AT YOUR RIGHT THUMB

KEEP YOUR LEFT SHOULDER STRAIGHT

DO NOT LET THE LEFT THIGH TURN IN

PRESS THE INNER EDGE OF YOUR LEFT HEEL DOWN ON THE FLOOR

UTTHITA TRIKONASANA – EXTENDED TRIANGLE POSTURE

उत्थित त्रिकोणासन

Utthita Trikonasana

ADVANCED WORK IN THE POSTURE

Keep your right arm steady, as it is the "brain" of the posture (*see page* 45). Work on your back. Imagine your body is being pulled in opposite directions from the spine. Check that both shoulders are equally stretched out. Make sure that your torso revolves slightly up and back. Keep the back of your neck in line with your spine, but relax your throat, keeping the muscles of your neck passive. Ensure that the tailbone and the back of your head align with each other, and that your whole body is balanced symmetrically in one plane.

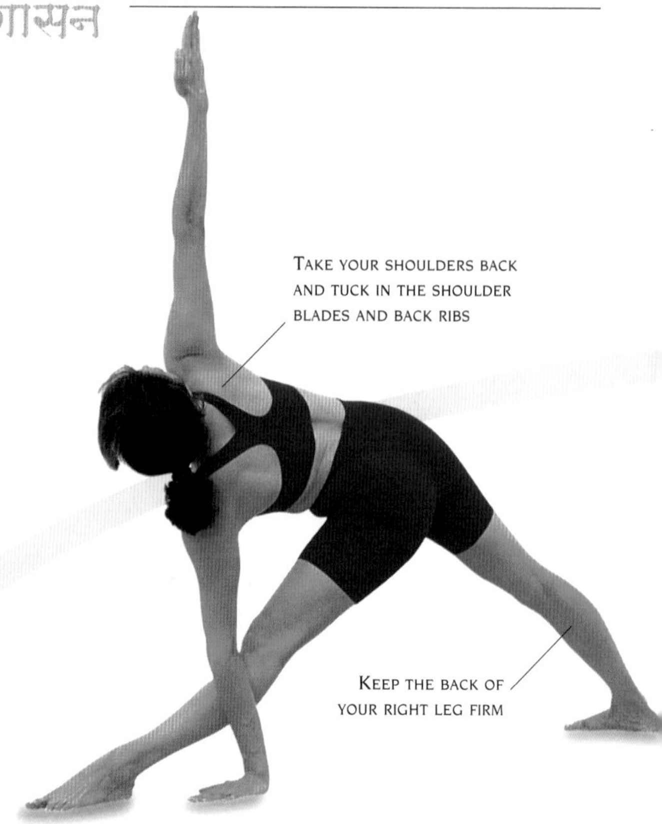

TAKE YOUR SHOULDERS BACK AND TUCK IN THE SHOULDER BLADES AND BACK RIBS

DO NOT LET YOUR ARM WAVER

KEEP THE BACK OF YOUR RIGHT LEG FIRM

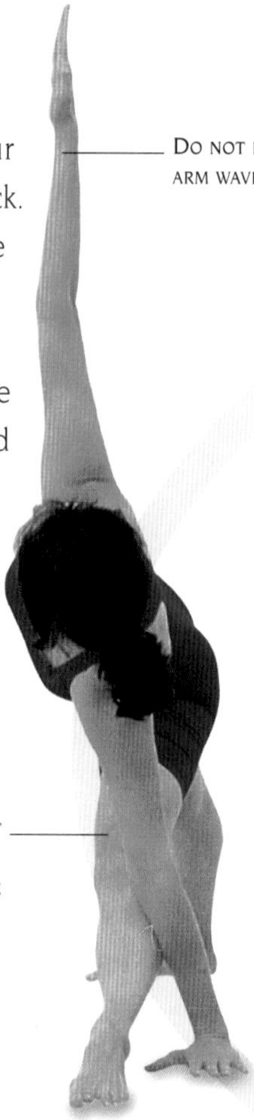

KEEP YOUR LEFT LEG ACTIVE, FIRM, AND STABLE

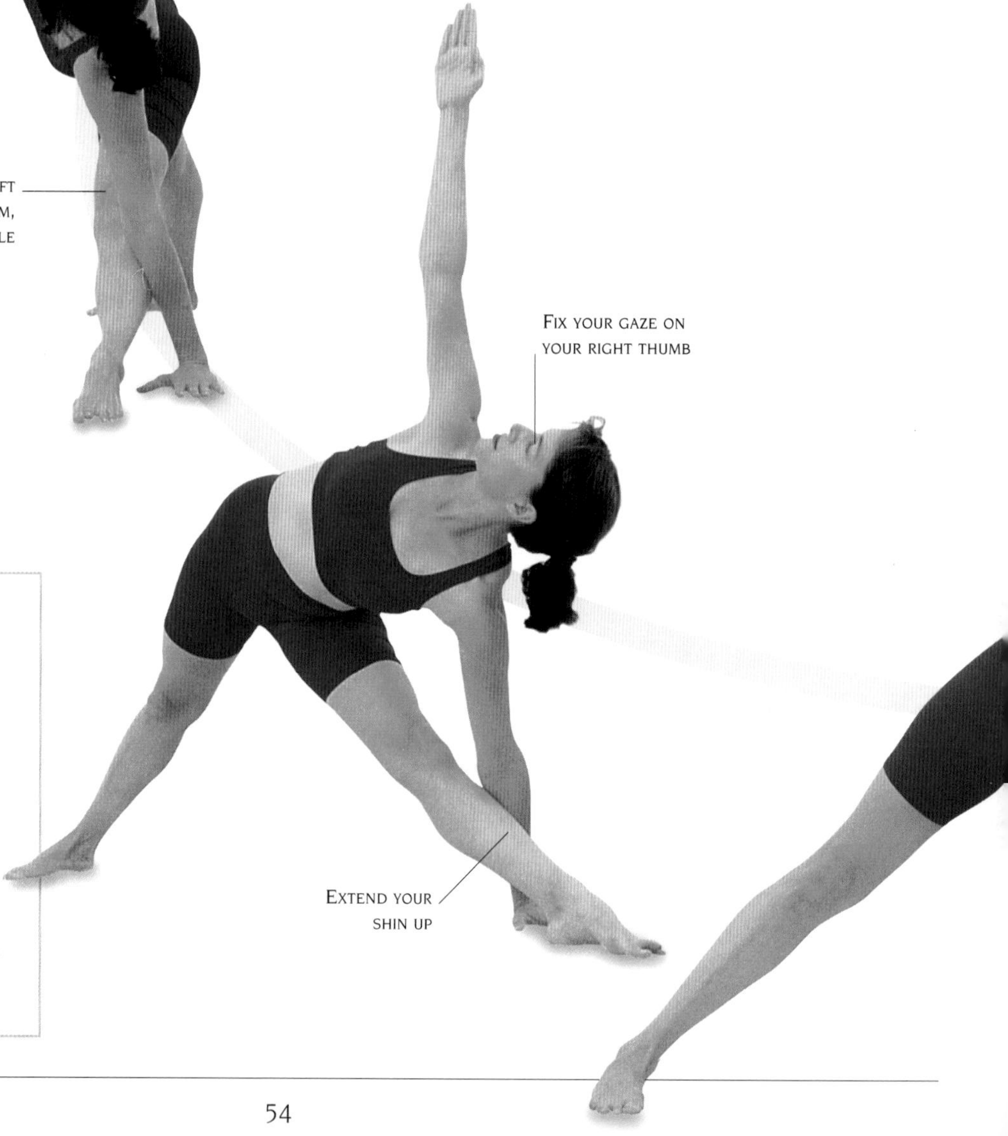

FIX YOUR GAZE ON YOUR RIGHT THUMB

EXTEND YOUR SHIN UP

COMING OUT OF THE POSTURE

◆

Inhale and lift your left palm from the floor. Stretch your right arm out to the side and straighten your torso gradually. Bring your arms down to your sides. Turn your feet to face forward. Repeat the posture on the other side. Then exhale and come back to Tadasana.

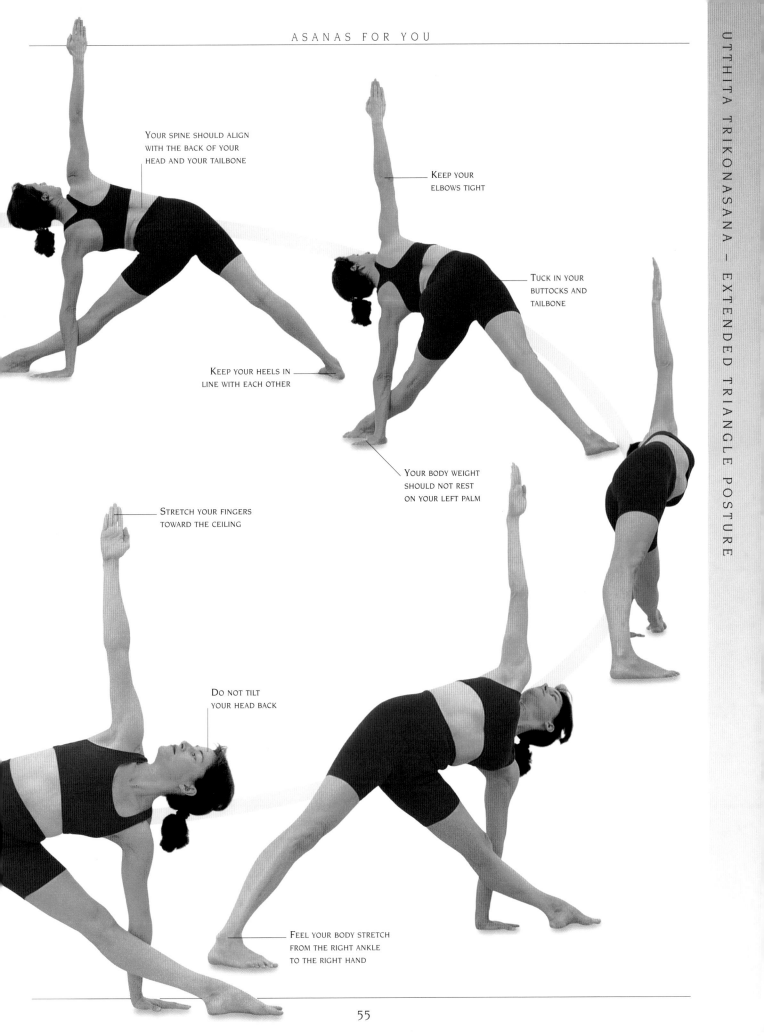

YOUR SPINE SHOULD ALIGN
WITH THE BACK OF YOUR
HEAD AND YOUR TAILBONE

KEEP YOUR
ELBOWS TIGHT

TUCK IN YOUR
BUTTOCKS AND
TAILBONE

KEEP YOUR HEELS IN
LINE WITH EACH OTHER

YOUR BODY WEIGHT
SHOULD NOT REST
ON YOUR LEFT PALM

STRETCH YOUR FINGERS
TOWARD THE CEILING

DO NOT TILT
YOUR HEAD BACK

FEEL YOUR BODY STRETCH
FROM THE RIGHT ANKLE
TO THE RIGHT HAND

UTTHITA TRIKONASANA – EXTENDED TRIANGLE POSTURE

वीरभद्रासन २

Virabhadrasana 2

- Warrior posture 2 -

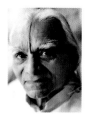

THIS POSTURE IS NAMED after Virabhadra, a legendary warrior. His story is told by the famous Sanskrit playwright, Kalidasa, in the epic, *Kumarasambhava*. Regular practice of this asana helps develop your strength and endurance. The steps exercise your limbs and torso vigorously, reducing stiffness in your neck and shoulders. It also makes your knee and hip joints more flexible.

CAUTIONS
◆

Do not practice if you have a cardiac condition, palpitations, heartburn, diarrhea, or dysentery. Women with menorrhagia and metrorrhagia should avoid this asana.

STRETCH YOUR TORSO UP

LOCK YOUR ELBOWS

KEEP YOUR LEFT KNEE FIRM

TURN THE RIGHT LEG OUT

1 Stand in Tadasana (*see page* 48) and inhale deeply. Jump your feet approximately 4ft (1.2m) apart. Your toes should point forward. Raise your arms out to the sides, in line with

your shoulders (*see inset*). Your palms should face the floor and be in line with each other. Keep your fingers straight and stretched out. Press the little toe of each foot down on the floor. Consciously pull the inner sides of your legs up toward your waist.

2 Exhale slowly and turn your right leg 90° to the right. Turn in your left foot slightly to the right. Ensure that your body weight is resting on your right heel and not on your toes. Keep your left leg stretched out and taut at the knee. To prevent this leg from slipping, make sure that your weight falls on the last two toes.

BEGINNERS Focus on turning the right thigh out correctly. The thigh should turn at the same time, and to the same extent, as your right foot.

3 Exhale and bend your right knee. Ensure that your right thigh is parallel to the floor. Keep the shin perpendicular to the floor, in line with your right heel. Pull the muscles of your right calf up. Turn your head to the right. Stretch the arches and toes of both feet. Hold the posture for 30 seconds. Breathe evenly.

INTERMEDIATES Bend your right knee from the buttock bone and consciously push the flesh and skin of the thigh toward the knee. Stretch your arms out fully. Imagine they are being pulled apart in a tug-of-war.

BENEFITS
◆

Improves breathing capacity by expanding the chest
◆

Helps in the treatment of a prolapsed or slipped disc
◆

Alleviates the condition of a broken, fused, or deviated tailbone
◆

Reduces fat around the hips
◆

Relieves lower backache

KEEP YOUR
BRAIN PASSIVE

STRETCH YOUR ARMS
AWAY FROM YOUR
SHOULDERS

EXPAND YOUR CHEST

CORRECTING YOURSELF

Do not allow the torso to either move right or tilt forward. To guard against this, make sure that your left armpit and your left hip are in a straight line.
Tuck in the left shoulder blade and keep your eyes on your right arm. Be conscious of the stretched side of your body.

THE RIGHT KNEE SHOULD
BE POSITIONED ABOVE
THE RIGHT HEEL

TIGHTEN THE MUSCLES
OF YOUR THIGHS

PRESS DOWN ON
YOUR RIGHT HEEL

57

वीरभद्रासन २

Virabhadrasana 2

ADVANCED WORK IN THE POSTURE

Do not bend your knee too rigidly and keep your bent leg relaxed. Consciously keep your brain passive. Your right buttock should be slightly lower than the right inner knee. Tighten your buttocks and broaden the hips. Press the outer edges of both your feet down onto the floor. Feel the energy rise from the ankle to the knee. Push your chest out and expand your chest cavity to its full extent. Keep the left knee taut and lifted up. If it drops, your chest will cave in. Maintain the stretch of your arms and shoulder blades away from your torso.

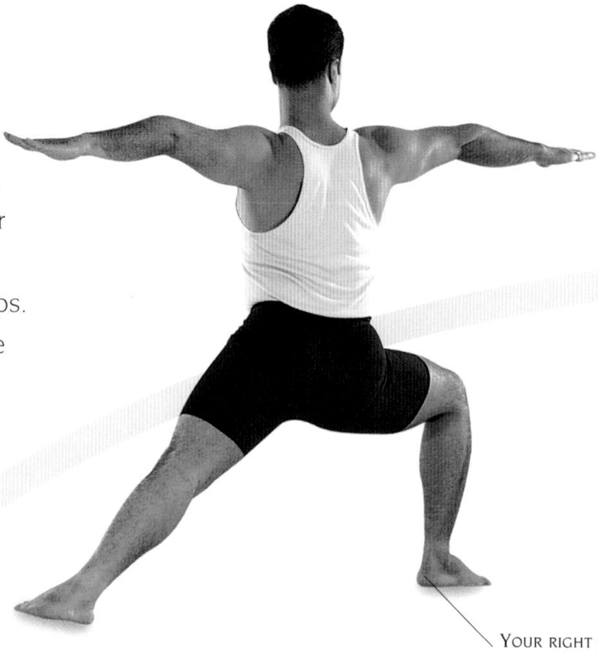

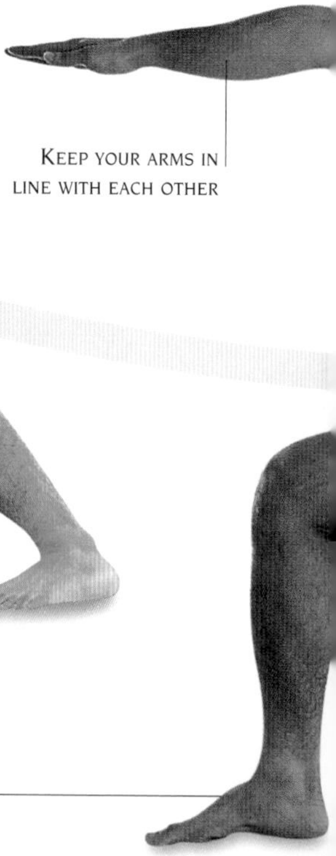

YOUR RIGHT HEEL SHOULD
BE IN LINE WITH YOUR
RIGHT KNEE

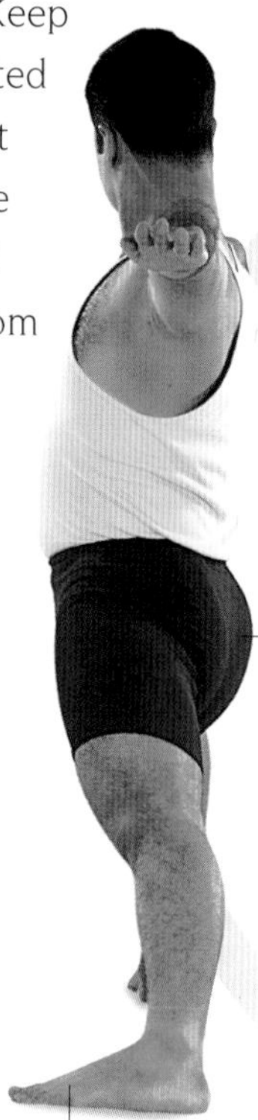

KEEP YOUR
BUTTOCKS TAUT

LOCK YOUR ELBOWS

KEEP YOUR TOES
SEPARATED AND ACTIVE

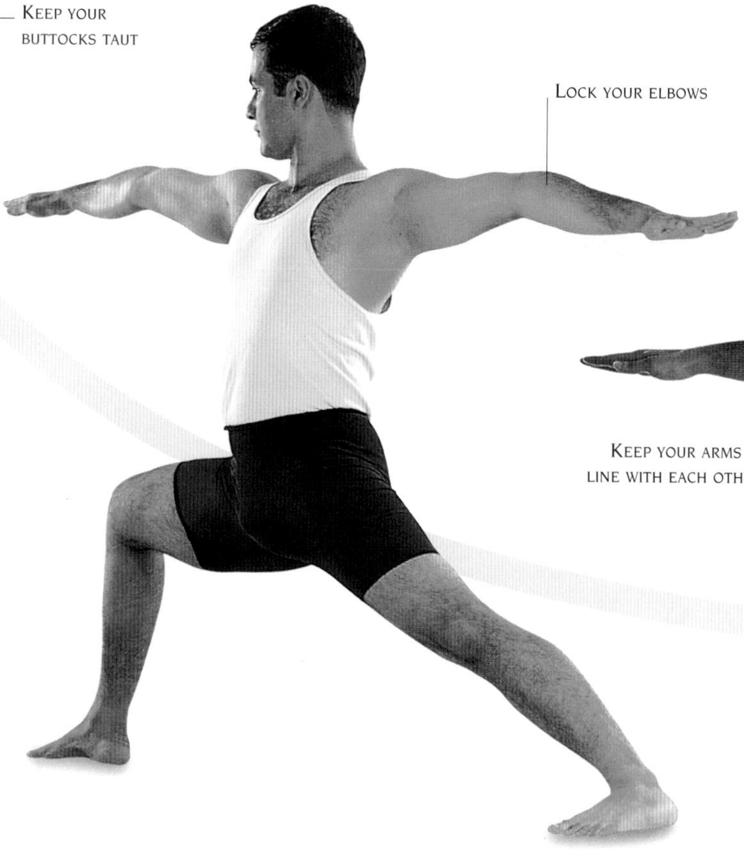

KEEP YOUR ARMS IN
LINE WITH EACH OTHER

COMING OUT OF THE POSTURE

◆

Inhale and straighten your right leg. Turn your feet so that they face forward. Repeat this posture on the other side. Then exhale and jump back to Tadasana.

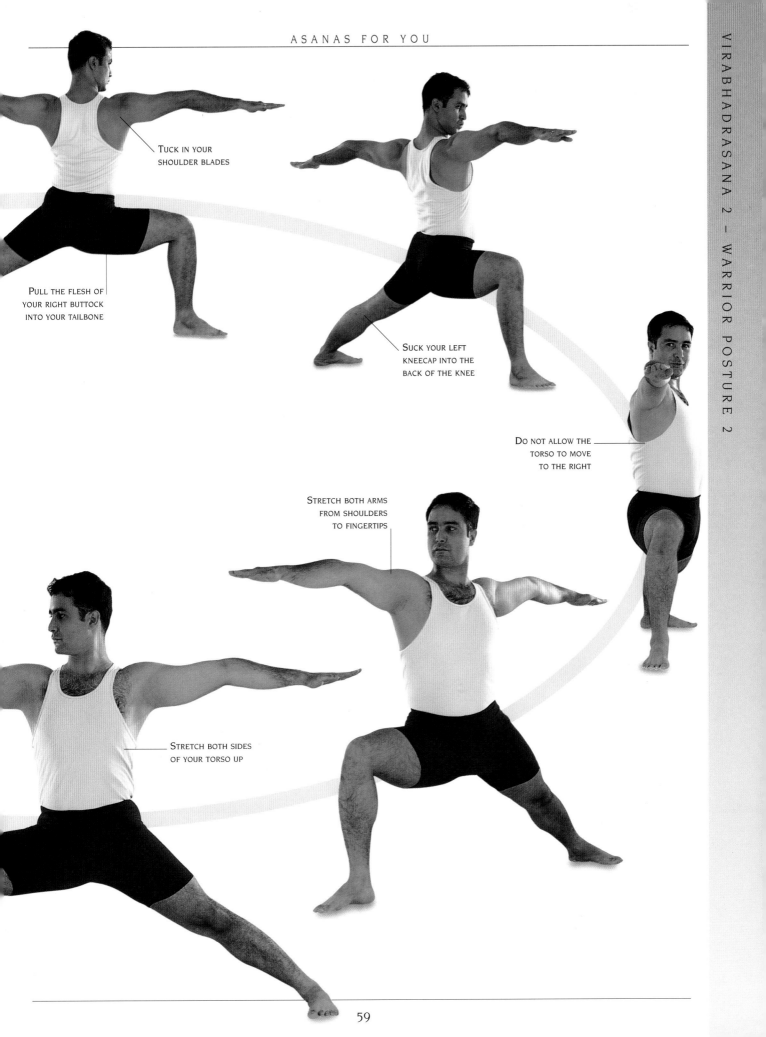

TUCK IN YOUR
SHOULDER BLADES

PULL THE FLESH OF
YOUR RIGHT BUTTOCK
INTO YOUR TAILBONE

SUCK YOUR LEFT
KNEECAP INTO THE
BACK OF THE KNEE

DO NOT ALLOW THE
TORSO TO MOVE
TO THE RIGHT

STRETCH BOTH ARMS
FROM SHOULDERS
TO FINGERTIPS

STRETCH BOTH SIDES
OF YOUR TORSO UP

उत्थित पार्श्वकोणासन

Utthita Parsvakonasana

- Extended side angle stretch -

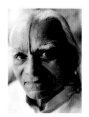

I N SANSKRIT, *utthita* means "stretch," *parsva* indicates "side" or "flank," while *kona* translates as "angle." In this asana, both sides of your body are stretched intensely, from the toes of one foot to the fingertips of the opposite hand. Remember to keep your body absolutely steady when practicing this asana.

CAUTIONS
◆

If you have high blood pressure, avoid this asana. If you have cervical spondylosis, do not turn your neck or look up.

BOTH PALMS SHOULD BE IN LINE WITH EACH OTHER

ROTATE YOUR RIGHT KNEE TOWARD THE RIGHT

KEEP YOUR LEFT KNEE FIRM

1 Stand in Tadasana (*see page* 48). Inhale, and jump your feet about 4ft (1.2m) apart. At the same time, raise both your arms out to the sides, to shoulder level. Your palms should face the floor. Stretch your arms from the back of the elbows. Ensure that your feet are in line with each other, toes pointing forward. Push down on the outer edges of your feet. Press the little toe of each foot onto the floor.

2 Exhale slowly, and simultaneously rotate your right leg and foot 90° to the right. At the same time, turn in the left foot slightly to the right. Stretch your left leg and tighten it at the knee. Ensure that your weight falls on the heel, not on the toes, of your right foot. Adjust the distance between your legs, if necessary. Make sure your feet remain in line with each other.

BEGINNERS As you rotate your right leg, focus on turning out your thigh. This reduces pressure on the right knee.

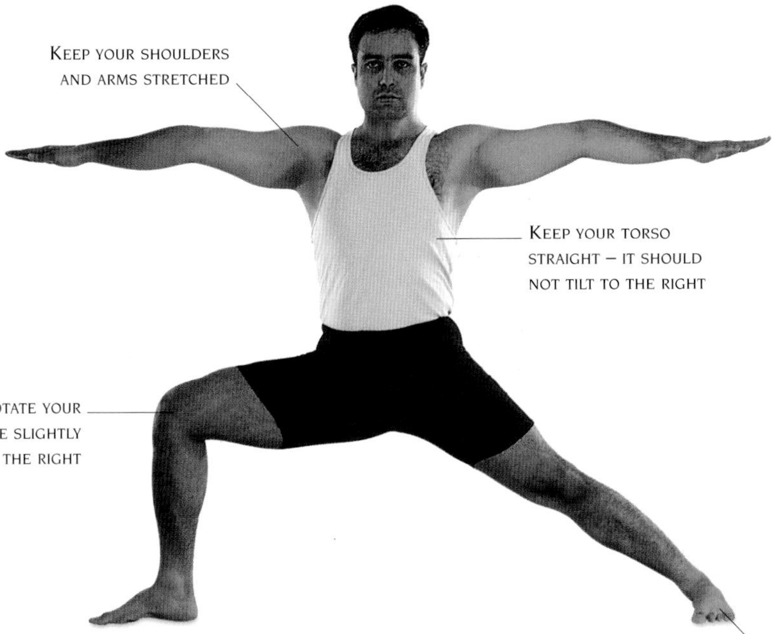

KEEP YOUR SHOULDERS
AND ARMS STRETCHED

KEEP YOUR TORSO
STRAIGHT – IT SHOULD
NOT TILT TO THE RIGHT

ROTATE YOUR
KNEE SLIGHTLY
TO THE RIGHT

BENEFITS
◆
Enhances lung capacity
◆
Tones the muscles of the heart
◆
Relieves sciatic and arthritic pain
◆
*Improves digestion and helps
the elimination of waste*
◆
Reduces fat on the waist and hips

PRESS DOWN ON THE
FOURTH AND FIFTH TOES
OF YOUR LEFT FOOT

3 Bend your right knee until your
thigh and calf form a right angle,
and your right thigh is parallel
to the floor. Take one or two breaths.

INTERMEDIATES Consciously pull your
left knee and ankle up. Open the back
of the left knee from the center to the
sides. Pull the muscles of both calves
toward your thighs.

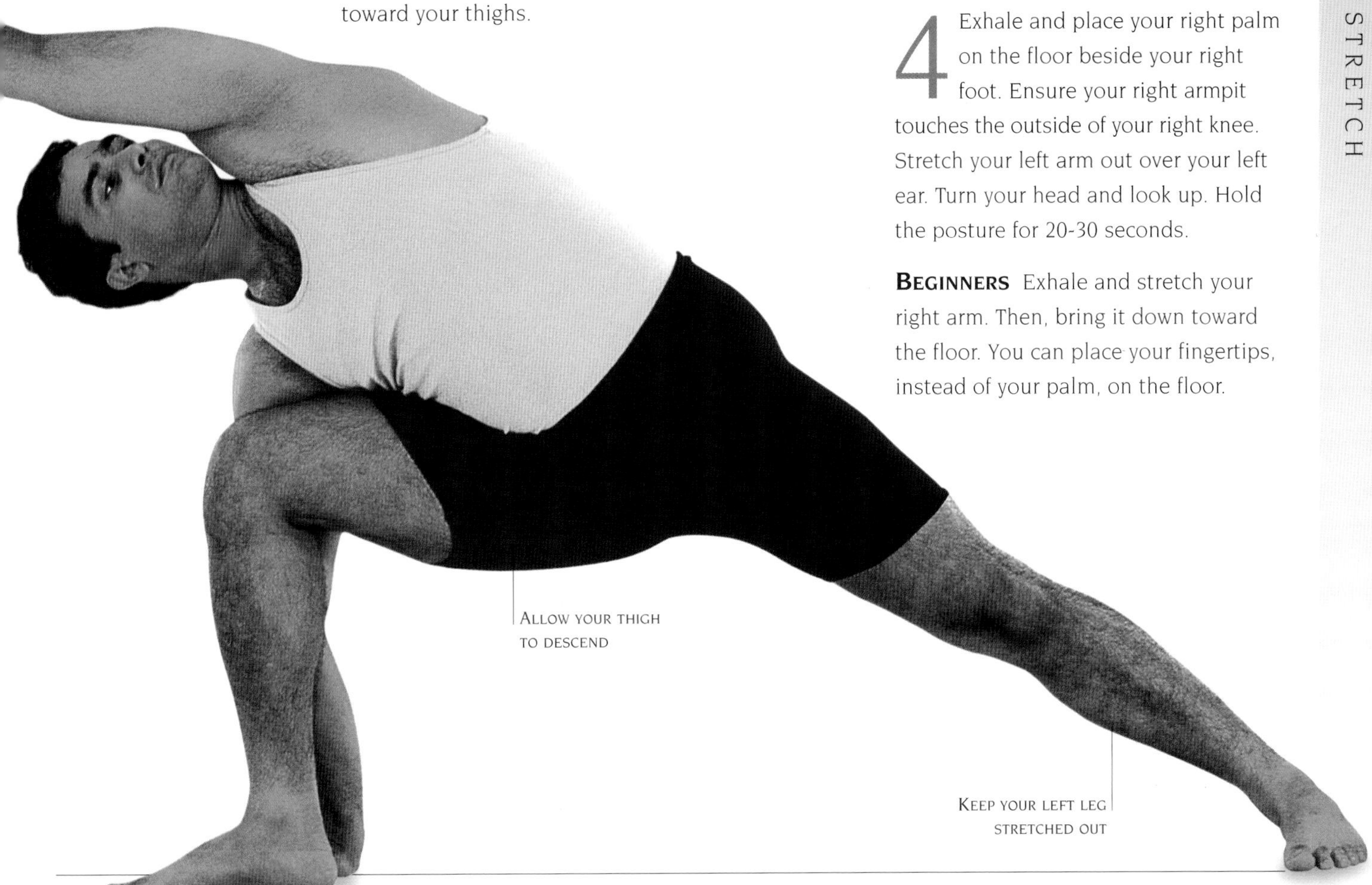

4 Exhale and place your right palm
on the floor beside your right
foot. Ensure your right armpit
touches the outside of your right knee.
Stretch your left arm out over your left
ear. Turn your head and look up. Hold
the posture for 20-30 seconds.

BEGINNERS Exhale and stretch your
right arm. Then, bring it down toward
the floor. You can place your fingertips,
instead of your palm, on the floor.

ALLOW YOUR THIGH
TO DESCEND

KEEP YOUR LEFT LEG
STRETCHED OUT

उत्थित पार्श्वकोणासन

Utthita Parsvakonasana

ADVANCED WORK IN THE POSTURE

Your left arm is the "brain" of the posture (*see page* 45), so keep it stable and do not allow it to move. Increase the intensity of the stretch in this arm, pushing it away from the left armpit. Bring your lower shoulder blades into your back. Lift your left thigh slightly. This will help the right hand descend more easily. Make sure you rest on the back of the right heel and do not allow dead weight to fall on your right thigh or palm. Keep your chest, hips, and left leg in line with each other. Stretch every part of your body, focusing especially on the spine. Feel a single, continuous stretch from your left ankle to your left wrist.

PUSH YOUR
SHOULDERS BACK

KEEP YOUR LEFT LEG
STRAIGHT AND EXTEND
THE HAMSTRINGS

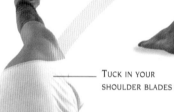

TUCK IN YOUR
SHOULDER BLADES

TURN THE LEFT SIDE
OF YOUR TORSO
UP AND BACK

TURN YOUR KNEE
TO THE RIGHT

COMING OUT OF THE POSTURE

◆

Inhale and lift your right hand from the floor. Bring your arms to your sides and straighten your right leg. Turn both feet so that they face forward. Repeat the posture on the other side. Then exhale and jump back to Tadasana.

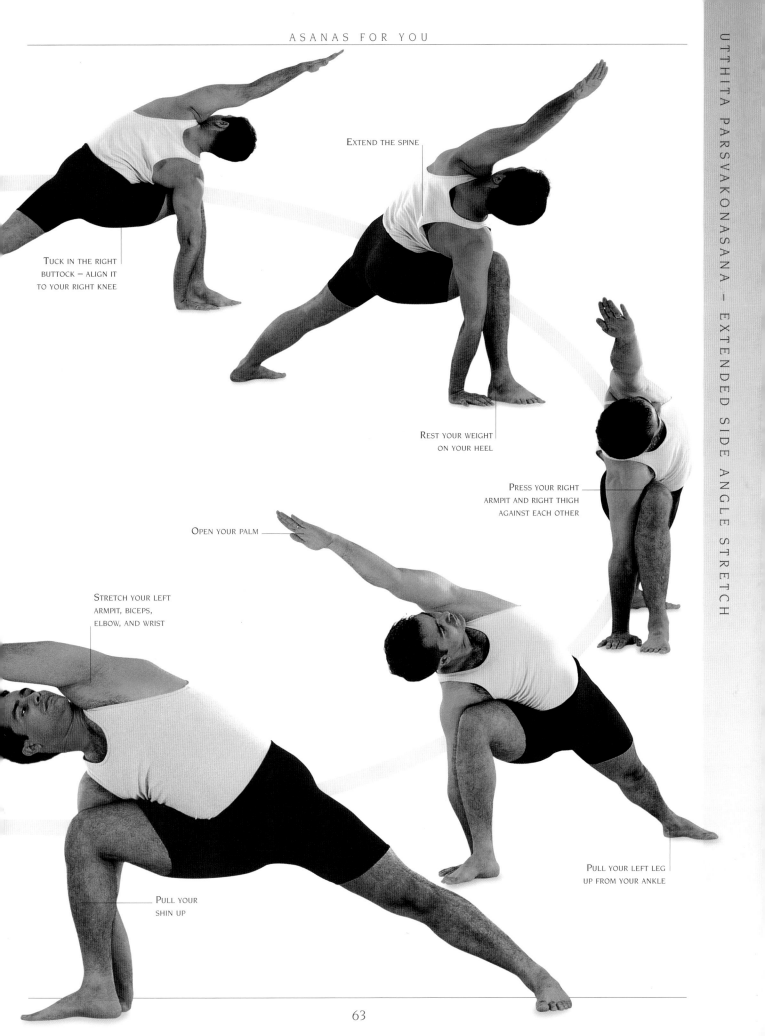

EXTEND THE SPINE

TUCK IN THE RIGHT
BUTTOCK – ALIGN IT
TO YOUR RIGHT KNEE

REST YOUR WEIGHT
ON YOUR HEEL

PRESS YOUR RIGHT
ARMPIT AND RIGHT THIGH
AGAINST EACH OTHER

OPEN YOUR PALM

STRETCH YOUR LEFT
ARMPIT, BICEPS,
ELBOW, AND WRIST

PULL YOUR
SHIN UP

PULL YOUR LEFT LEG
UP FROM YOUR ANKLE

UTTHITA PARSVAKONASANA – EXTENDED SIDE ANGLE STRETCH

पार्श्वोत्तानासन

Parsvottanasana

- Intense chest stretch -

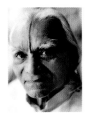

THIS ASANA GIVES an intense stretch to your chest. *Parsva* means "side" or "flank" in Sanskrit, while *uttana* indicates the great intensity of the final stretch. Regular practice of Parsvottanasana stimulates and tones the kidneys, an effect you can feel once you are comfortable in the final posture. The asana also helps to remove stiffness in the neck, shoulders, and elbows.

CAUTIONS
◆

If you have high blood pressure or a cardiac condition, omit Step 4. If you have dysentery or an abdominal hernia, practice this asana up to Step 4.

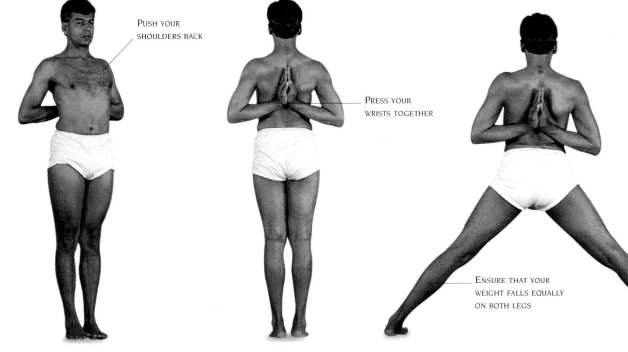

PUSH YOUR SHOULDERS BACK

PRESS YOUR WRISTS TOGETHER

ENSURE THAT YOUR WEIGHT FALLS EQUALLY ON BOTH LEGS

1 Stand in Tadasana (*see page* 48). Loosen your arms by turning them inside and out several times. Join your fingertips together behind your  back with your fingers pointing down toward your feet. Then rotate your wrists (*see inset*) until your fingers point to the ceiling.

BEGINNERS If joining your palms is too difficult, take your arms behind your back, bend your elbows, and rest each palm on the opposite elbow.

2 Move your joined palms up to the middle of your back. The little fingers of each hand should touch your back. Then move your hands up your back (*see inset*) until they rest between your shoulder blades. Press your fingers together. Press your palms together by pushing your elbows in. This will help to push your shoulders back and expand your chest even further.

3 Inhale and jump up, landing with your feet about 4ft (1.2m) apart. If your legs feel overstretched or uncomfortably close together, adjust the distance accordingly. When you feel that your body weight is distributed equally and comfortably on both legs, you have the distance right. Pause for a few seconds and exhale slowly.

DO NOT TILT YOUR NECK TOO FAR BACK

4 Inhale, and turn your right foot 90° to the right. Turn the left foot 75-80° to the right. At the same time, rotate to the right from the waist and hips. Ensure that your torso faces front and is in line with your right leg. Rest your weight on the heel of your right foot. Tighten your right knee and extend your chest, waist, and hips. Then tilt your head and chest back and look up at the ceiling, making sure that you do not strain your throat. Press your palms to your back. Do not allow them to slide down.

STRETCH YOUR RIGHT FOOT SO THAT IT IS COMPLETELY FLAT ON THE FLOOR

WIDEN YOUR ELBOWS

BENEFITS

◆

Cools the brain and soothes the nerves

◆

Relieves arthritis of the neck, shoulders, elbows, and wrists

◆

Strengthens the abdominal organs

◆

Improves digestion

◆

Tones the liver and spleen

◆

Reduces menstrual pain

5 Exhale, extend the spine, and bend forward from the top of both your thighs. As you bend, lead with your sternum and do not allow your right knee to bend as you come forward. Take care to bend equally from both sides of the waist. Rest your chin on your right knee. Stay in the posture for 20-30 seconds.

BEGINNERS If you find the final stretch difficult, then place your palms on the floor on either side of the right foot. Take care to stretch your back and neck gradually.

TURN IN YOUR LEFT KNEECAP SLIGHTLY

KEEP THE RIGHT LEG FULLY STRETCHED

पार्श्वोत्तानासन

Parsvottanasana

ADVANCED WORK IN THE POSTURE

Maintain the stretch of your upper body, from the pelvis to the collar bones, while holding the posture. Elongate both sides of your waist evenly, to increase the stretch of your thighs. Bend down from your groin, keeping the perineum area passive. To ensure that your torso rests on the center of your right thigh, move your abdomen slightly to the right, until your navel rests on the center of your right thigh. Tighten the leg muscles and feel the stretch along the back of both legs. Push your spine down even further over your right leg. Move both your shoulders back, until both sides of your chest are equally expanded. Breathe evenly.

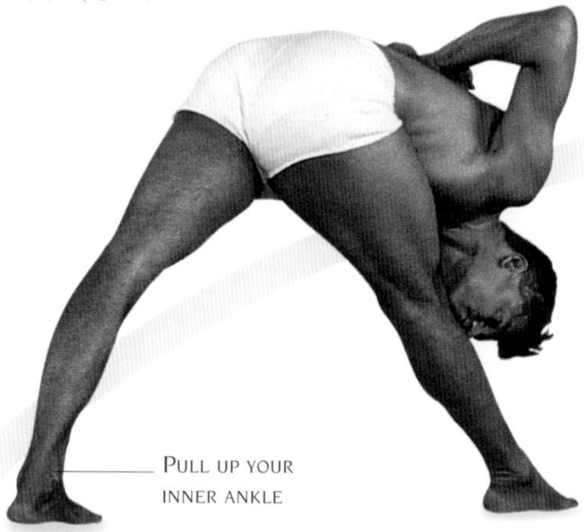

PULL UP YOUR INNER ANKLE

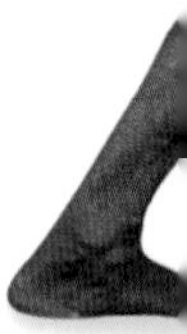

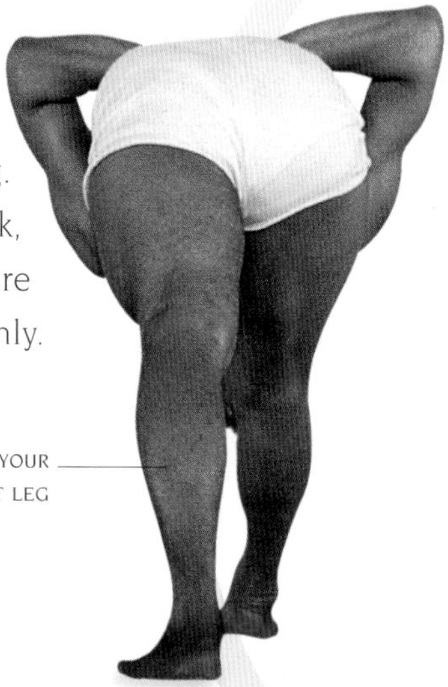

STRETCH YOUR LEFT LEG

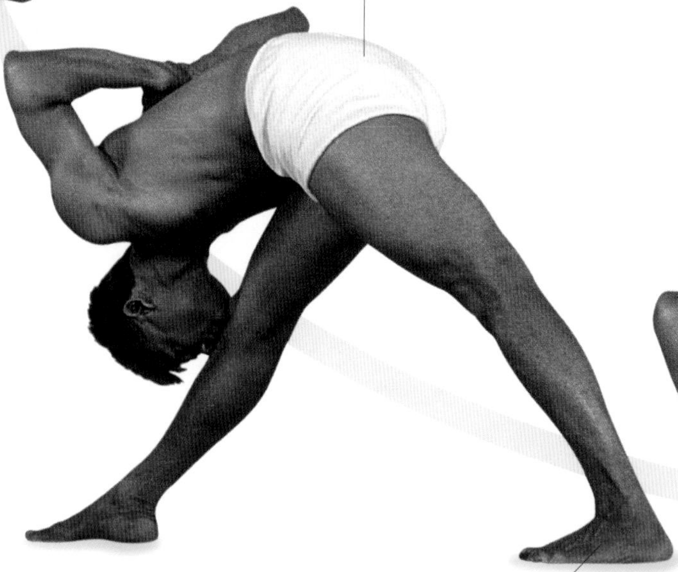

KEEP YOUR BUTTOCKS PARALLEL TO EACH OTHER

PRESS THE OUTER EDGE OF YOUR LEFT FOOT TO THE FLOOR

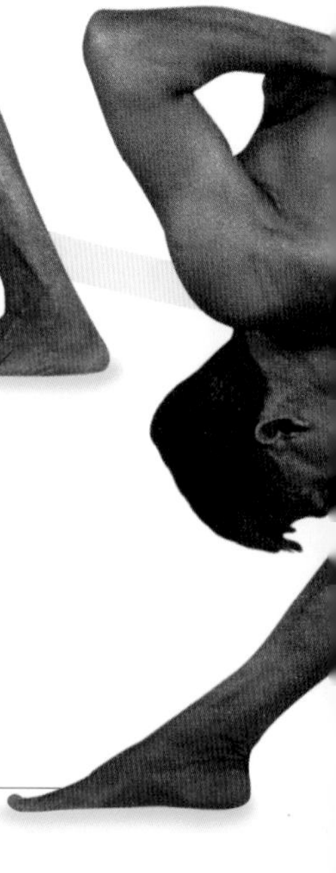

COMING OUT OF THE POSTURE

◆

Inhale and lift your torso. Come back to a standing position, but raise your head gradually. Repeat the posture on the other side. Stretch out your arms to shoulder level and jump your feet together. Stand in Tadasana.

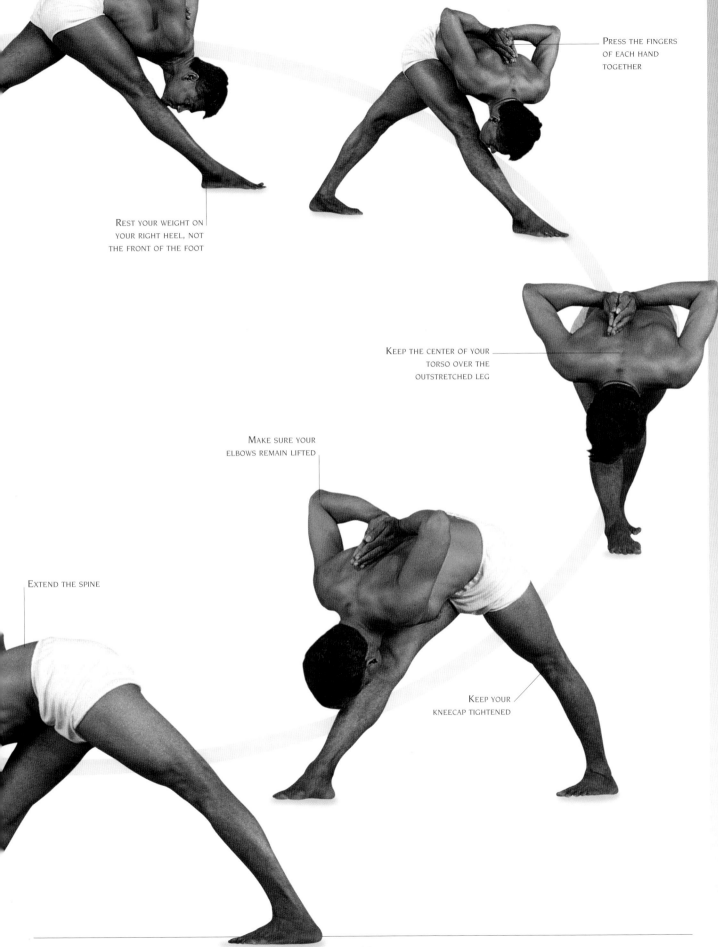

REST YOUR WEIGHT ON YOUR RIGHT HEEL, NOT THE FRONT OF THE FOOT

PRESS THE FINGERS OF EACH HAND TOGETHER

KEEP THE CENTER OF YOUR TORSO OVER THE OUTSTRETCHED LEG

MAKE SURE YOUR ELBOWS REMAIN LIFTED

EXTEND THE SPINE

KEEP YOUR KNEECAP TIGHTENED

PARSVOTTANASANA – INTENSE CHEST STRETCH

अधोमुख श्वानासन

Adhomukha Svanasana

- Downward-facing dog posture-

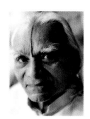

IN THIS ASANA, your body takes the shape of a dog stretching itself. *Adhomukha* means to have your "face downward" in Sanskrit, and *svana* translates as "dog." The asana helps runners, since it reduces stiffness in the heels and makes the legs strong and agile. Holding the posture for one minute restores energy when you are tired. This asana gently stimulates your nervous system and regular practice will rejuvenate your whole body.

CAUTIONS
◆

If you have high blood pressure or frequent headaches, support your head with a bolster (*see page* 167). If you are prone to dislocation of the shoulders, ensure that your arms do not rotate out. Do not practice this asana in an advanced stage of pregnancy.

1 Stand in Tadasana (*see page* 48). Exhale, and bend from the waist, placing each palm onto the floor beside each foot.

BEGINNERS Exhale, and bend from your waist. Bend both knees and place your palms on the floor next to your feet.

STRAIGHTEN YOUR ARMS

2 Bend your knees and step back approximately 4ft (1.2m), one leg at a time. Keep your palms about 3-4ft (1m) apart. Make sure that the distance between your feet is the same as that between your palms.

3 Position your right leg in line with your right arm, and your left leg in line with your left arm. Stretch your fingers and toes. Raise your heels, tighten the muscles at the top of your thighs, and pull in your kneecaps. Then stretch the arches of your feet and bring your heels down onto the floor again.

KEEP YOUR ARMS FULLY STRETCHED

KEEP YOUR FEET PARALLEL TO EACH OTHER

THE GURU'S ADVICE

"To make sure that my student's arms are straight, I stand on his hands to keep them firmly placed on the floor. Then I press his shoulder blades in, creating a right-angled triangle presentation of the posture. In this position, you should feel an intense stretch from your buttocks, along the dorsal and thoracic spine, right down to your palms."

BENEFITS

◆

Calms the brain and gently stimulates the nerves

◆

Slows down the heartbeat

◆

Reduces stiffness in the shoulder blades and arthritis in the shoulder joints

◆

Strengthens the ankles and tones the legs

◆

Relieves pain in the heels and softens calcaneal spurs

◆

Checks heavy menstrual flow

◆

Helps to prevent hot flashes during menopause

4 Pull your inner arms up from the elbows to the shoulders. Move your torso toward your legs. Feel the stretch from your palms to your heels. Now exhale, stretch the base of your neck, and lower the crown of your head onto the floor. Hold the posture for 15-20 seconds.

INTERMEDIATES Before you lower your head, move the deltoids deep into the shoulder joints and lift your shoulder blades. Press both palms down onto the floor and pull your sternum up toward your diaphragm.

PUSH YOUR BUTTOCKS UP

STRETCH BOTH LEGS EQUALLY

KEEP YOUR FEET FLAT ON THE FLOOR WITH THE TOES POINTING STRAIGHT AHEAD

REST ON THE FRONT OF YOUR CROWN

अधोमुख श्वानासन

Adhomukha Svanasana

ADVANCED WORK IN THE POSTURE

Move your legs as far back as possible. Ensure that both thighs are stretched equally. The inner and outer back edges should be parallel to each other. If your thighs are not parallel, they tend to shorten and lose their stretch. Similarly, keep your spine stretched out; do not compress it. Feel the energy in the spine flowing up, from the neck to the buttocks, and not the other way around. Tuck in your shoulder blades and broaden your chest. As the chest opens out fully, your breathing becomes deep. Be aware of that depth.

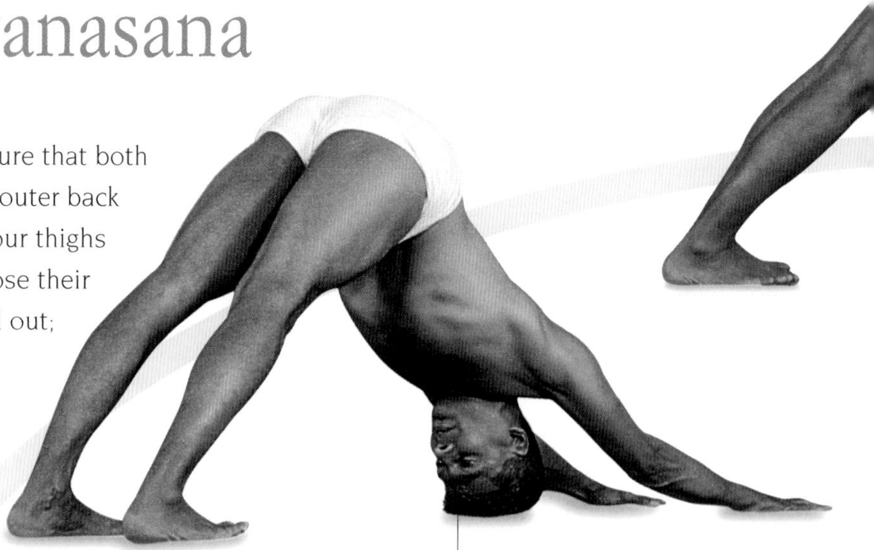

REST ON THE FRONT YOUR CROWN

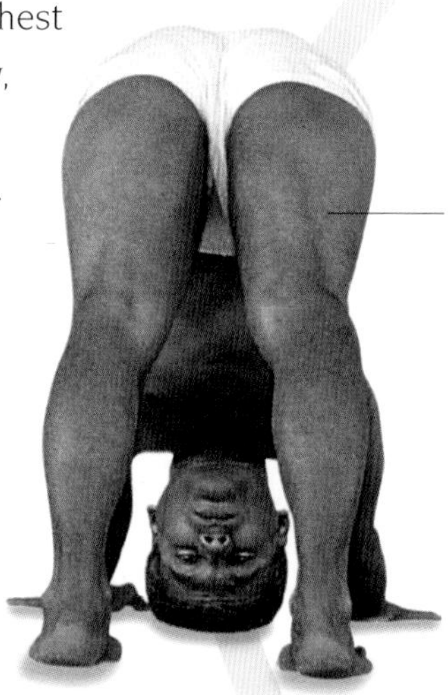

KEEP YOUR THIGHS PARALLEL TO EACH OTHER

" The long and practice of asanas will bring

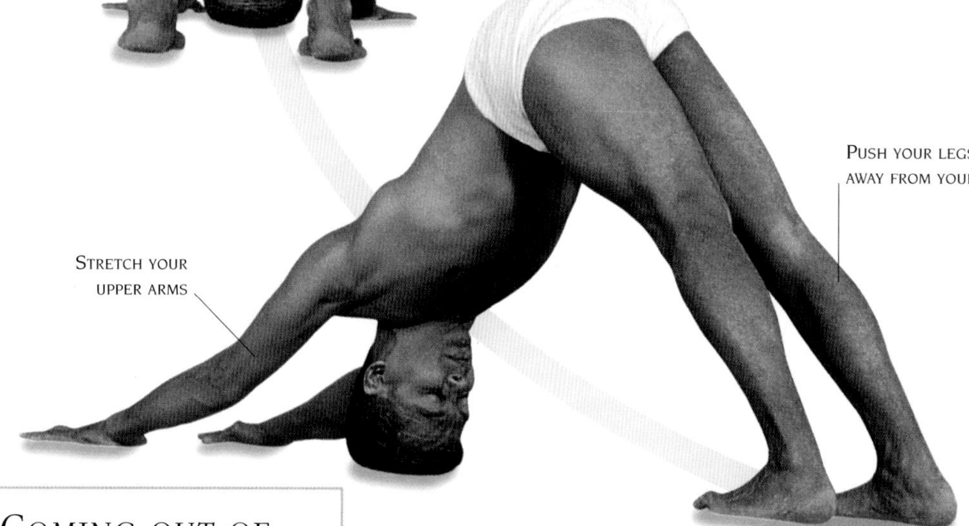

PUSH YOUR LEGS AWAY FROM YOUR BODY

STRETCH YOUR UPPER ARMS

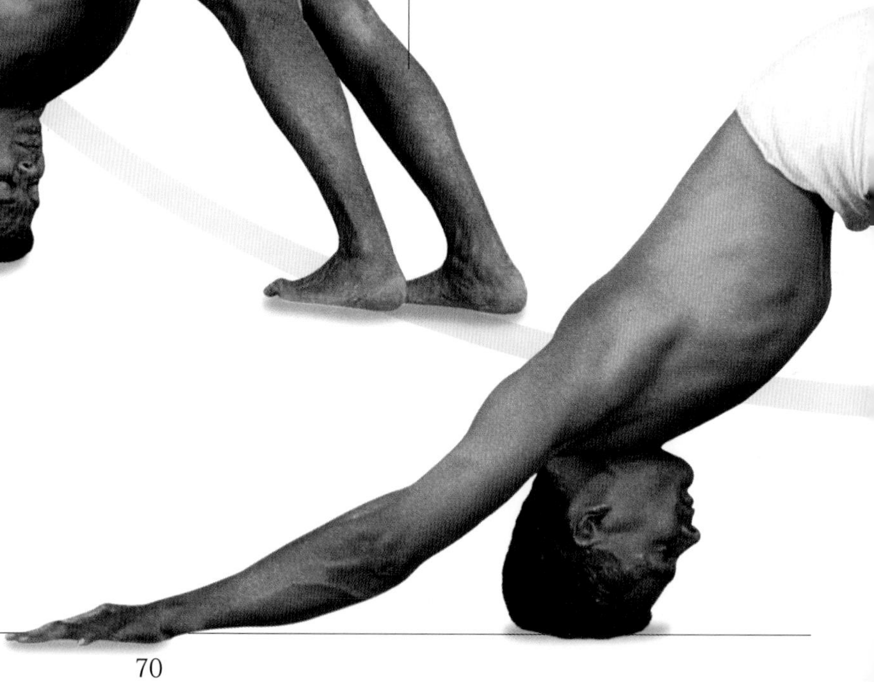

COMING OUT OF THE POSTURE

◆

Inhale and gradually lift your head off the floor. Walk your feet toward your palms and come back to Tadasana.

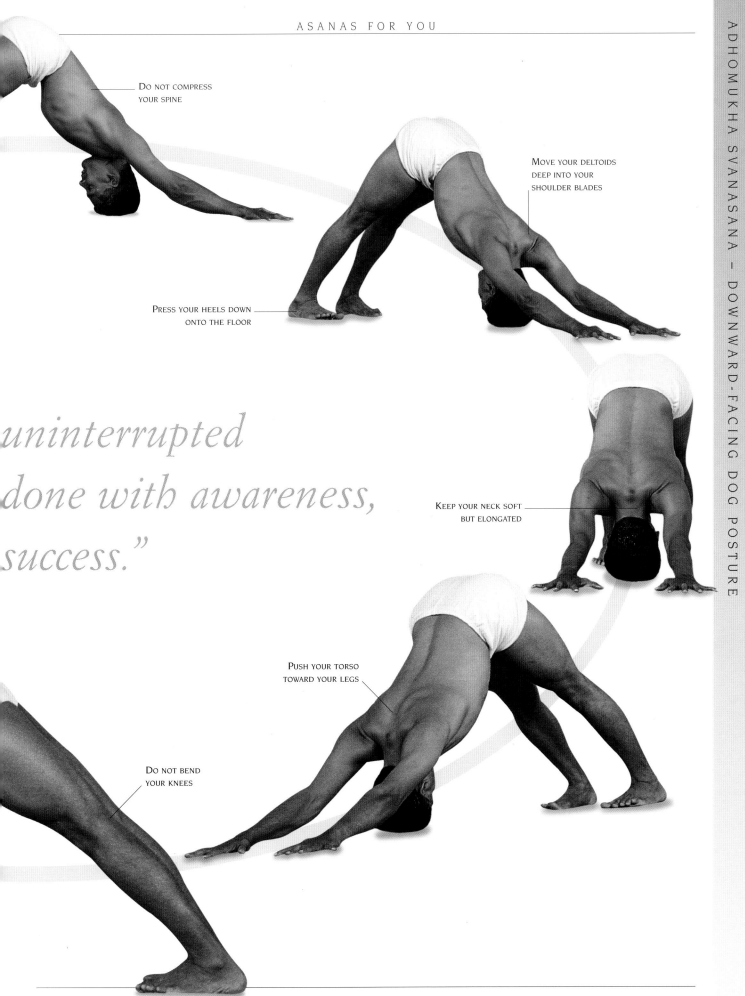

DO NOT COMPRESS
YOUR SPINE

MOVE YOUR DELTOIDS
DEEP INTO YOUR
SHOULDER BLADES

PRESS YOUR HEELS DOWN
ONTO THE FLOOR

uninterrupted
done with awareness,
success."

KEEP YOUR NECK SOFT
BUT ELONGATED

PUSH YOUR TORSO
TOWARD YOUR LEGS

DO NOT BEND
YOUR KNEES

उत्तानासन

Uttanasana

- Intense forward stretch posture -

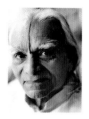

THE SPINE RECEIVES a deliberate and intense stretch in this asana. The word *ut* means "deliberate" or "intense" in Sanskrit, while *tana* connotes "stretch." The practice of Uttanasana helps the body and the brain recover from mental and physical exhaustion. This asana can help those who are prone to anxiety or depression since it rejuvenates the spinal nerves and brain cells. It also slows down the heartbeat.

CAUTIONS
◆

If you have a spinal disc disorder, stop at Step 3. Ensure that your spine is concave throughout the asana. Those prone to acidity or dizziness should practice this asana with the legs positioned slightly apart.

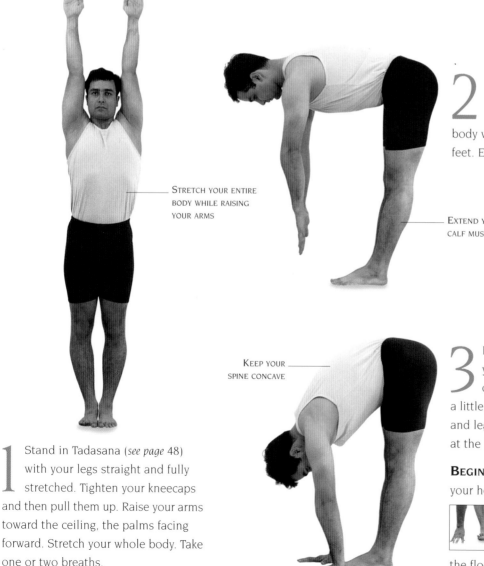

STRETCH YOUR ENTIRE
BODY WHILE RAISING
YOUR ARMS

2 Exhale, and bend forward from the waist. Keep your legs fully stretched. Make sure that your body weight is placed equally on both feet. Extend your toes.

EXTEND YOUR
CALF MUSCLES

KEEP YOUR
SPINE CONCAVE

1 Stand in Tadasana (*see page* 48) with your legs straight and fully stretched. Tighten your kneecaps and then pull them up. Raise your arms toward the ceiling, the palms facing forward. Stretch your whole body. Take one or two breaths.

3 Bend your torso further and place your palms onto the floor in front of your feet. Separate your ankles a little, to free your lower back, buttocks, and legs. Consciously stretch the skin at the backs of your knees and thighs.

BEGINNERS Lift your toes and press your heels down on the floor as you

bend (see inset). Instead of your palms, you can rest your fingertips on the floor, until you are more flexible.

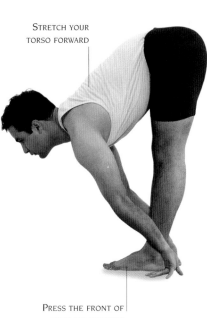

STRETCH YOUR
TORSO FORWARD

PRESS THE FRONT OF
YOUR SOLES DOWN
ON THE FLOOR

4 Move your hands back and place them next to your heels. Rest on your fingers and thumbs, with the palms raised off the floor. Keep your thighs fully stretched. Feel the energy flow along the back of your legs, into the waist, and down your spine. Pull your kneecaps into your knees, keeping both knees parallel to each other and fully opened out at the back. The pressure on the inner and outer edges of your feet should be equal.

CORRECTING YOURSELF

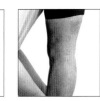

WRONG *If your knees bend, the tailbone juts out, affecting the posture.*

RIGHT *Stretch your thighs, keeping the kneecaps locked and pushed up.*

PUSH YOUR
HIPS FORWARD

EXTEND YOUR THIGHS
FROM THE KNEES
TO THE HIPS

STRETCH YOUR ARMS
FROM YOUR SHOULDERS

5 Exhale and push your torso closer to your legs until your face rests on the knees. Push your torso and abdomen further down toward the floor until your chin touches both knees. Your chin should not touch your chest, since this will cause your neck and throat to tighten leading to pressure on the head. Hold the posture for 30-60 seconds, breathing evenly.

BENEFITS
◆
Relieves mental and physical exhaustion
◆
Slows down the heartbeat
◆
Tones the liver, spleen, and kidneys
◆
Relieves stomach ache
◆
*Reduces abdominal and back pain
during menstruation*

Uttanasana

उत्तानासन

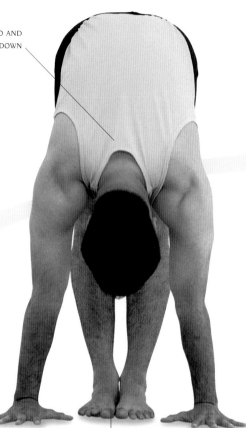

PUSH YOUR TORSO AND
SPINE DOWN

ADVANCED WORK IN THE POSTURE

When you place your fingers on the floor, turn your arms out and stretch them down. Imagine you are pushing the skin of your arms down from your armpits to your fingertips. Focus on your ribs. Consciously stretch each rib, from the bottom of your ribcage right up to your armpits. Then descend even further from your armpits. This will open the back of your inner thighs. Feel a continuous stretch from your heels to the crown of your head.

OPEN OUT THE
BACKS OF YOUR KNEES

KEEP THE INNER SIDES
OF YOUR ANKLES, KNEES,
AND THIGHS TOGETHER

COMING OUT OF THE POSTURE

◆

Inhale and raise your head without lifting your palms off the floor. Press your fingers into the floor and descend your armpits. Then raise your torso gradually. Always be sure to come up with your back straight. Stand in Tadasana.

"Your body exists
your mind exists in
they come together

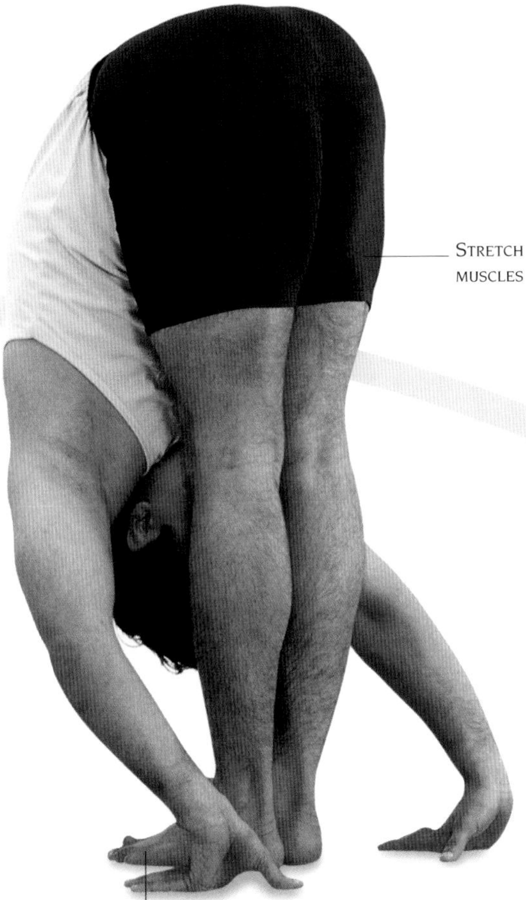

STRETCH AND OPEN THE
MUSCLES OF YOUR THIGHS

KEEP YOUR HIPS
PARALLEL TO THE FLOOR

EXTEND YOUR TOES FROM
THE ARCHES OF YOUR FEET

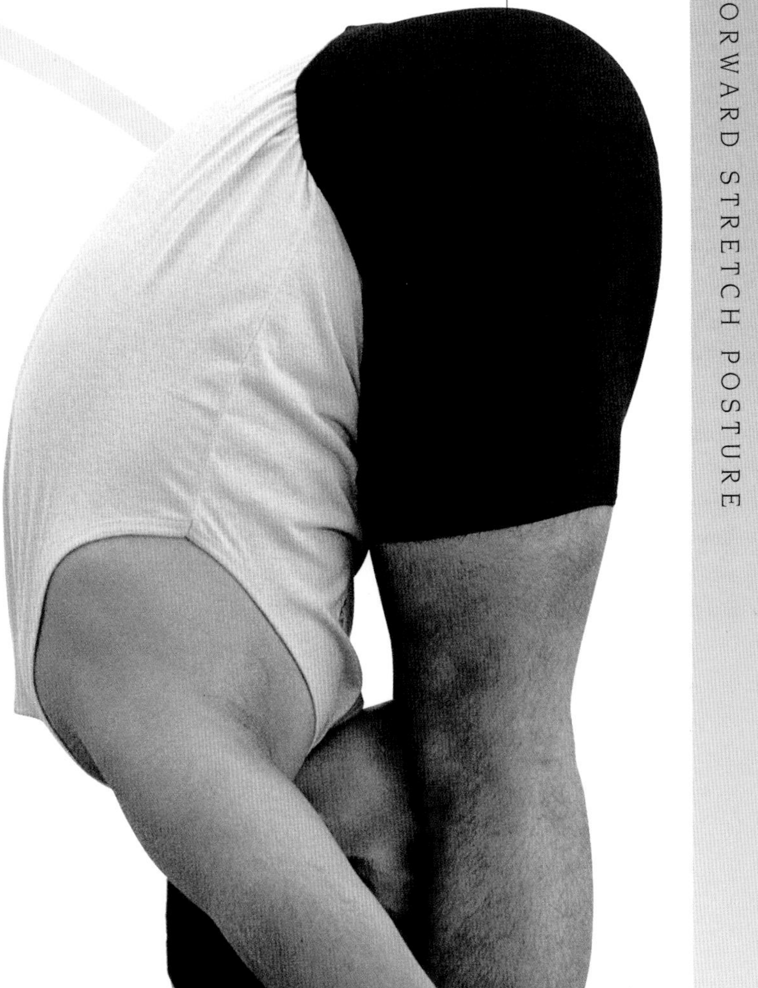

in the past and

the future. In yoga,

in the present."

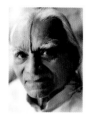

वीरभद्रासन १
Virabhadrasana 1

- Warrior posture 1 -

THIS ASANA, BASED ON a warrior posture, is a more intense version of Virabhadrasana 2 (*see page* 56). Both asanas are named after the mythic warrior-sage, Virabhadra. This vigorous asana strengthens your spine and increases the flexibility of your knees and thighs. The arms receive an intense stretch, and this expands the muscles of your chest and enhances the capacity of your lungs.

CAUTIONS
◆
Do not practice this asana if you have high blood pressure or a cardiac condition.

KEEP YOUR PALMS FACING DOWN AND IN LINE WITH EACH OTHER

LOCK YOUR ELBOWS

PULL UP YOUR PELVIS

1 Stand in Tadasana (*see page* 48). Inhale and jump, landing with your feet about 4ft (1.2m) apart. Your feet should be in line, the toes pointing forward. Raise your arms up to shoulder level, parallel to the floor. Lock your elbows. Press the little toes of both feet onto the floor. The outer edges of both feet should rest on the floor.

INTERMEDIATES For a more effective stretch, focus on the inner sides of your legs. Imagine that you are pulling the skin of both legs up from your heels to your waist.

2 Turn your wrists until your palms face the ceiling. Raise both arms until they are perpendicular to the floor and parallel to each other. Lift your shoulder blades and push them into your body (*see inset*).

INTERMEDIATES Your elbows are the "brain" of your arms (*see page* 45). Stretch from your elbows to your fingertips.

3 Exhale, and turn your torso and your right leg 90˚ to the right. Then turn your left leg to the right. Rotate your torso from the chest as well as the waist. The more you rotate to the right and stretch your upper arms, the more effective the posture.

INTERMEDIATES Be conscious of your left leg, and concentrate on the stretch from the back of your heel to the back of your thigh.

THE GURU'S ADVICE

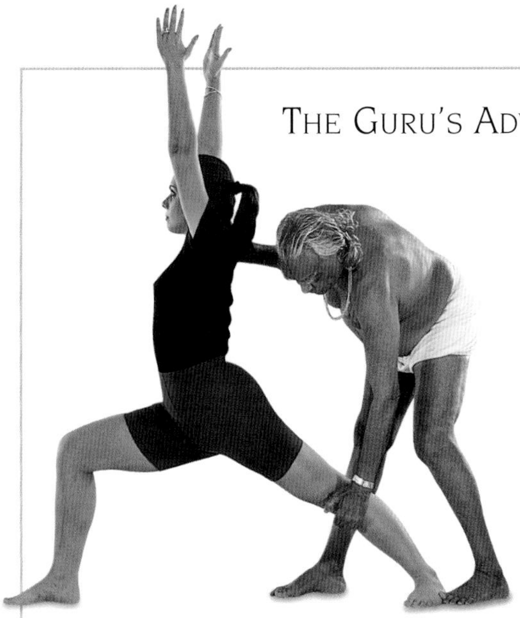

"You must maintain the lift of the left knee. Simultaneously, adjust your shoulder blades by pushing them in, and then lifting them."

BENEFITS

◆

Relieves backache, lumbago, and sciatica

◆

Strengthens the back muscles

◆

Tones the abdominal muscles

◆

Relieves acidity and improves digestion

◆

Strengthens the bladder and corrects a displaced uterus

◆

Relieves menstrual pain and reduces heavy menstruation

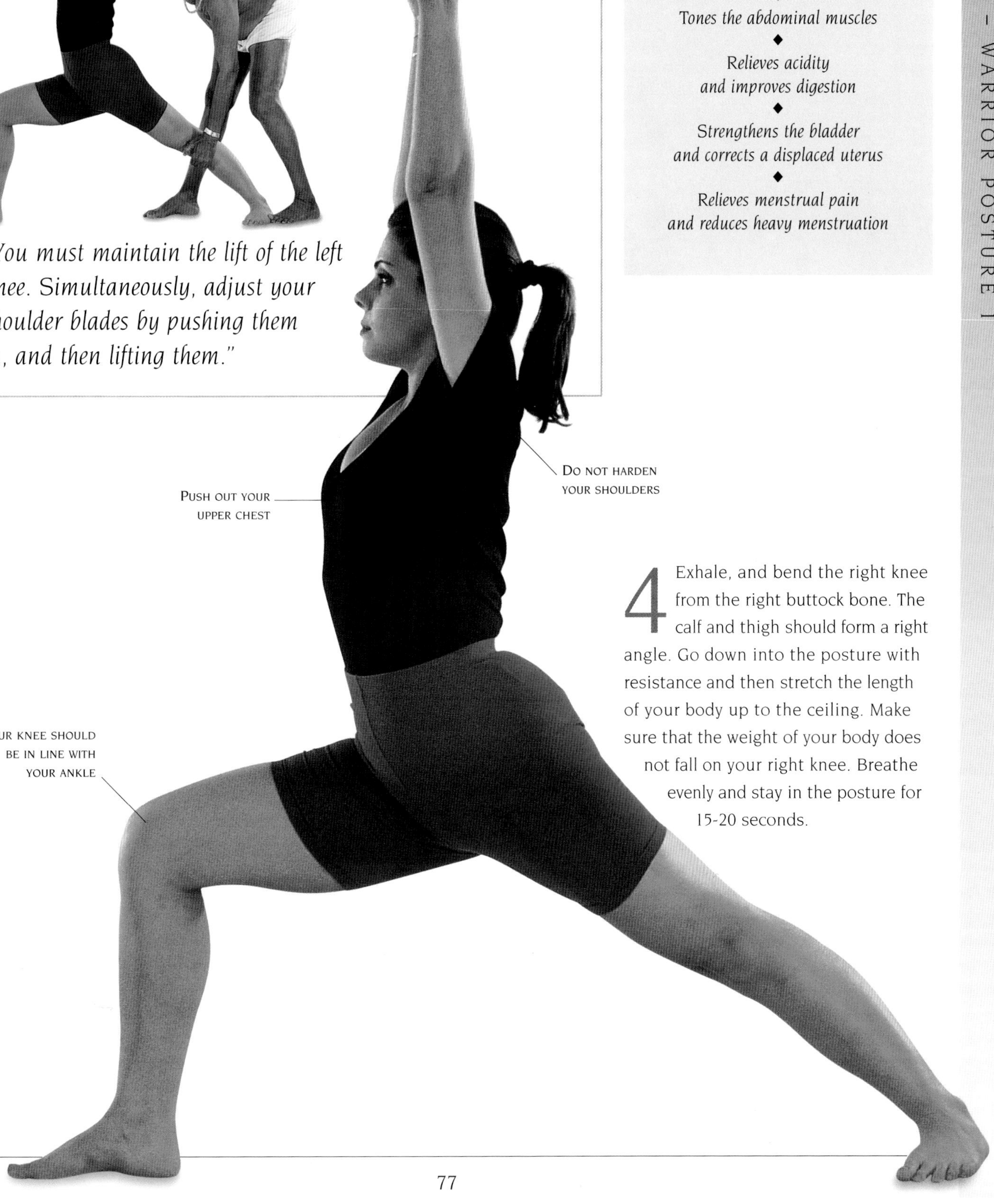

DO NOT HARDEN YOUR SHOULDERS

PUSH OUT YOUR UPPER CHEST

YOUR KNEE SHOULD BE IN LINE WITH YOUR ANKLE

4 Exhale, and bend the right knee from the right buttock bone. The calf and thigh should form a right angle. Go down into the posture with resistance and then stretch the length of your body up to the ceiling. Make sure that the weight of your body does not fall on your right knee. Breathe evenly and stay in the posture for 15-20 seconds.

वीरभद्रासन १

Virabhadrasana 1

ADVANCED WORK IN THE POSTURE

Feel the stretch in your back to experience the posture. Push your shoulder joints into the armpits, stretching your arms up higher. Ensure that the upper part of your body is symmetrical with both armpits parallel to each other. Your face, chest, and right knee should be in line with your right foot. To avoid straining your right knee, turn your kneecap out toward the little toe of your right foot. Your weight should rest on the inner edge of your left buttock and on the outer heel of the left foot. Focus on your left side as it controls the harmony of the posture. Feel the energy flow up your left leg.

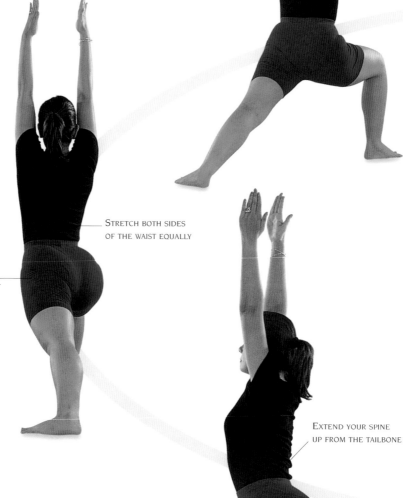

STRETCH YOUR ARMS FROM THE SHOULDER BLADES

STRETCH BOTH SIDES OF THE WAIST EQUALLY

TURN YOUR LEFT BUTTOCK OUT SLIGHTLY

EXTEND YOUR SPINE UP FROM THE TAILBONE

KEEP THE MUSCLES OF THE RIGHT THIGH RELAXED

COMING OUT OF THE POSTURE

◆

Inhale and stretch your arms out to your sides. Straighten your right knee and bring both your feet together, facing forward. Repeat the posture on the other side. Then exhale and jump back to Tadasana.

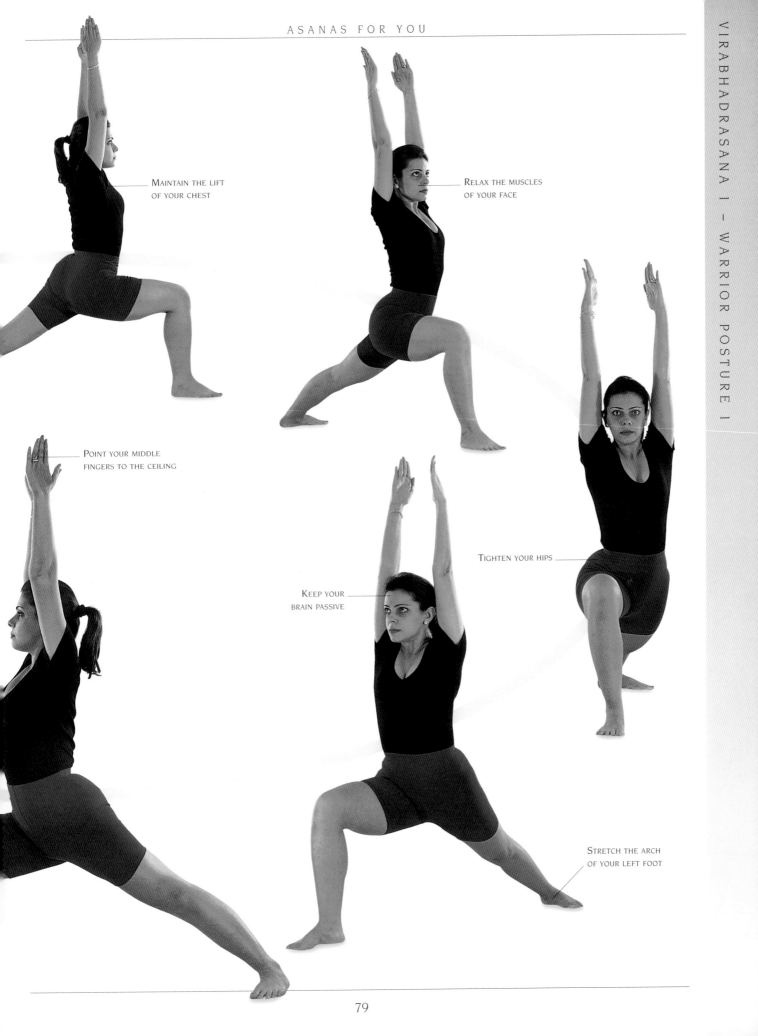

MAINTAIN THE LIFT
OF YOUR CHEST

RELAX THE MUSCLES
OF YOUR FACE

POINT YOUR MIDDLE
FINGERS TO THE CEILING

KEEP YOUR
BRAIN PASSIVE

TIGHTEN YOUR HIPS

STRETCH THE ARCH
OF YOUR LEFT FOOT

Sitting Asanas

"Classic postures, when practiced with discrimination and awareness, bring the body, mind, and consciousness into a single, harmonious whole."

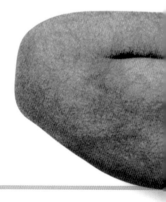

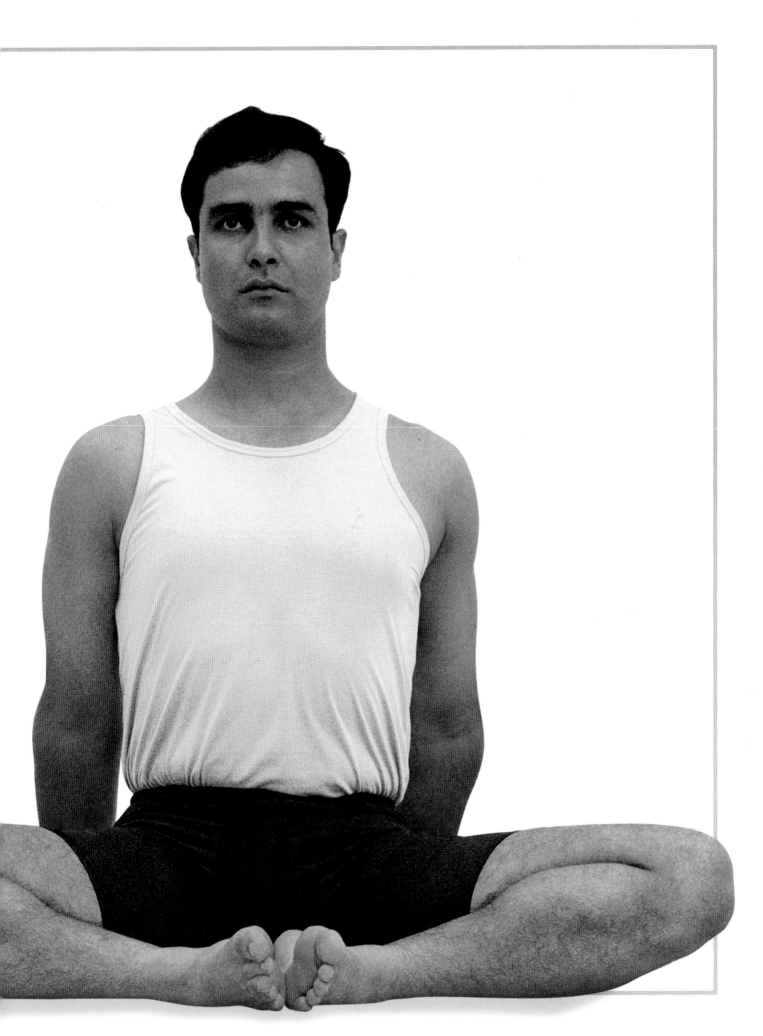

दंडासन

Dandasana

- Staff posture -

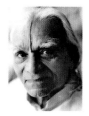

Dandasana is the basic sitting posture for all forward bends. *Danda* means "staff" or "walking stick" in Sanskrit, and regular practice of this asana improves your posture when seated. Your legs are rested during this asana, and it is recommended for people with arthritis or rheumatism of the knees and ankles. If you are prone to anxiety or mood swings, practicing this asana helps increase your will power and enhance your emotional stability.

CAUTIONS
◆

If your spine has a tendency to sag, or if you are experiencing a severe attack of asthma, practice this asana with the length of your spine supported against a wall.

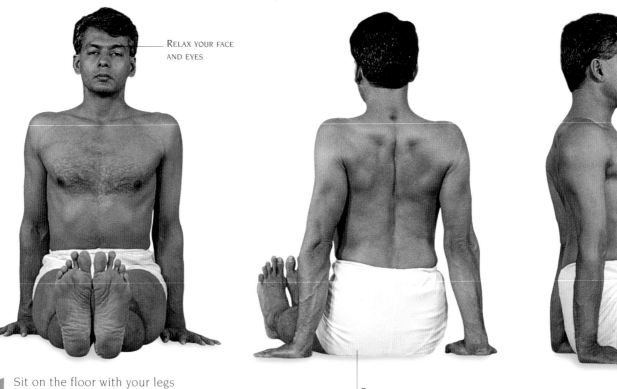

RELAX YOUR FACE AND EYES

REST ON YOUR BUTTOCK BONES

SPREAD OUT THE SOLES OF YOUR FEET

1 Sit on the floor with your legs stretched out. Move the flesh of each buttock out to the side with your hands (*see inset*), so that you are resting on the buttock bones. Keep your thighs, knees, ankles, and feet together. Place your palms on the floor beside your hips with your fingers pointing forward. Lift your chest. Lock your elbows and straighten your arms.

BENEFITS

◆

Relieves breathlessness, choking, and throat congestion in asthmatics

◆

Strengthens the muscles of the chest

◆

Tones the abdominal organs and lifts sagging abdominal walls

◆

Reduces heartburn and flatulence

◆

Tones the spinal and leg muscles

◆

Lengthens the ligaments of the legs

2 Tighten your quadriceps and pull them toward your groin. Press your thighs down onto the floor, and counter that pressure by lifting your waist. Ensure that your diaphragm is free of tension. Lift your ribcage and keep your spine firm. Guard against digging your lower spine into the floor. Focus on keeping your head, neck, and buttocks in a straight line. Hold the posture for 20-30 seconds.

KEEP YOUR HEAD AND NECK ERECT

MOVE YOUR SHOULDERS BACK

DO NOT LET YOUR ABDOMEN SAG

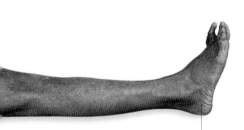

REST ON THE CENTER OF YOUR HEELS

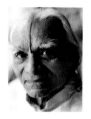

वीरासन

Virasana

- Hero posture -

I N THIS ASANA, you assume the posture of a seated warrior. *Vira* in Sanskrit means "hero" or "warrior." Regular practice of this asana helps to develop your strength and endurance. The asana stretches the chest and increases your capacity for deep breathing. Virasana relieves stiffness in the joints and improves the flexibility of your whole body.

CAUTIONS
◆

If the ligaments of your knee are injured, use a blanket to support your legs (*see page* 188), or sit on your heels (*see* Step 2). Do not practice this posture if you have a cardiac condition.

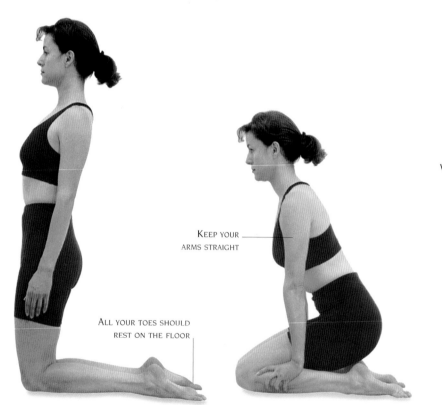

KEEP YOUR ARMS STRAIGHT

ALL YOUR TOES SHOULD REST ON THE FLOOR

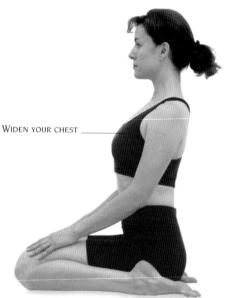

WIDEN YOUR CHEST

1 Kneel on the floor with your knees together. Spread your feet about 12-18in (40cm) apart, with your soles facing the ceiling.

INTERMEDIATES Adjust your ankles so that they stretch evenly from the arch to the toes and from the arch to the heels. Feel the energy flow smoothly in both directions.

2 Lean forward and rest your palms on your shins. Lower your buttocks toward the floor. Make sure that the inner side of each calf touches the outer side of each thigh. Turn your calf muscles out and ensure that you turn your thigh muscles in.

BEGINNERS If you cannot rest your buttocks on the floor, place one sole on top of the other and rest your buttocks on them. Separate your feet.

3 Rest your buttocks on the floor. Do not sit on your feet. Place both palms on your thighs close to the knees. Rest your weight on your thighs. Raise your waist and the sides of your torso, and press your shins firmly down on the floor.

BEGINNERS Place your palms on your knees and push your thighs down. Lift your torso from the base of the pelvis.

INTERMEDIATES Imagine that your legs are tied to the floor, then lift your torso. Feel the energy flow up from the bottom of your chest.

EXTEND YOUR SPINE
FROM THE BASE
OF YOUR PELVIS

BENEFITS

◆

Relieves gout

◆

Eases stiffness in the shoulders, neck, hip joints, knees, and groin

◆

Alleviates arthritis of the elbows and fingers

◆

Relieves backache

◆

Reduces the pain of broken, deviated, or fused tailbones

◆

Corrects herniated discs

◆

Improves circulation in the feet

◆

Relieves calcaneal spurs

4 Raise your arms to shoulder level. Stretch them forward, parallel to the floor. With your palms facing you (*see inset below*), firmly interlock your fingers. Do not leave any gaps between the base of your fingers and the knuckles. Rotate your wrists and palms outward (*see inset left*), facing your palms away from your torso. Keep your spine steady.

ENSURE THAT YOUR ARMS
ARE PERPENDICULAR
TO THE FLOOR

LIFT YOUR STERNUM

5 Raise your arms from the armpits until the palms face the ceiling. Keep your neck erect, your chest expanded, and your elbows straight. Make sure that your head does not tilt back, and your body does not lean forward. Breathe evenly, and hold the posture for 1 minute. With practice, increase the length of time spent in the posture to 5 minutes.

KEEP YOUR KNEES
PRESSED DOWN FIRMLY

वीरासन

Virasana

ADVANCED WORK IN THE POSTURE

The intelligence of the body is energy, while the intelligence of the brain is consciousness. This energy moves with each action. When you stretch your arms up it is a physical action. Lifting the arms from the armpits after locking the elbows and deltoids is an action done by the physiological body (*see page* 42). When you raise your arms, you will feel the energy move to the front of your legs. With every move, the energy in your legs flows to a different position. As the mind moves with this energy, focus on your legs. Imagine you are releasing the energy of your legs into the floor as you stretch your arms up even further. This will calm your mind and free your body of tension.

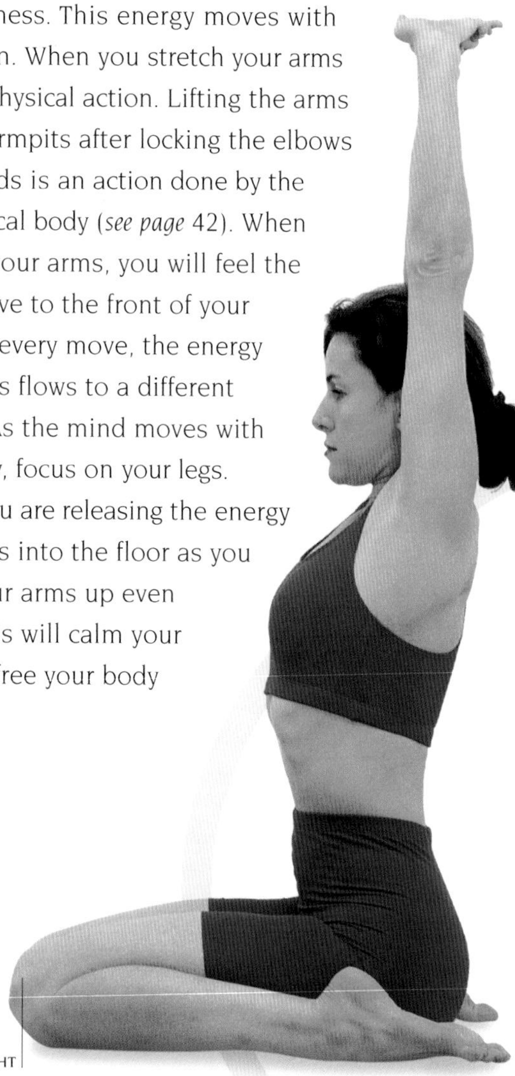

TUCK IN YOUR
SHOULDER BLADES

STRETCH AND STRAIGHTEN
YOUR SPINE BY CONTRACTING
YOUR BUTTOCKS

REST YOUR WEIGHT
ON YOUR KNEES

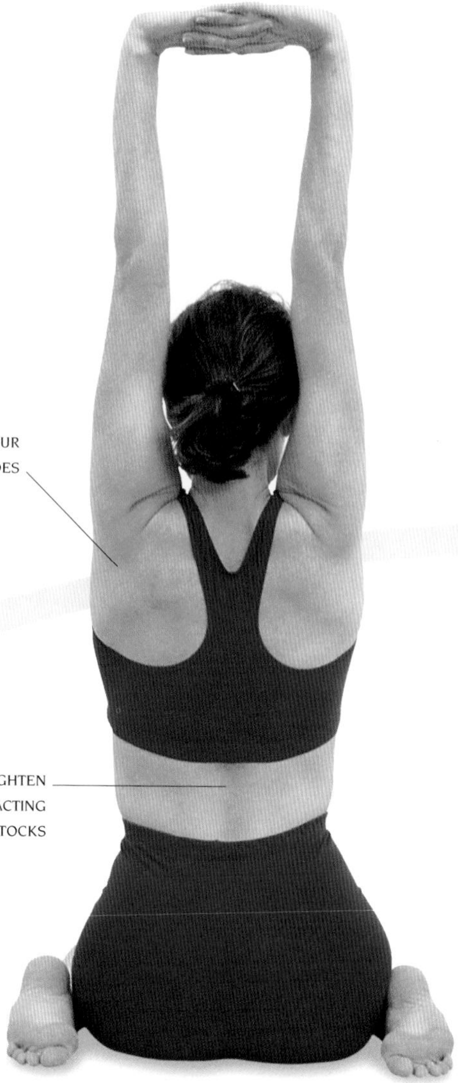

COMING OUT OF THE POSTURE

◆

Bring your arms down to your sides. Place your palms on the floor and raise your buttocks. Kneel and then straighten your legs one by one.

"The practice

change a person's

a positive

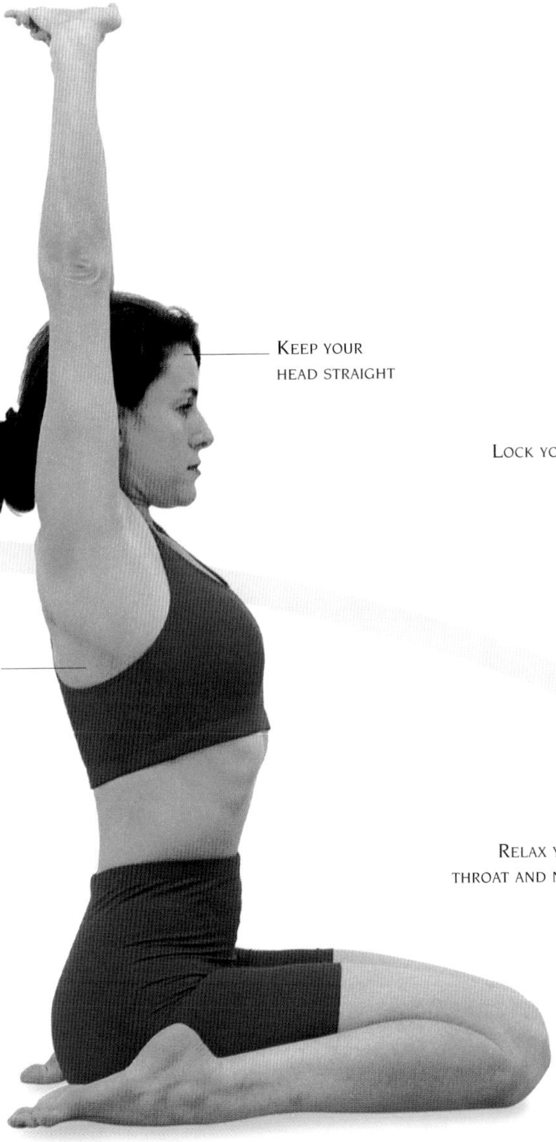

KEEP YOUR
HEAD STRAIGHT

LOCK YOUR ELBOWS

DO NOT ALLOW
YOUR BODY TO
LEAN FORWARD

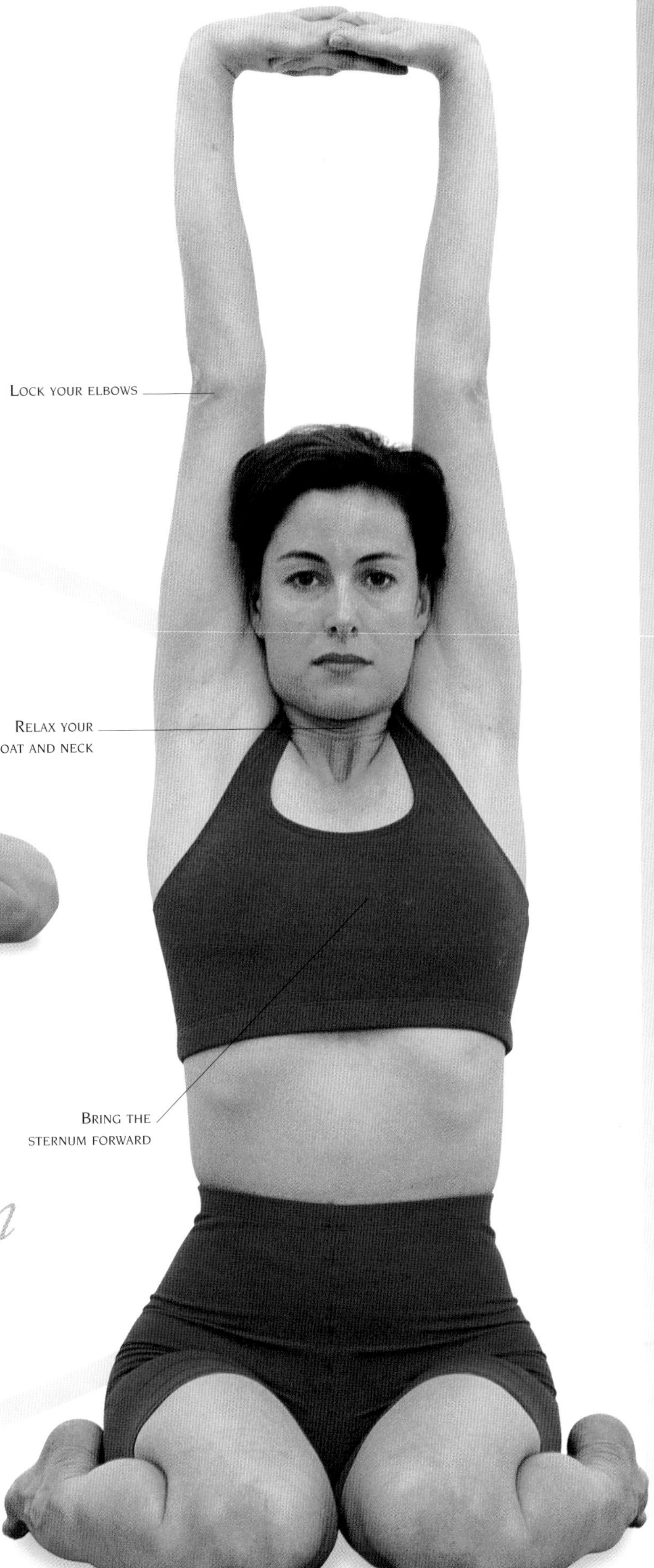

RELAX YOUR
THROAT AND NECK

of yoga helps to

BRING THE
STERNUM FORWARD

mental attitude in

way."

बद्ध कोणासन
Baddhakonasana

- Bound angle posture -

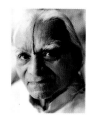

IN SANSKRIT, *baddha* means "bound" or "caught" and *kona* translates as "angle." Regular practice of Baddhakonasana increases the flow of blood to the abdomen, pelvis, and back. It helps to treat arthritis of the knee, hip, and pelvic joints. Pregnant women will experience less pain during labor and will be free of varicose veins if they hold the posture for a few minutes each day. You can practice this asana at any time, even just after a meal.

CAUTIONS
◆

Do not practice this asana if you have a displaced or prolapsed uterus.

DO NOT RAISE YOUR SHOULDERS

RELAX YOUR SHOULDERS AND NECK

1 Sit in Dandasana (*see page* 82). Bend your right knee and hold your right ankle and heel with both hands. Draw your right foot toward your groin. Keep your left leg straight, resting on the floor.

PRESS YOUR LEFT HEEL DOWN FIRMLY

3 Hold your feet firmly near the toes with both hands. Pull your heels even closer to your groin. Stretch your spine up. Widen your thighs and push your knees down toward the floor. Look straight ahead. Stay in this position for 30-60 seconds.

INTERMEDIATES Maintain your hold on your feet. The firmer your grip, the better the lift of the torso. Stretch out both sides of your chest.

2 Bend your left knee the same way as your right knee. Pull your left foot toward your groin, until the soles of both feet touch each other. Make sure that both heels touch the groin. Rest the outer edges of both feet on the floor.

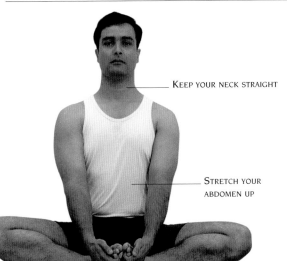

KEEP YOUR NECK STRAIGHT

STRETCH YOUR
ABDOMEN UP

BENEFITS

◆

*Keeps the kidneys
and prostate gland healthy*

◆

*Helps to treat
urinary tract disorders*

◆

Reduces sciatic pain

◆

Prevents hernia

◆

*Relieves heaviness and pain in
the testicles if practiced regularly*

◆

Keeps the ovaries healthy

◆

Corrects irregular menstruation

◆

*Helps to open blocked
fallopian tubes and reduces
vaginal irritation*

4 Push both your knees down by pressing your thighs firmly down on the floor. Stretch your knees away from the torso (*see inset*). This will

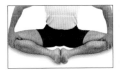

also help to bring them down to the floor. Then pull your heels back to the groin and relax your groin. Press your ankles and shins down onto the floor and push your soles lightly toward each other. Straighten both your arms by stretching your torso up even further. Breathe evenly.

BEGINNERS It is difficult at first to bring your knees down onto the floor. Focus on your groin and consciously relax it.

5 Take your hands behind your back and place both palms onto the floor. Make sure you keep your fingers pointing toward your buttocks. Push your shoulders back. Stay in this posture for 30-60 seconds, breathing deeply.

ENSURE BOTH SIDES OF
YOUR TORSO ARE PARALLEL

PRESS YOUR KNEES
TO THE FLOOR

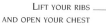

Baddhakonasana

ADVANCED WORK IN THE POSTURE

Once you are comfortable in the final posture, learn to open your chest, stretching it out from all sides. Imagine that your legs are tied to the floor raising your front ribs and lifting up your torso without disturbing the position of your lower limbs. Then focus on your kidneys. Imagine you are pulling them into your body. Keep your back absolutely straight. Inhale and exhale deeply, feeling your energy flow from the bottom of your chest, over your shoulders and down along the spine into the abdomen in one continuous, cyclical flow. Gradually increase the length of time you stay in this posture to 5 minutes.

LIFT YOUR RIBS AND OPEN YOUR CHEST

KEEP YOUR GROIN RELAXED

PRESS YOUR THIGH AND CALF TOGETHER

" All of us have divinity in us fanned into

COMING OUT OF THE POSTURE

◆

Relax your arms and bring them forward to rest on either side of your body. Raise one knee at a time, then straighten your legs one by one. Return to Dandasana.

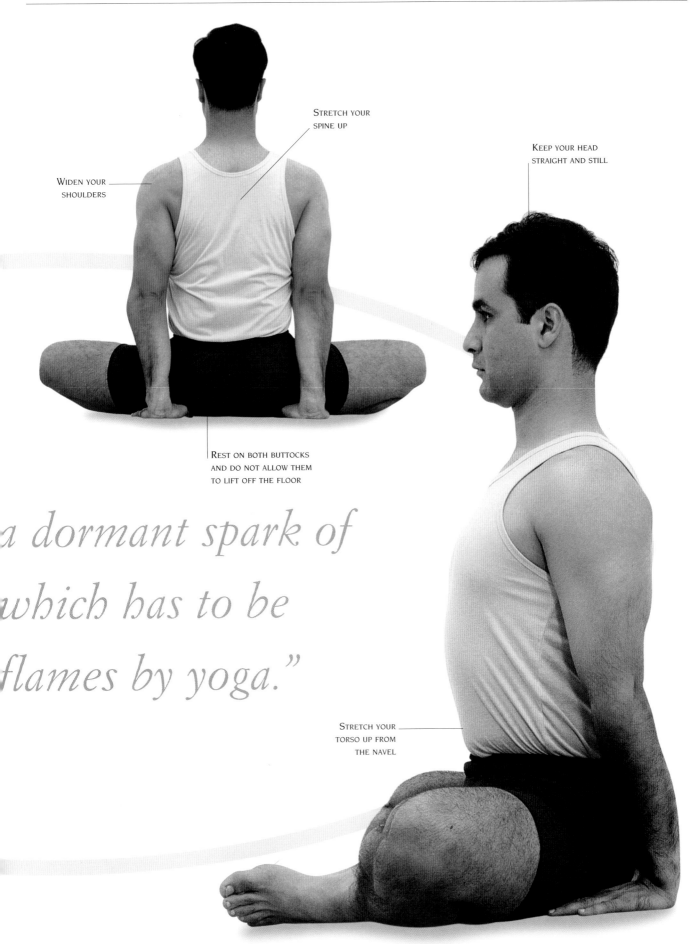

WIDEN YOUR
SHOULDERS

STRETCH YOUR
SPINE UP

KEEP YOUR HEAD
STRAIGHT AND STILL

REST ON BOTH BUTTOCKS
AND DO NOT ALLOW THEM
TO LIFT OFF THE FLOOR

a dormant spark of
which has to be
flames by yoga."

STRETCH YOUR
TORSO UP FROM
THE NAVEL

Forward Bends

"Practice asanas by creating space in the muscles and skin, so that the fine network of the body fits into the asana."

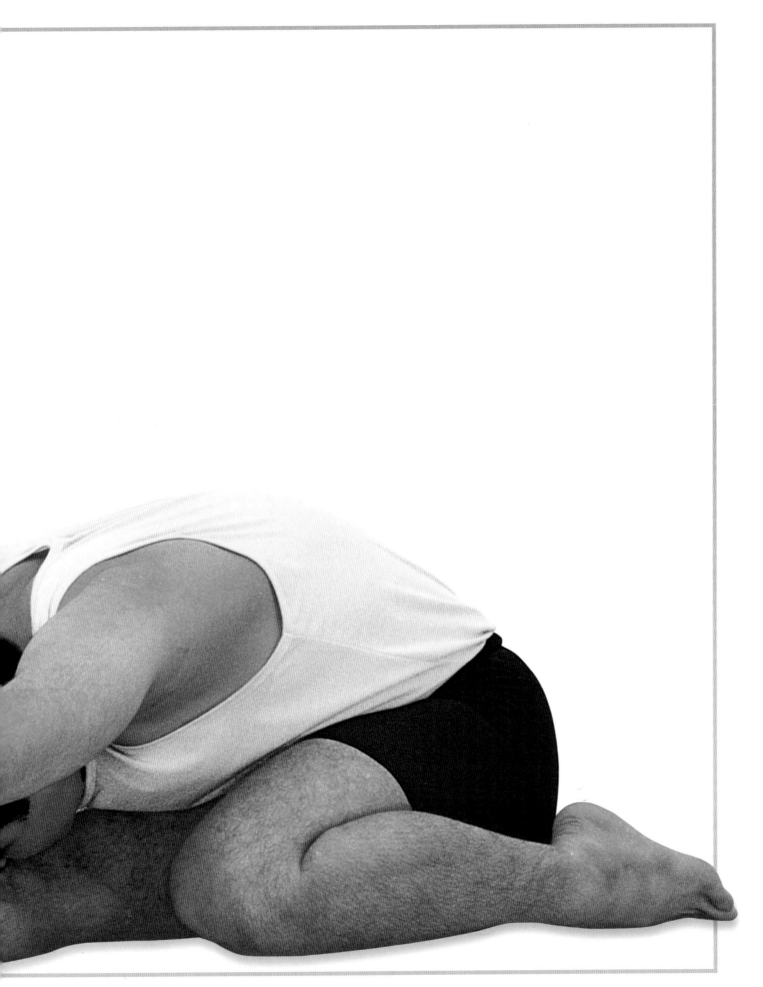

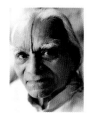

जानु शीर्षासन
Janu Sirsasana

- Head on knee posture -

IN SANSKRIT, THE WORD for "knee" is *janu*, while "head" translates as *sirsa*. Practicing this "head on knee" posture has a dynamic impact on the body and has many benefits. It stretches the front of the spine and eases stiffness in the muscles of the legs and the hip joints. It increases the flexibility of all the joints of the arms, from the shoulders to the knuckles. Forward bends like Janu Sirsasana rest the frontal brain and heart.

CAUTIONS

◆

To protect your hamstring muscles from damage, always open out the knee of the outstretched leg completely, extending it evenly on all sides. Do not allow the thigh of the same leg to lift off the floor.

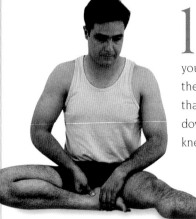

1 Sit in Dandasana (*see page* 82). Bend your right knee and move it to the right. Pull your right foot toward your perineum until the big toe touches the inside of your left thigh. Make sure that your bent knee is pressed firmly down onto the floor. Push back the bent knee until the angle between your legs is more than 90°. Keep your left leg straight. It should rest on the exact center of the left calf.

EXTEND THE LENGTH OF YOUR SPINE

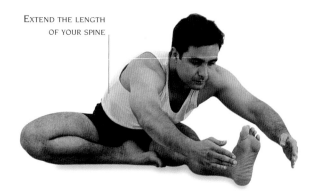

STRETCH YOUR ARMS FROM THE ARMPITS TO THE FINGERTIPS

2 Stretch your left foot so that it feels as if the sole has widened, but keep your toes pointing straight up. Push the right knee even further away from your body. Then lift your arms straight up above your head with the palms facing each other. Stretch your torso up from the hips. Continue the stretch through your shoulders and arms.

3 Exhale, and bend forward from your hips, keeping the lower back flat. For a more effective stretch, push your torso down toward your waist to relax the spinal muscles. Stretch your arms toward your left foot and hold the toes.

BEGINNERS If you cannot reach your toes, stretch as far along the leg as you can, holding on to your knee, shin, or ankle. Gradually, with practice, you will learn to stretch each part of your body separately: the buttocks, the back, the ribs, spine, armpits, elbows, and arms. Focus on keeping your left thigh, knee, and calf on the floor. Always press down on your thigh, not on your calf.

BENEFITS

◆

Eases the effects of stress on the heart and the mind

◆

Stabilizes blood pressure

◆

Gradually corrects curvature of the spine and rounded shoulders

◆

Eases stiffness in the shoulder, hip, elbow, wrist, and finger joints

◆

Tones the abdominal organs

◆

Relieves stiffness in the legs and strengthens their muscles

4 Now increase the stretch. Exhale and extend your arms beyond your left foot. Hold your right wrist with your left hand. Adjust your position. Stretch the spine and press the right knee down onto the floor. Keep your arms straight and lift your chest. Hold this position for 15 seconds.

KEEP YOUR NECK ELONGATED AND RELAXED

PUSH YOUR RIGHT KNEE FURTHER BACK

5 Exhale and stretch your torso further toward the toes. Bring your forehead to your left knee, or as close to it as possible. Hold the posture for 30-60 seconds.

INTERMEDIATES Try to rest your nose on your knee, then your lips, and finally, rest your chin on your leg just beyond the kneecap.

CORRECTING YOURSELF

When in the final posture, visualize the shape of your back. If it is rounded, as shown here, only a small part of the spine at the level of the shoulders is being stretched. Lengthen and flatten the lower spine and extend your arms out from your shoulder blades.

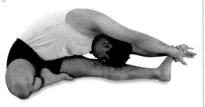

PUSH YOUR TORSO TOWARD YOUR LEFT FOOT

REST THE CHEST ON YOUR LEFT THIGH

जानु शीर्षासन

Janu Sirsasana

ADVANCED WORK IN THE POSTURE

When you are holding this posture, your sternum and abdomen should rest on the left thigh as though the leg and torso were one. One side of your back and torso might stretch more than the other. This is usually the same side as the outstretched leg. Be conscious of this, and try to equalize the stretch on both sides. Keep your elbows out, widening them to increase the expansion of your chest.

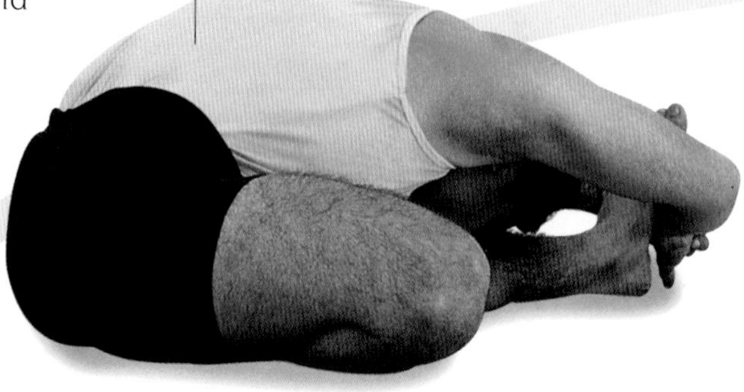

DO NOT ALLOW THE RIGHT SIDE OF YOUR BACK TO JUT UP

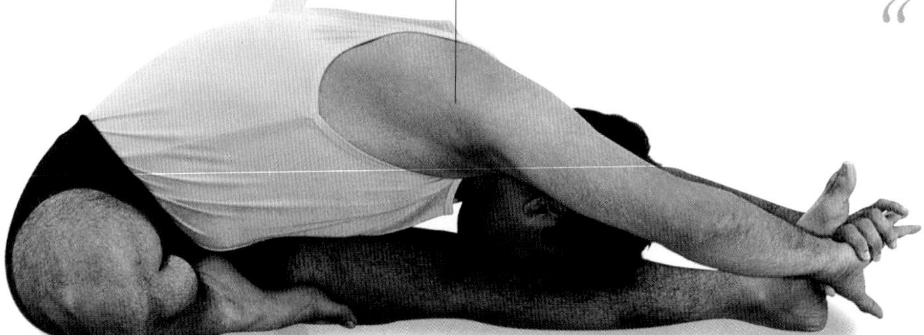

STRETCH THE ARMS FROM THE ARMPITS

"The intensit

increase and

momen.

PRESS YOUR KNEE TO THE FLOOR

HOLD YOUR RIGHT WRIST LIGHTLY

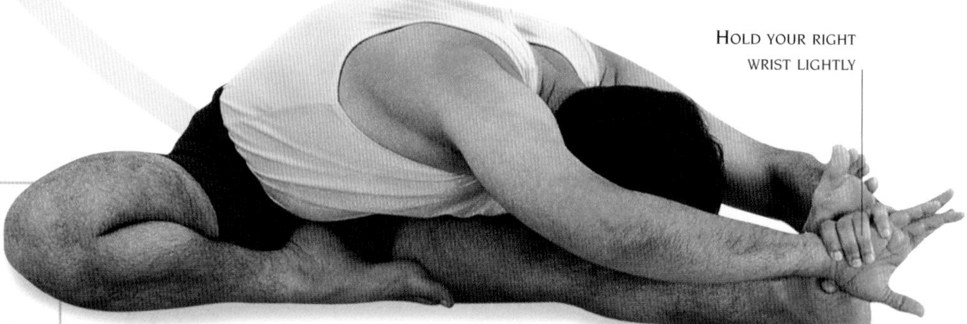

COMING OUT OF THE POSTURE

◆

Inhale, then lift your head and torso slightly. After a few seconds release your hands and sit up. Stretch out your right leg and sit in Dandasana. Now repeat the posture on the other side.

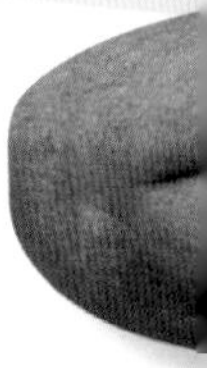

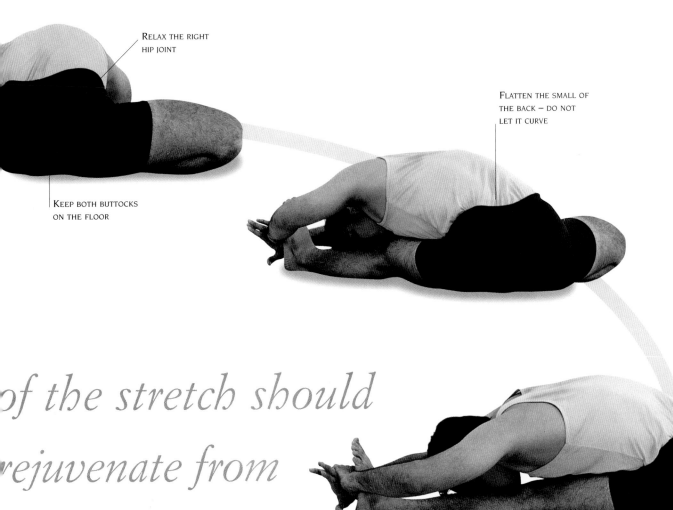

RELAX THE RIGHT HIP JOINT

KEEP BOTH BUTTOCKS ON THE FLOOR

FLATTEN THE SMALL OF THE BACK – DO NOT LET IT CURVE

of the stretch should

rejuvenate from

to moment."

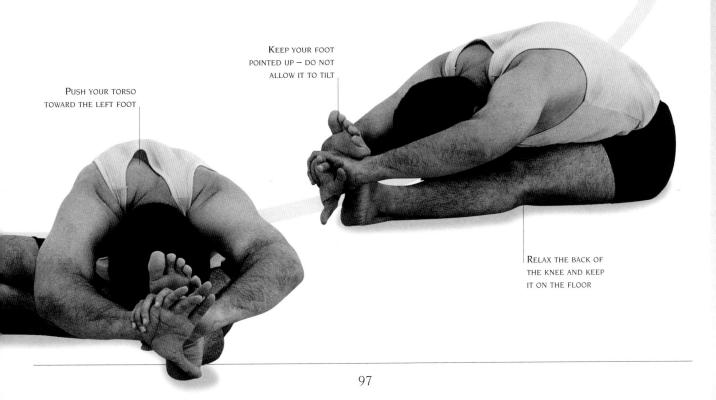

PUSH YOUR TORSO TOWARD THE LEFT FOOT

KEEP YOUR FOOT POINTED UP – DO NOT ALLOW IT TO TILT

RELAX THE BACK OF THE KNEE AND KEEP IT ON THE FLOOR

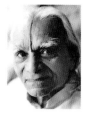

त्र्यंग मुखैकपाद पश्चिमोत्तानासन

Trianga Mukhaikapada Paschimottanasana

- Three limbs intense west stretch posture -

I N SANSKRIT, the literal meaning of *trianga* is "three parts of the body." In this asana, the "three parts" comprise the buttocks, knees, and feet. The back of the body, which is known in Sanskrit as the *paschima* or "west," is stretched over *eka pada* or "one foot," and the *mukha* or "face" rests on the leg. Regular practice of this asana makes the whole body supple and agile.

CAUTIONS

◆

Do not practice this asana during, or immediately after, an asthmatic attack. Avoid this asana if you have diarrhea. Do not twist your torso or allow it to lean toward the outer side of your extended leg, as this could strain your spine or abdominal organs.

1 Sit in Dandasana (*see page* 82). Bend your right leg back toward your right hip. Use your right hand to pull the ankle into place. Keep your left leg stretched out, making sure that it rests on the center of your left calf and heel.

3 Raise your arms up toward the ceiling. Extend your torso up and feel the stretch from your waist to your fingertips.

BEGINNERS To maintain your balance, keep the weight of your body on the bent knee. This will ensure that your torso does not tilt toward the left.

2 Keep your thighs together. Press your right knee down onto the floor. The inner side of your right calf should touch the outer side of your right thigh. Balance equally on both buttocks. Make sure that your right buttock rests squarely on the floor (*see inset*). Rest your palms, fingers pointing forward, on the floor beside your hips.

PUSH DOWN ON YOUR BENT KNEE

STRETCH THE BACK OF YOUR LEFT LEG FROM THIGH TO HEEL

STRAIGHTEN AND STRETCH YOUR TOES

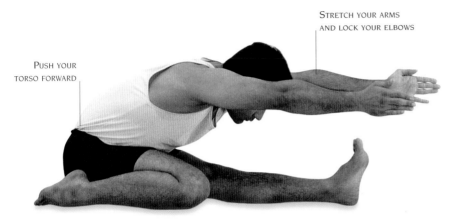

PUSH YOUR
TORSO FORWARD

STRETCH YOUR ARMS
AND LOCK YOUR ELBOWS

BENEFITS

◆

*Tones and stimulates the
abdominal organs*

◆

*Assists digestion and counters
the effects of excess bile secretion*

◆

Reduces flatulence and constipation

◆

Creates flexibility in the knee joints

◆

*Corrects dropped arches
and flat feet*

4 Exhale and bend forward from the waist. Stretch both arms beyond your left foot, with the palms facing each other. Ensure your thighs and knees are pressed together. Rest on both buttocks. The essence of the posture is getting this balance right.

INTERMEDIATES While you are getting into the posture, the torso has a tendency to tilt to the left. To guard against this, shift your weight to your right. This will bring the center of gravity to the middle of your right thigh. Then equalize your weight on both buttocks.

5 Exhale, widen your elbows, and push your torso toward your left foot. Press both your wrists against the sole of your left foot. Then hold your right wrist with your left hand. First touch your forehead to your left knee, then place your nose, lips, and finally, your chin, beyond your left knee. Push your left buttock out and rest on the inside of your left buttock bone. Hold the posture for 30-60 seconds.

BEGINNERS Stretch forward as far as you can. With practice, you will learn to hook your wrists around your foot.

DO NOT LET YOUR TORSO
TILT TO THE LEFT

EXTEND YOUR
SHOULDERS AND KEEP
YOUR NECK RELAXED

TRIANGA MUKHAIKAPADA PASCHIMOTTANASANA – THREE LIMBS INTENSE WEST STRETCH POSTURE

 त्र्यंग मुखैकपाद पश्चिमोत्तानासन

Trianga Mukhaikapada Paschimottanasana

ADVANCED WORK IN THE POSTURE

In the final stretch, make sure that your body weight is distributed evenly over your legs and buttocks. Keep your sternum in contact with your thighs. Both arms should be equally stretched forward. Make sure that the weight on the knee of the outstretched leg is equal to the weight borne by the bent knee. Focus on maintaining the center of gravity of this posture at the middle of the right thigh. Extend the right side of your torso from the pelvic rim toward your head. Elongate the right side of your chest and waist and expand the side of the ribs resting on the bent knee, stretching your torso further forward.

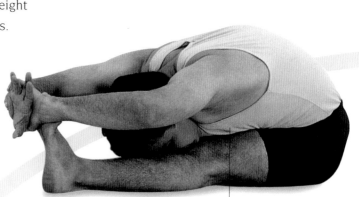

REST YOUR STERNUM ON YOUR THIGHS

KEEP THE MUSCLES OF YOUR NECK SOFT

"A yogi's brair

bottom of the

of his

POINT YOUR TOES STRAIGHT UP

COMING OUT OF THE POSTURE

◆

Inhale, raise your head and torso, and wait for a few seconds. Keep your back concave. Release your hands, then sit up and straighten your right leg. Repeat the posture on the other side. Return to Dandasana.

ENSURE THAT YOUR BENT KNEE REMAINS PRESSED ONTO THE FLOOR

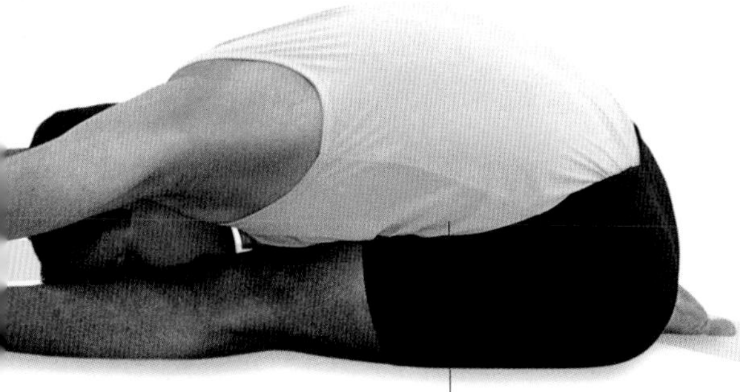

ENSURE THAT BOTH
SIDES OF YOUR BACK
ARE EVENLY STRETCHED

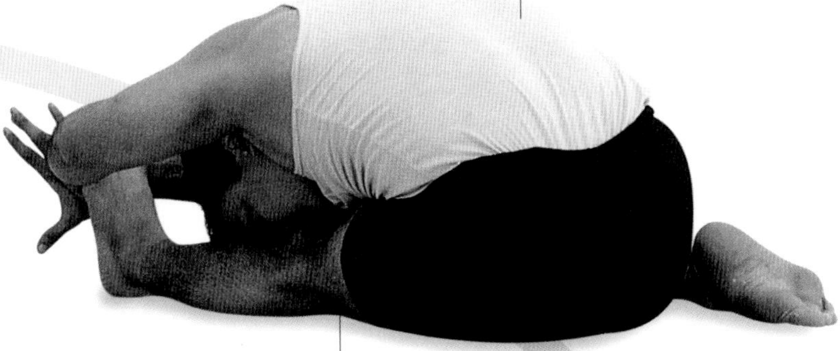

PUSH YOUR WAIST TOWARD
THE QUADRICEP MUSCLES
OF YOUR THIGHS

PRESS YOUR INNER THIGHS
DOWN ONTO THE FLOOR

extends from the
foot to the top
head."

KEEP BOTH HIPS
PARALLEL TO EACH OTHER

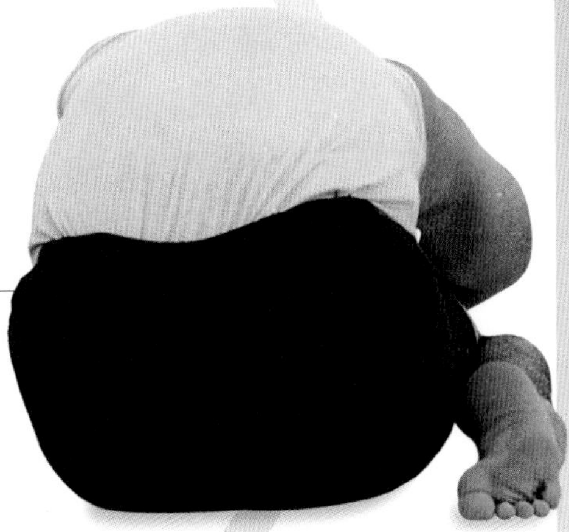

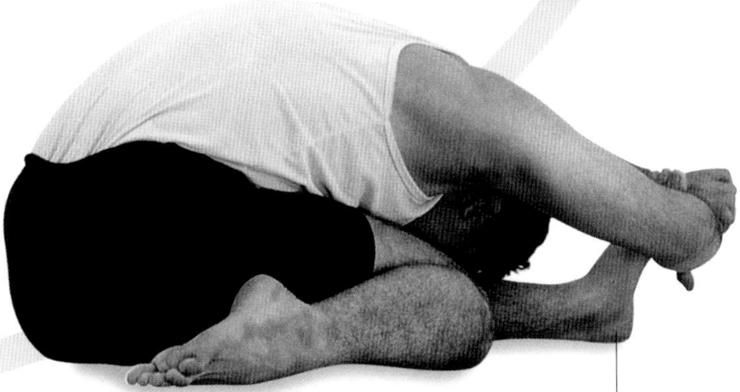

STRETCH BOTH ARMS
EVENLY FROM THE ARMPITS

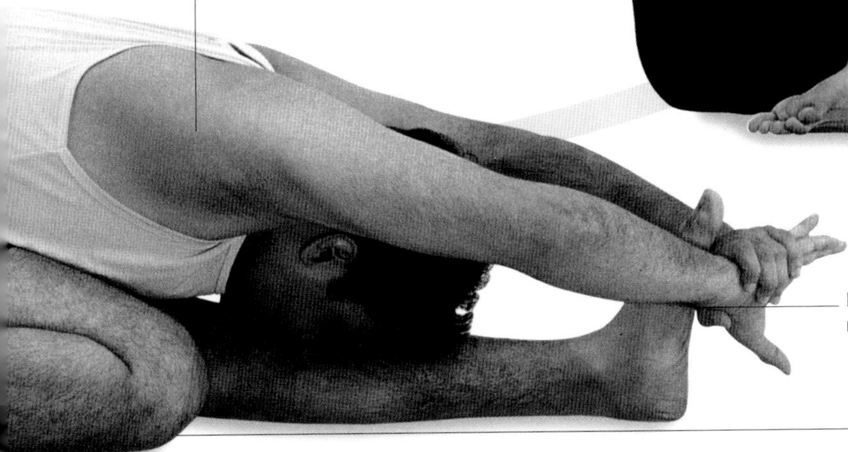

REST ON THE
CENTER OF YOUR HEEL

PRESS BOTH WRISTS
FIRMLY AGAINST YOUR SOLES

पश्चिमोत्तानासन

Paschimottanasana

- Intense west stretch posture -

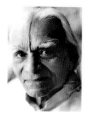

THE BACK OF YOUR BODY, from your heels to your head, is known as *paschim*, which means "west" in Sanskrit. U*t* indicates "intense," while *tan* means "stretch." This asana stretches the length of your spine allowing the life-force to flow to every part of your body. Resting your forehead on your knees calms the active front brain and keeps the meditative back brain quiet, yet alert.

CAUTIONS

◆

Do not practice this asana during, or just after, an asthmatic attack. Avoid this posture if you have diarrhea. Do not allow your thighs to lift off the floor, as the muscles at the backs of your knees might rupture.

KEEP YOUR HEAD STRAIGHT

STRETCH YOUR LEGS OUT

1 Sit in Dandasana (*see page* 82). Keep your legs together. Stretch your heels, ensuring that both are evenly pressed down. Put your palms

on the floor beside your hips. Take a few deep breaths. Now stretch your arms above your head (*see inset*) with the palms facing each other. Stretch your spine up.

2 Exhale and stretch your arms toward your feet. Grip the big toe of your left foot with the thumb and first two fingers of your left hand.

Do the same to your right toe with your right hand (*see inset*). Press your thighs down on the floor. The pressure on your thighs should be greater than that on your calves. This helps you stretch more effectively.

BEGINNERS Focus on keeping your thighs flat on the floor. You must not allow them to lift off the floor. This is more important than holding your toes.

HOLD YOUR TOES FIRMLY

DO NOT RAISE THE BUTTOCK BONES OFF THE FLOOR

PRESS YOUR SHINS AND THIGHS FIRMLY ONTO THE FLOOR

BENEFITS

◆

Rests and massages the heart

◆

Soothes the adrenal glands

◆

Tones the kidneys, bladder, and pancreas

◆

Activates a sluggish liver and improves the digestive system

◆

Helps to treat impotence

◆

Stimulates the ovaries, uterus, and the entire reproductive system

THE GURU'S ADVICE

"Stretch from the seat of the buttocks and feel the lightness in your buttocks. This is the heart of the perfect posture."

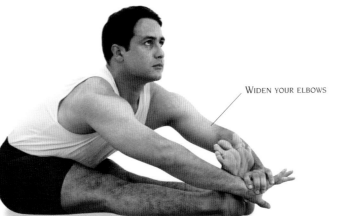

3 Make sure that you are sitting on your inner buttock bones and that your weight is distributed equally on them. Do not allow either buttock to rise off the floor. Then hold your right wrist with your left hand.

INTERMEDIATES Hold the soles of your feet with the interlocked fingers of both hands. Breathe evenly.

WIDEN YOUR ELBOWS

STRETCH YOUR ARMS FROM YOUR SHOULDER BLADES

4 Exhale and lift your torso. Bend forward from your lower back keeping your spine concave. Stretch forward from both sides of the waist. First, place your forehead firmly on your knees, and then push it toward your shins. Widen and lift your elbows, but do not allow them to rest on the floor. Hold the posture for 1 minute.

BEGINNERS Rest your forehead on a folded blanket placed on your shins.

पश्चिमोत्तानासन

Paschimottanasana

ADVANCED WORK IN THE POSTURE

As you bend keep your diaphragm as soft as dough. For a more effective stretch bring your diaphragm closer to your chest as you lower your head. The front of your chest is the "brain" of this posture (*see page* 45). Bring it close to your thighs. Check that both sides of your chest are evenly stretched so that there is a symmetry in the final posture. Press your forehead onto your shins. Consciously descend your mind into the posture. Focus on your back. Extend the skin of your back toward your head. Descend your spine completely. This will bring lightness and calm to the brain. Rejuvenate the stretch constantly. With practice, increase the duration of the posture to 5 minutes.

KEEP THE MUSCLES OF YOUR NECK PASSIVE

DO NOT LET YOUR ELBOWS MOVE DOWN

" The movement of intelligence of the and keep pace

PUSH YOUR FEET AND HANDS AGAINST EACH OTHER

COMING OUT OF THE POSTURE
◆

Inhale, then raise your head and torso, keeping your back concave. Wait for a few seconds, then release your hands. Sit up and come back to Dandasana.

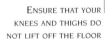

KEEP YOUR SPINE STRETCHED

ENSURE THAT YOUR KNEES AND THIGHS DO NOT LIFT OFF THE FLOOR

RAISE THE INNER SIDES OF YOUR UPPER ARMS

he body and the
rain should synchronize
with each other."

COMPRESS YOUR HIPS AND KEEP THEM PARALLEL TO EACH OTHER

STRETCH FORWARD FROM THE BASE OF YOUR SPINE

KEEP YOUR ARMPITS ACTIVE AND STRETCH THEM FORWARD

REST ON BOTH BUTTOCKS EQUALLY

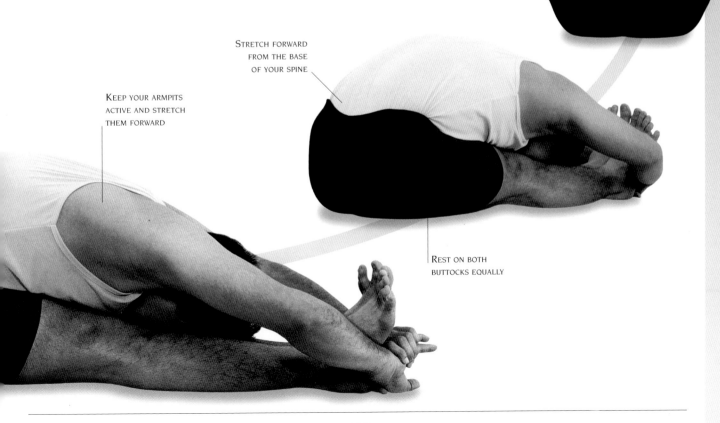

Twists

"If you practice yoga every day with perseverance, you will be able to face the turmoil of life with steadiness and maturity."

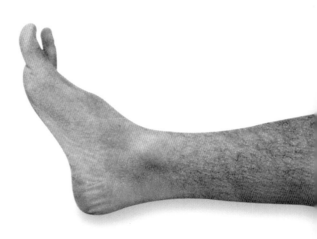

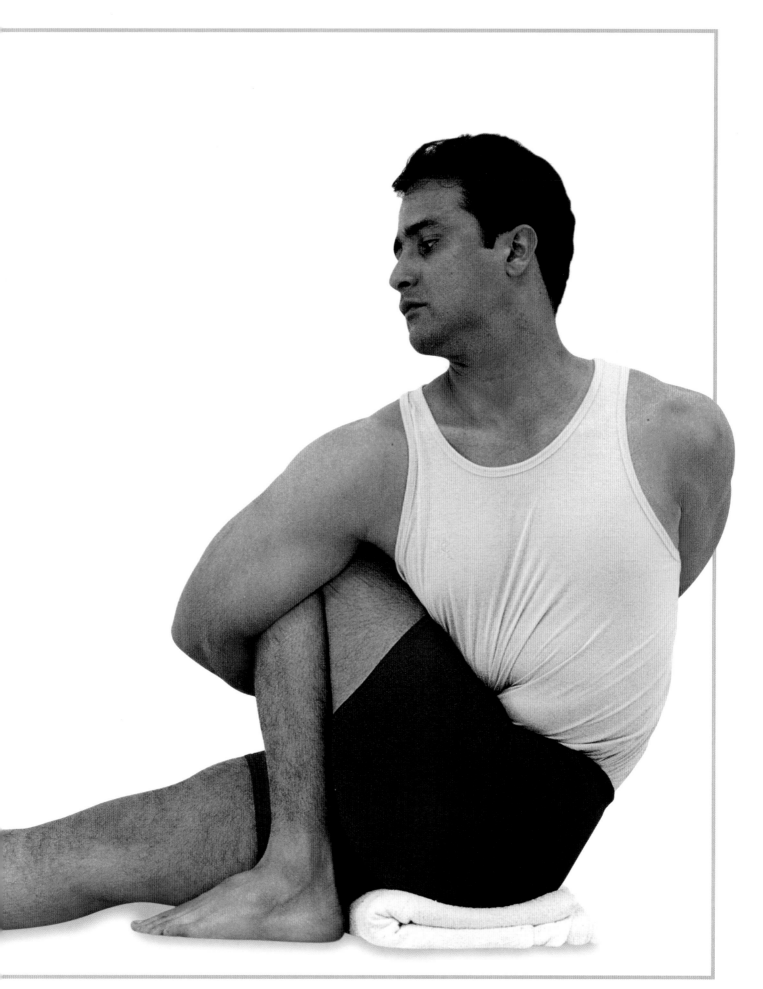

भरद्वाजासन
Bharadvajasana

- Torso stretch -

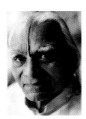

THIS ASANA IS NAMED after the ancient sage, Bharadvaja, who was the father of the great warrior, Dronacharya. Both are major characters in the Indian epic, *Mahabharata*. Regular practice of this asana teaches you to rotate your spinal column effectively, which increases the flexibility of your back and torso, and prepares you for the more advanced twists. It also massages, tones, and rejuvenates your abdominal organs.

CAUTIONS
◆

Do not practice this asana if you have high blood pressure, eye strain, a stress-related headache, or migraine. The asana should not be attempted if you have diarrhea or dysentery. Avoid this asana during menstruation.

DO NOT MOVE
YOUR HEAD

TAKE THE LEFT
SHOULDER BACK

1 Sit in Dandasana (*see page* 82). Place your palms flat on the floor behind your buttocks with your fingers pointing forward. Bend your knees, and with your legs together, move your shins to the left. Make sure that your thighs and knees are facing forward. Breathe evenly.

KEEP YOUR
FEET RELAXED

2 Hold your ankles and bring your shins further to the left until both feet are beside your left hip. The front of your left ankle should rest on the arch of your right foot (*see inset*).

Extend the toes of your left foot and keep your right ankle pressed down onto the floor. Rest your buttocks on the floor, not on your feet. Lift your torso stretching your spine fully up. Pause for a few breaths.

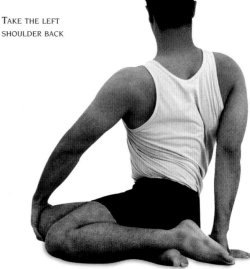

3 Exhale and then turn your chest and abdomen to the right, moving your left shoulder forward to the right and your right shoulder back. Place your left palm on your right knee and rest your right palm on the floor. Revolve your right shoulder blade to the back and tuck in your left shoulder blade. Take one or two breaths.

BENEFITS

◆

*Relieves pain in the neck, shoulders,
and back*

◆

*Helps to keep the spine
and shoulders supple*

◆

*Eases a painful, stiff, sprained,
or fused lumbar spine*

◆

*Reduces discomfort
in the dorsal spine area*

◆

*Increases the flexibility of the back
and hips*

4 Press your right shin to the floor. This will help to lift your torso and turn it even further to the right. Rotate until the left side of your body is in line with your right thigh. Turn your head and neck to the right. Inhale, and holding your breath, firmly press the fingertips of your right hand down onto the floor. Then exhale and simultaneously raise and rotate your spine strongly to the right. Look over your right shoulder. Hold the posture for 30-60 seconds.

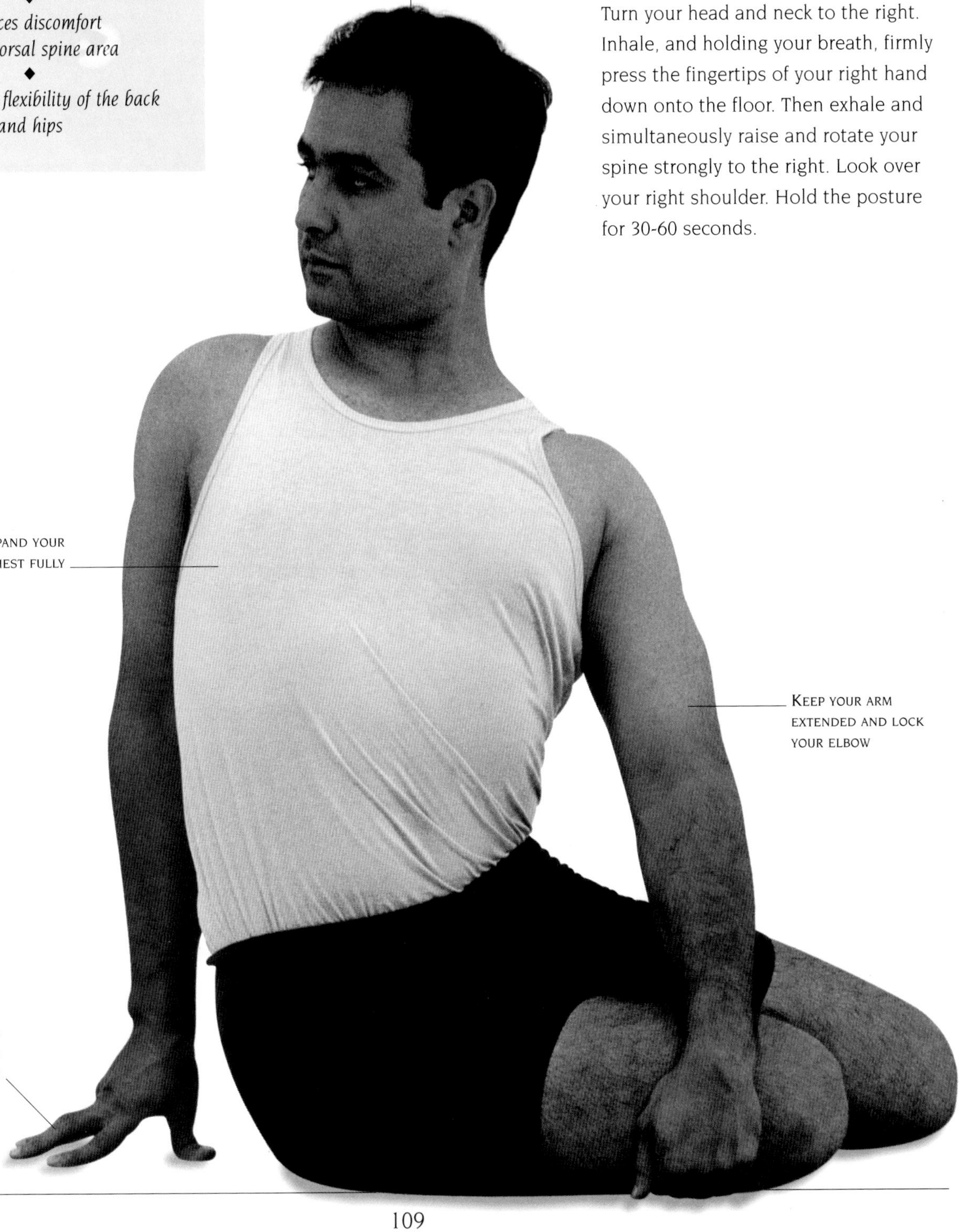

TURN YOUR HEAD
TO THE RIGHT

EXPAND YOUR
CHEST FULLY

KEEP YOUR ARM
EXTENDED AND LOCK
YOUR ELBOW

PRESS YOUR
FINGERTIPS TO
THE FLOOR

भरद्वाजासन

Bharadvajasana

ADVANCED WORK IN THE POSTURE

Once you have turned your neck and head to the right and rotated your torso, tuck in both your shoulders. Lift your sternum, keeping the spine erect as it turns on its axis. Do not change the position of your knees while turning, since they tend to move with the body. Ensure that your body does not lean back. Maintain the turn of your head and neck to the right. Keep the left hip and the left shoulder in line when you revolve your torso. Twist the spine strongly, turning it as far to the right as you can. Focus on the skin of your back. Try, consciously, to push your skin down from your neck, and pull the skin up from your lower back. Breathe evenly.

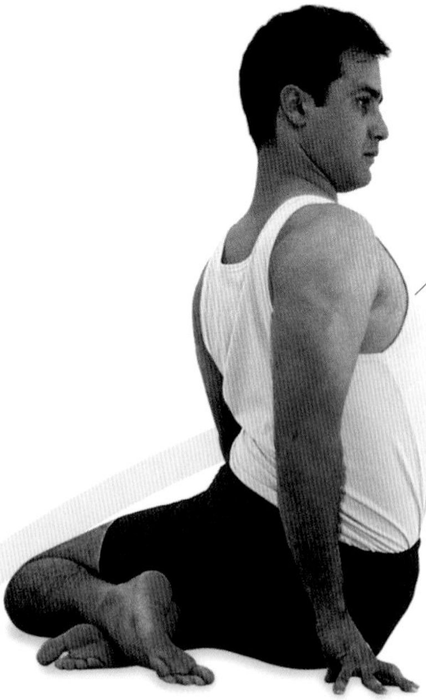

KEEP BOTH SIDES OF YOUR RIBCAGE PARALLEL

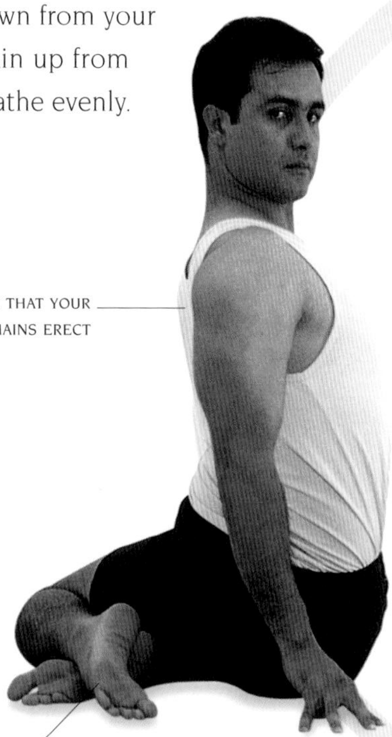

ENSURE THAT YOUR SPINE REMAINS ERECT

REST YOUR LEFT FOOT ON THE ARCH OF THE RIGHT FOOT

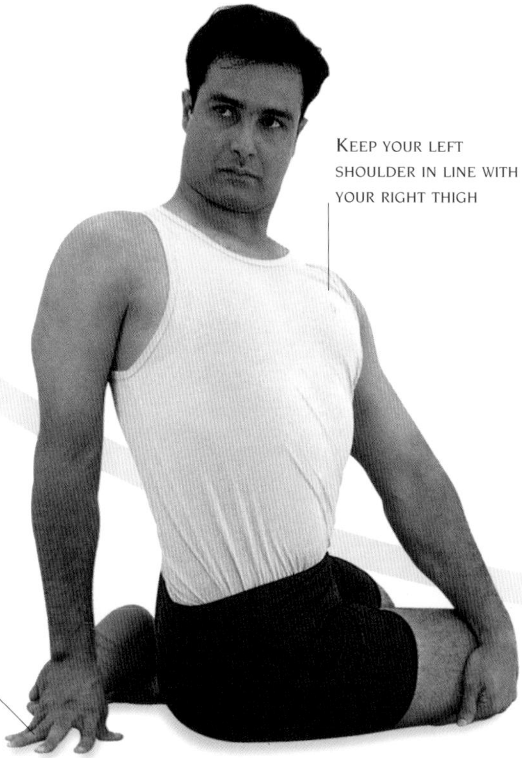

KEEP YOUR LEFT SHOULDER IN LINE WITH YOUR RIGHT THIGH

STRETCH THE FINGERS OUT FULLY

COMING OUT OF THE POSTURE

◆

Release your hands and bring your torso to the front. Straighten your legs. Repeat the posture on the other side. Come back to Dandasana.

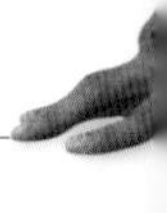

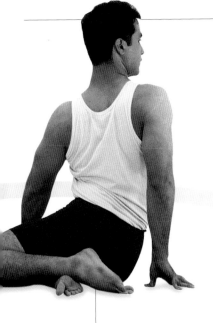

RELAX THE MUSCLES
OF YOUR NECK

TUCK IN YOUR RIGHT
SHOULDER BLADE

REST BOTH FEET
ON THE FLOOR

DO NOT ALLOW YOUR
TORSO TO LEAN BACK

LOOK OVER YOUR
RIGHT SHOULDER

KEEP BOTH SIDES OF
THE CHEST LEVEL

PRESS YOUR KNEES
DOWN AND KEEP THEM
FACING FORWARD

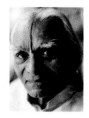

मरीच्यासन
Marichyasana

- Spinal twist -

THIS ASANA IS DEDICATED to the sage, Marichi. His father was Brahma, creator of the universe, and his grandson was the sun god, Surya, the giver of life. Regular practice of the asana stretches your entire body and rejuvenates it. Marichyasana increases your levels of energy. The asana also massages and tones your abdominal organs.

CAUTIONS
◆
Do not practice this asana if you have diarrhea or dysentery, or during a cold. Avoid this posture if you have a headache, migraine, insomnia, or when you are feeling fatigued. Do not practice during menstruation.

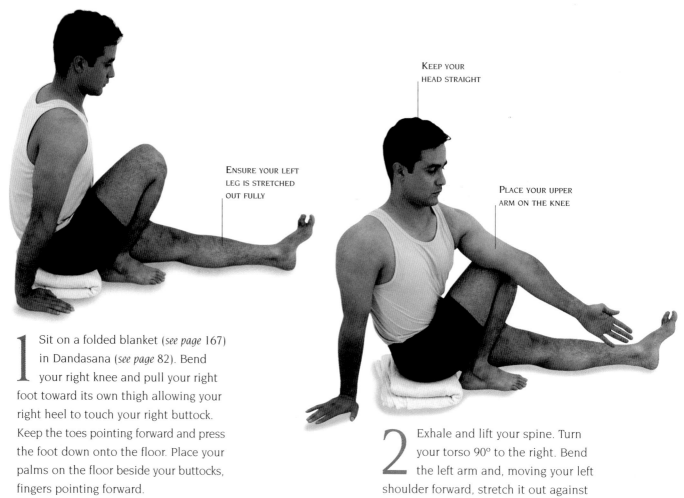

KEEP YOUR
HEAD STRAIGHT

ENSURE YOUR LEFT
LEG IS STRETCHED
OUT FULLY

PLACE YOUR UPPER
ARM ON THE KNEE

1 Sit on a folded blanket (*see page* 167) in Dandasana (*see page* 82). Bend your right knee and pull your right foot toward its own thigh allowing your right heel to touch your right buttock. Keep the toes pointing forward and press the foot down onto the floor. Place your palms on the floor beside your buttocks, fingers pointing forward.

2 Exhale and lift your spine. Turn your torso 90° to the right. Bend the left arm and, moving your left shoulder forward, stretch it out against your right thigh. Extend this arm from the armpit to the elbow. This is crucial to the final stretch. Do not allow your left leg to tilt left. Your weight should not fall on your right palm.

BENEFITS

◆

Increases energy levels

◆

*Tones and massages the
abdominal organs*

◆

*Improves the functioning of the liver,
spleen, pancreas, kidneys,
and intestines*

◆

Reduces fat around the waistline

◆

Alleviates backache

◆

Relieves lumbago

3 Press your right ankle down on the floor and turn your torso further to the right. Push your left armpit against the outer side of the right knee. This will help you rotate your torso more effectively. Ensure that you turn from your waist and not the chest. Exhale and encircle your right knee with your left arm.

PRESS YOUR RIGHT
FOOT DOWN ONTO
THE FLOOR

THERE SHOULD BE NO
GAP BETWEEN YOUR
ARMPIT AND THIGH

4 Exhale and lift your right palm off the floor. Take your right arm behind your back. Bend it and bring it toward the left hand. First hold the fingers, then the palm, and finally the wrist, of the left hand with your right hand (*see inset*). Lift your torso and rotate further to the right. Turn your head to the left and look over your shoulder. Hold the posture for 20-30 seconds.

INTENSIFY THE STRETCH
OF YOUR LEFT LEG

मरीच्यासन

Marichyasana

ADVANCED WORK IN THE POSTURE

This asana requires spinal action. Do not turn from your arms, but from your spine. The torso has a tendency to lean to the right in this posture so consciously keep the left side of your body higher than the right. Stretch and lift the front of your spine. Bring your waist, and not just your chest, close to the middle of your right thigh. The entire length of the left side of your torso should be in contact with your right thigh. Bring your arms closer to each other and intensify your grip. The upper part of your right arm is the "brain" of the pose (*see page* 45) so keep it completely stable.

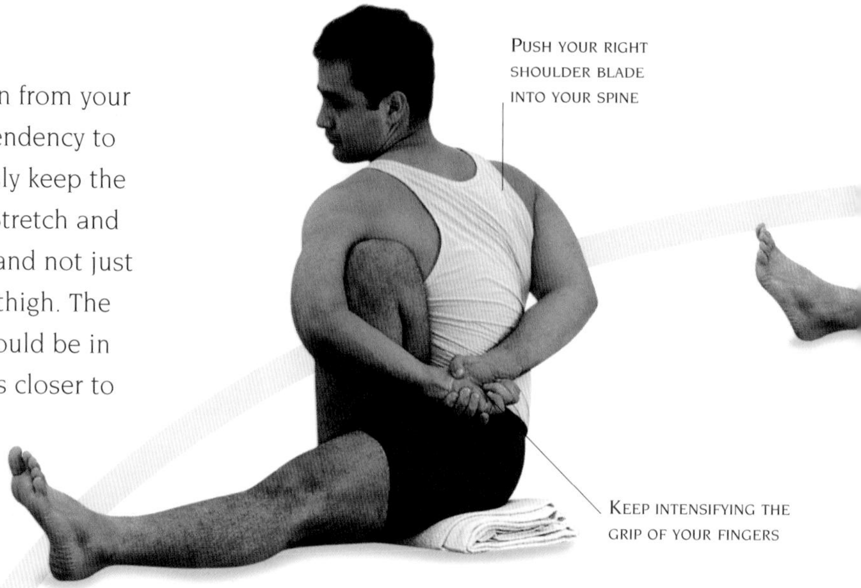

PUSH YOUR RIGHT
SHOULDER BLADE
INTO YOUR SPINE

KEEP INTENSIFYING THE
GRIP OF YOUR FINGERS

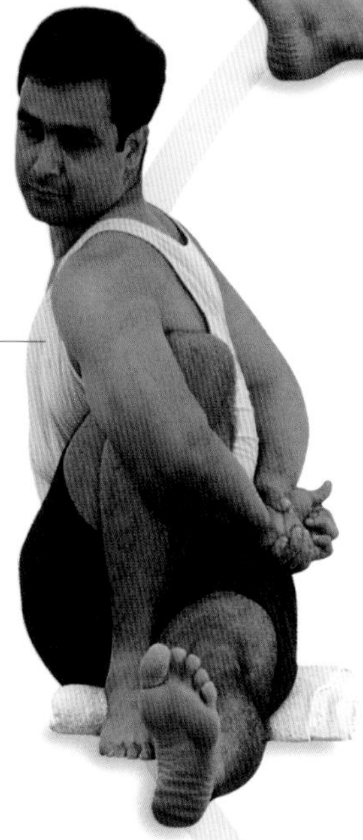

MOVE YOUR WHOLE
BODY CLOSER TO
THE BENT KNEE

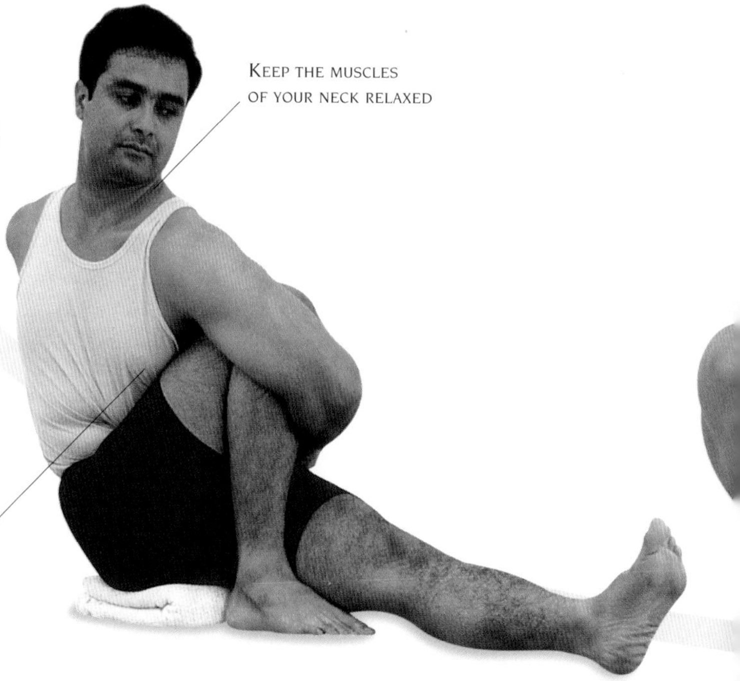

KEEP THE MUSCLES
OF YOUR NECK RELAXED

YOUR CHEST SHOULD
TOUCH THE LENGTH OF
YOUR RIGHT THIGH

COMING OUT OF THE POSTURE

◆

Inhale and holding your breath, rotate your spine to straighten it. Turn your head to face front. Release your hands and straighten your leg. Repeat the posture on the other side. Return to Dandasana.

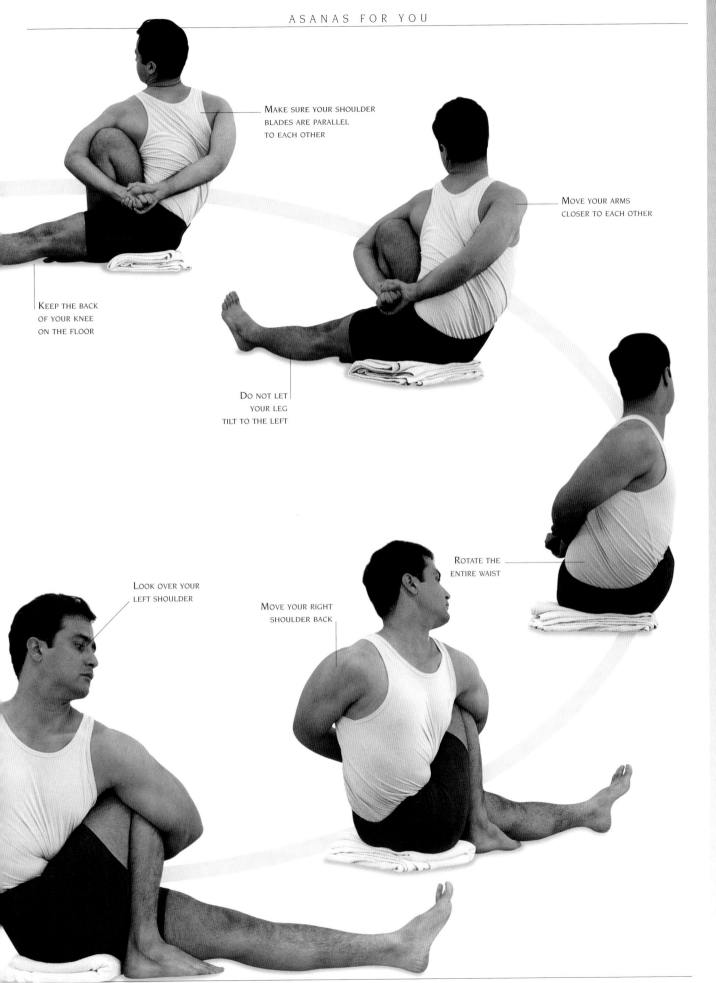

MAKE SURE YOUR SHOULDER
BLADES ARE PARALLEL
TO EACH OTHER

MOVE YOUR ARMS
CLOSER TO EACH OTHER

KEEP THE BACK
OF YOUR KNEE
ON THE FLOOR

DO NOT LET
YOUR LEG
TILT TO THE LEFT

ROTATE THE
ENTIRE WAIST

LOOK OVER YOUR
LEFT SHOULDER

MOVE YOUR RIGHT
SHOULDER BACK

Inversions

"The practice of asanas purges the body of its impurities, bringing strength, firmness, calm, and clarity of mind."

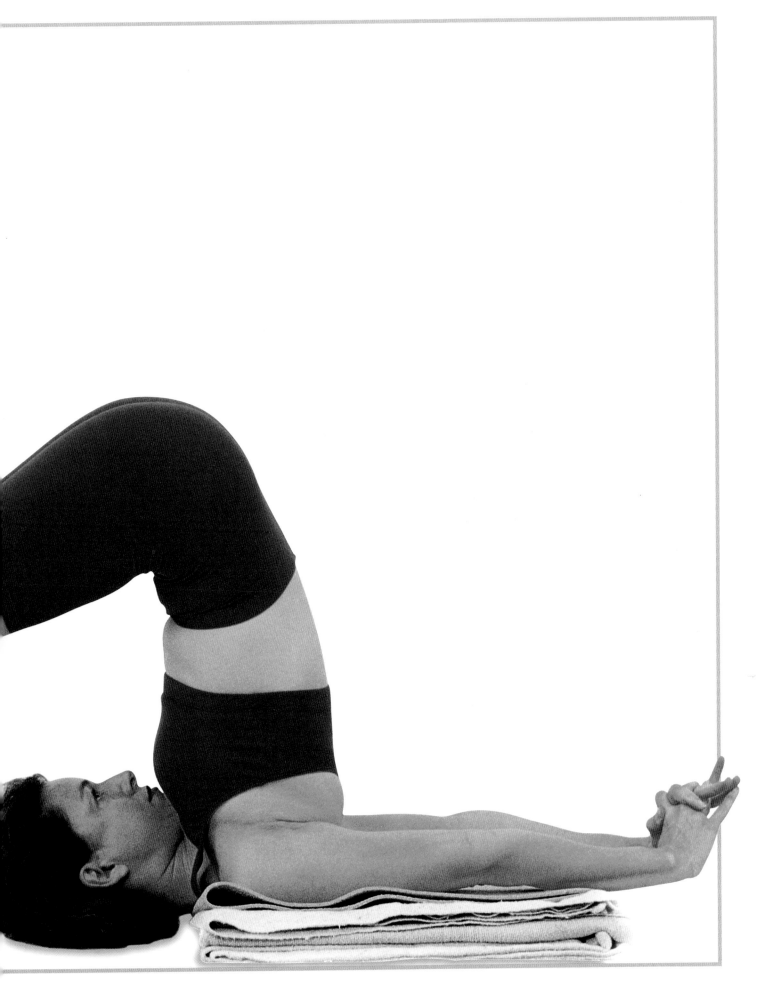

सालंब शीर्षासन
Salamba Sirsasana

- Headstand -

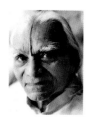

THE HEADSTAND IS ONE of the most important yogic asanas. The inversion in the final posture brings a rejuvenating supply of blood to the brain cells. Regular practice of this asana widens your spiritual horizons. It enhances clarity of thought, increases your concentration span, and sharpens memory. This asana helps those who get mentally exhausted easily. In Sanskrit, *sirsa* translates as "head," and *salamba* means "supported."

CAUTIONS
◆

Do not practice this asana if you have high blood pressure, cervical spondylosis, a cardiac condition, a backache, headache, or migraine. Do not start your yoga session with this posture if you have low blood pressure. Perform the asana only once in a session and do not repeat it if you fall. Your body should not be overworked. Do not practice this asana during menstruation.

KEEP YOUR SHOULDERS
PARALLEL TO EACH OTHER

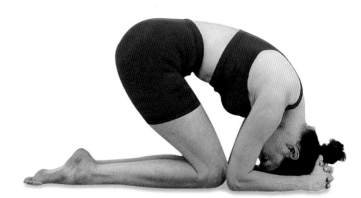

1 Kneel on the floor in Virasana (*see page* 84). Clasp the inside of your left elbow with your right hand and the inside of your right elbow with your left hand. Now lean forward and place your elbows on the floor. Ensure that the distance between your elbows is not wider than the breadth of the shoulders. Release your hands and interlock your fingers to form a cup with your hands (*see inset*). Keep your fingers firmly locked, but not rigid. Place your joined hands on the floor.

2 Place the crown of your head on the floor, so that the back of the head touches your cupped palms. Check that only the crown is resting on the floor, not the forehead or the back of the head. In the final posture, your weight must rest exactly on the center, not the back or front. Otherwise, the pressure will fall on your neck or eyes, causing your spine to bend. Make sure that your little fingers touch the back of the head, but are not underneath it. Hold this position for a few seconds breathing evenly.

KEEP YOUR THIGHS,
KNEES, AND HEELS
TOGETHER

ENSURE THAT YOUR ELBOWS
ARE PRESSED DOWN
ON THE FLOOR

3 Push up on the balls of your feet and straighten your knees. Keep your heels raised off the floor. To ensure that your torso is perpendicular to the floor, walk your feet toward your head, until the back of your body forms a vertical line from your head to the back of the waist.

4 Exhale and bring your knees toward the chest. Then press your toes down onto the floor, and push your legs up off the floor. This action resembles a hop and gives you the thrust to raise your legs. Bring your heels close to your buttocks.

BEGINNERS Practice this asana against a wall (*see box below*).

SALAMBA SIRSASANA AGAINST A WALL

BEGINNERS Practice against a corner where two walls meet at a right angle until you gain the confidence to practice without support. Place a folded blanket against the corner. Then follow Steps 1-3 (*see left and above*). Ensure that your cupped hands are placed not more than 2-3in (5-8cm) from the corner. If not, your weight will fall on your elbows, causing your spine to bend and your eyes to protrude. Follow Steps 4, 5, and 6 shown here. Initially, ask someone to help you raise your legs off the floor. To come out of the posture, follow the instructions on page 122 or reverse Steps 4-6.

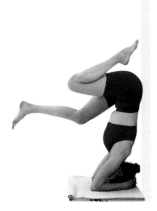

4 *Once your torso is positioned perpendicular to the floor, rest your hips against the corner. Now bend your left knee and raise your left foot off the floor. Then swing it up and rest the foot on the corner, above your left buttock. Repeat with the right leg.*

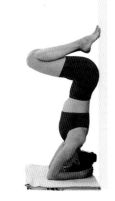

5 *In this position, your hips and the balls of your feet rest against the corner. Adjust your body in the posture. Press your elbows to the floor and stretch your upper arms. Follow the stretch through the armpits and along the torso to the waist.*

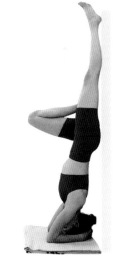

6 *Straighten your legs one by one until your hips, legs, and heels rest against the corner. With practice, bring your hips away from the wall and let your head, arms, and torso bear your weight. Constant support of the wall will bend your spine.*

सालंब शीर्षासन

Salamba Sirsasana

KEEP YOUR HEELS
CLOSE TO THE BACKS
OF YOUR THIGHS

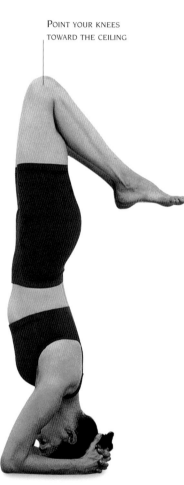

EXTEND YOUR TOES

POINT YOUR KNEES
TOWARD THE CEILING

5 Press your elbows to the floor and lift your shoulders up, away from the floor (*see inset*). Exhale, and gently swing your knees up in a smooth

arc, until both your thighs are parallel to the floor. In this position the entire upper body, from the head to the waist and hips, should be perpendicular to the floor. Do not move your elbows until you come out of the final posture.

6 Continue to move the knees up, slowly bringing them to point toward the ceiling. Keep the heels close to the buttocks. Focus on your balance and do not allow your torso to move during this action. Steps 5, 6, and 7 constitute a gentle and continuous movement, as you raise your legs toward the ceiling.

7 Once your knees are pointing to the ceiling, hold the posture for a few breaths. Make sure that the spine is straight. Ensure that your thighs are positioned perpendicular to the floor and your lower legs bent toward your back. Your shoulders should not tilt. Pause and get used to the feel of the position.

8 Straighten your knees to bring the lower legs in line with the thighs so that your body forms a vertical line. Point your toes toward the ceiling. Tighten both knees as in Tadasana (*see page* 48) and keep your thighs, knees, and toes together. The entire body should be balanced on the crown, not on the forearms and hands, which should simply support the balance in the posture. Stretch your upper arms, torso, and waist up, along the legs to the toes, ensuring that your torso does not tilt. Steadiness and a constant lift of the shoulders ensure stability in the posture. Hold the posture for 5 minutes breathing evenly.

STRETCH THE BACKS OF YOUR KNEES AND THIGHS

TIGHTEN THE QUADRICEP MUSCLES

EXPAND YOUR CHEST

BENEFITS
◆

Builds stamina

◆

Alleviates insomnia

◆

Reduces the occurrence of heart palpitations

◆

Helps to cure halitosis

◆

Strengthens the lungs

◆

Improves the function of the pituitary and pineal glands

◆

Increases the hemoglobin content in the blood

◆

Relieves the symptoms of colds, coughs, and tonsillitis

◆

Brings relief from digestive and eliminatory problems, when practiced in conjunction with Salamba Sarvangasana

CORRECTING YOURSELF

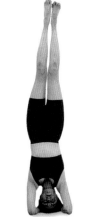

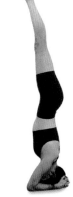

You may find that your legs lose alignment with the torso either by wavering to the right or left. Check the position of your elbows and tighten your knees.

If you do not stretch the dorsal area and chest your legs will swing forward and your buttocks jut back. When this happens, your weight falls on your elbows, not your head.

सालंब शीर्षासन

Salamba Sirsasana

ADVANCED WORK IN THE POSTURE

As you hold the posture stretch your whole body from the upper arms to the toes. Lift and widen the sternum expanding your chest equally on all sides. Tighten your knees and bring your legs to the median plane. This will ensure that they are perpendicular to the floor. Pull the abdominal muscles in and toward the waist to extend the lower spine. You must practice this asana from the spine, not the brain. Balance is the key to this asana, not strength. You must develop the skill to balance effortlessly on the small surface area of the crown. This brings a feeling of lightness to the brain and complete relaxation to each part of the body.

EXTEND THE BACKS OF THE KNEES AND STRETCH YOUR SHINS

STRETCH THE BICEPS AND DELTOIDS UP

LENGTHEN THE SPINE FROM THE NECK TO THE TAILBONE

ELONGATE THE INNER SIDES OF YOUR LEGS

COMING OUT OF THE POSTURE
◆

Keep your legs straight and close together. Lower them until your toes rest on the floor. Bend the knees, kneel, and sit on your calves. Rest your forehead on the floor. Stay in this position for a few seconds before sitting up in Virasana.

RELAX THE FINGERS BUT KEEP THEM FIRMLY LOCKED

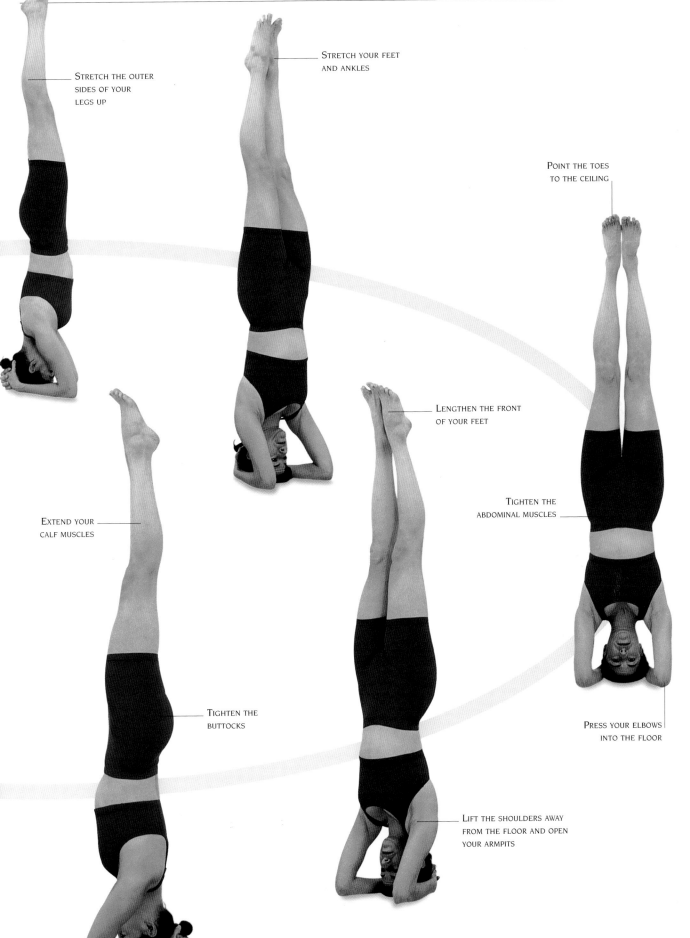

STRETCH THE OUTER SIDES OF YOUR LEGS UP

STRETCH YOUR FEET AND ANKLES

POINT THE TOES TO THE CEILING

EXTEND YOUR CALF MUSCLES

LENGTHEN THE FRONT OF YOUR FEET

TIGHTEN THE ABDOMINAL MUSCLES

TIGHTEN THE BUTTOCKS

LIFT THE SHOULDERS AWAY FROM THE FLOOR AND OPEN YOUR ARMPITS

PRESS YOUR ELBOWS INTO THE FLOOR

सालंब सर्वांगासन

Salamba Sarvangasana

- Shoulderstand -

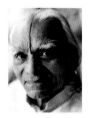

PRACTICING THIS ASANA integrates your mind with your body and soul. Your brain feels bright yet calm, your body feels light and infused with radiance. The inverted posture allows fresh, healthy blood to circulate around your neck and chest. This alleviates bronchial disorders and stimulates the thyroid and parathyroid glands. *Salamba* means "propped up" in Sanskrit, while *sarvanga* indicates "all the limbs" of the body.

CAUTIONS

◆

Do not practice this posture if you have diarrhea, or during menstruation. People with high blood pressure should only attempt this asana immediately after holding the final posture of Halasana (*see page* 130) for at least 3 minutes.

LIFT YOUR STERNUM

KEEP YOUR TOES, HEELS, AND ANKLES TOGETHER

REST ON THE BACK OF YOUR HEAD

1 Place a mat on 3 folded blankets, (*see page* 167) one on top of the other, on the floor. Lie down with your neck, shoulders, and back on the blankets. Rest your head on the floor. Stretch your legs and tighten your knees. Push the inner sides of your legs toward your heels. Press the outer sides of

your shoulders down on the blankets. Raise your upper spine, but push your lower spine down on the blankets. Stretch your arms out close to your body, palms facing the ceiling. Make sure that your wrists touch your body. Raise and expand your sternum without moving your head.

2 Roll your shoulders back and pull in your shoulder blades. Turn your upper arms out slightly and stretch the inner sides of your arms toward the little fingers of each hand. Exhale and bend your knees.

RELAX THE MUSCLES OF YOUR FACE

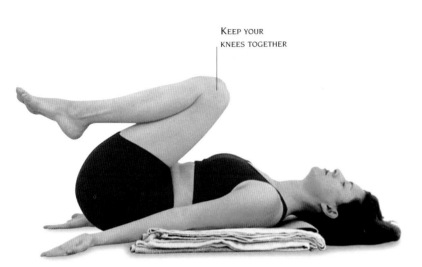

KEEP YOUR
KNEES TOGETHER

BENEFITS

◆

Alleviates hypertension

◆

Relieves insomnia and soothes
the nerves

◆

Improves the functioning of the thyroid
and parathyroid glands

◆

Alleviates asthma, bronchitis,
and throat ailments

◆

Relieves breathlessness and palpitations

◆

Helps to treat colds and sinus blockages

◆

Improves bowel movements
and relieves colitis

◆

Helps to treat hemorrhoids

◆

Alleviates urinary disorders

◆

Helps to treat hernia

◆

Helps to treat a prolapsed uterus and
reduces uterine fibroids

◆

Relieves congestion and heaviness in the
ovaries and helps to treat ovarian cysts

◆

Reduces menstrual cramps and helps
to regulate menstrual flow

3 Without moving the upper part of your body, exhale and raise your hips and buttocks off the floor. Bring your knees over your chest.

BEGINNERS If you find it difficult at first to raise your hips off the floor, ask a helper to hold your ankles and push your bent legs toward your head. At the same time, lift your hips and back off the floor and come to the final posture. Keep your body firm, and rest your back against your helper's knees. Alternatively, once you have been helped to raise your legs off the floor, follow Steps 5, 6, and 7 on the next page.

TIGHTEN YOUR
BUTTOCKS

KEEP YOUR SHINS
PRESSED TOGETHER

4 Place your palms on your hips and keep your elbows pressed firmly down on the blankets. Lift your torso until your buttocks are perpendicular to the floor. Bring your knees toward your head.

सालंब सर्वांगासन

Salamba Sarvangasana

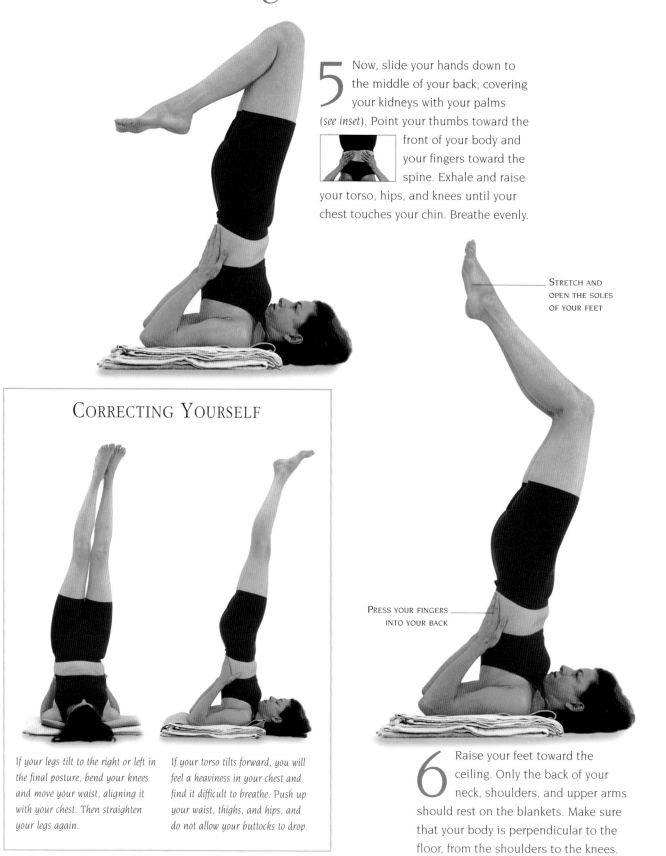

5 Now, slide your hands down to the middle of your back, covering your kidneys with your palms (*see inset*). Point your thumbs toward the front of your body and your fingers toward the spine. Exhale and raise your torso, hips, and knees until your chest touches your chin. Breathe evenly.

STRETCH AND
OPEN THE SOLES
OF YOUR FEET

CORRECTING YOURSELF

If your legs tilt to the right or left in the final posture, bend your knees and move your waist, aligning it with your chest. Then straighten your legs again.

If your torso tilts forward, you will feel a heaviness in your chest and find it difficult to breathe. Push up your waist, thighs, and hips, and do not allow your buttocks to drop.

PRESS YOUR FINGERS
INTO YOUR BACK

6 Raise your feet toward the ceiling. Only the back of your neck, shoulders, and upper arms should rest on the blankets. Make sure that your body is perpendicular to the floor, from the shoulders to the knees.

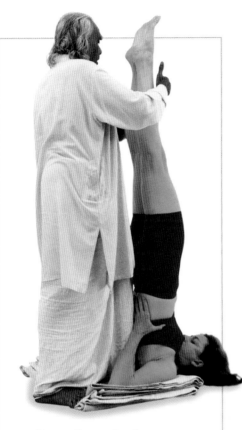

THE GURU'S ADVICE

"Do not throw the legs back, but raise them slowly. Turn the inner calves outward and extend the skin of the outer legs up toward the heels."

7 Press both palms into your back and straighten and stretch your body from the armpits to the toes. Your spine must be absolutely straight. Keep both elbows close to your body, since this keeps your chest expanded. To raise your torso further, release your palms, then press them into your back again. This will push your chest up further. Lift your body from the back of your neck, not your throat. Push both shoulders back to relax and stretch your neck. Extend your inner and outer legs toward the ceiling. Do not allow your legs to waver back and forth. Hold the posture for 2-3 minutes. Continue to breathe evenly.

STRETCH YOUR LEGS
FROM YOUR GROIN
TO YOUR TOES

PULL UP YOUR
PELVIC RIM

KEEP YOUR PALMS
CLOSE TO YOUR
SHOULDER BLADES

KEEP YOUR EYES
ON YOUR CHEST

REST YOUR ELBOWS
SQUARELY ON THE BLANKETS

सालंब सर्वांगासन

Salamba Sarvangasana

ADVANCED WORK IN THE POSTURE

Create life in your spine. The energy in your spine should flow into your body through your fingers. Keep your eyes on your sternum since this reinforces your will power and steadies your mind. Press your thumbs into the muscles of your back to push them toward the spine. This compresses the back. In the asana your back should be narrow and your chest broad. Do not allow your elbows to spread out. Bring them together since too wide a distance between them makes your chest concave. Keep the bridge of your nose aligned with the middle of your sternum. Move your shoulders back. Focus on your inner legs and stretch them toward the ceiling. This is a subtle and difficult action, but can be achieved over time. With practice, increase the duration of the posture to 5 minutes. Breathe evenly.

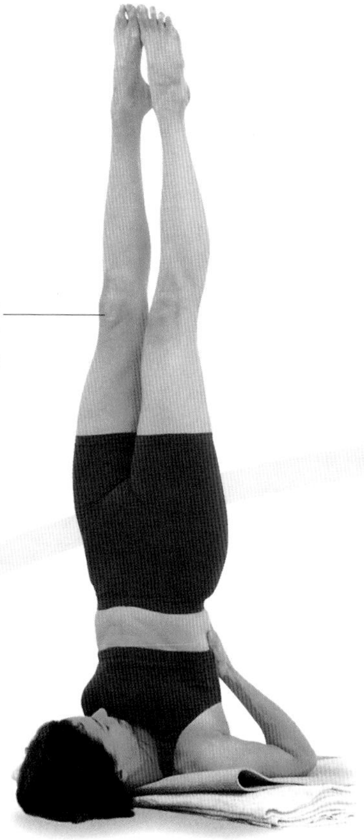

CONTRACT YOUR KNEECAPS EVENLY FROM ALL SIDES

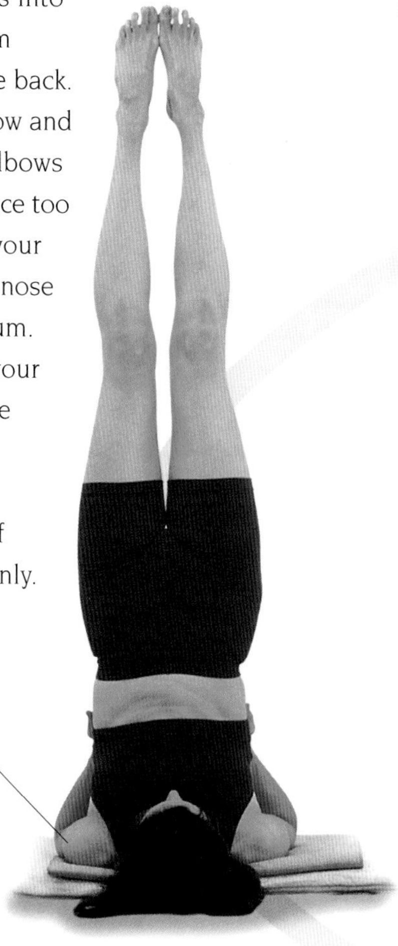

KEEP YOUR SHOULDERS BACK, AWAY FROM YOUR HEAD

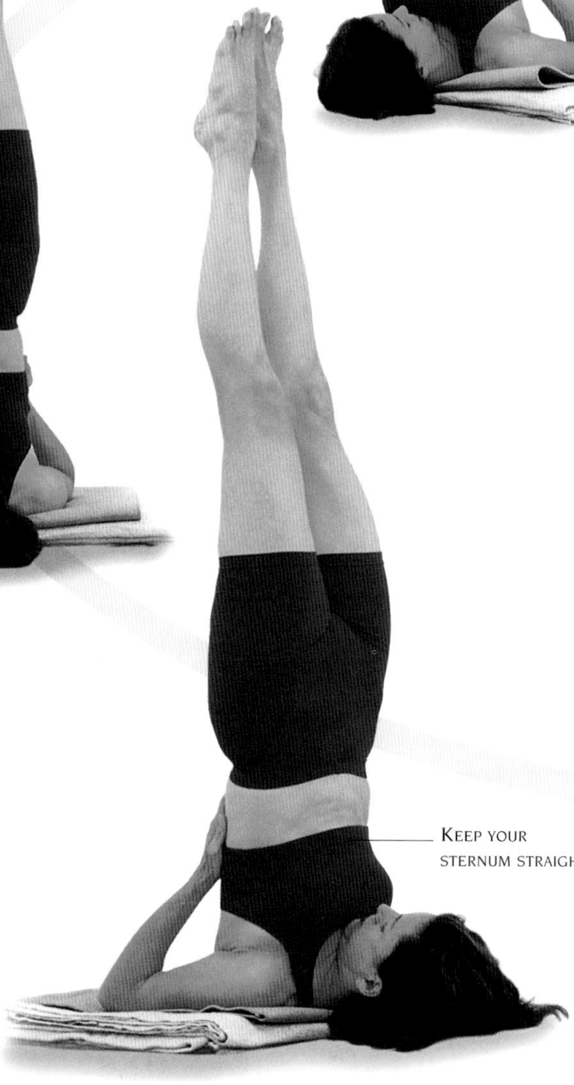

KEEP YOUR STERNUM STRAIGHT

COMING OUT OF THE POSTURE
◆

Exhale and bend your legs at the knees. Bring your thighs toward the stomach, then gently lower your buttocks and back toward the floor. Release the hands and bring them to your sides. Lie on the floor and relax your whole body.

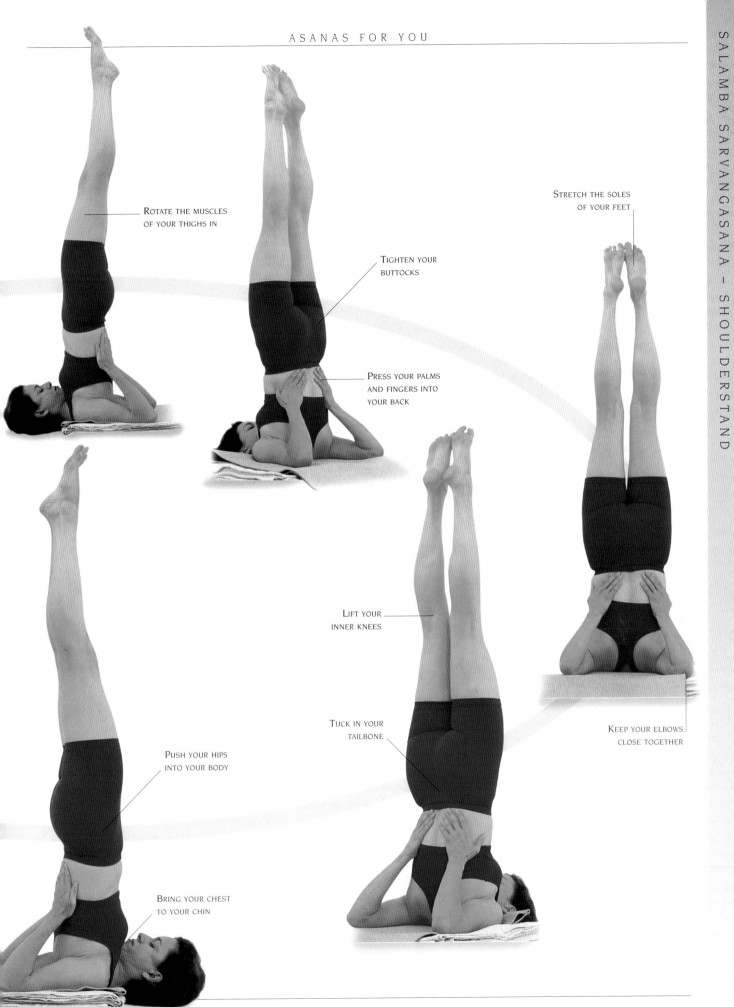

ROTATE THE MUSCLES
OF YOUR THIGHS IN

TIGHTEN YOUR
BUTTOCKS

PRESS YOUR PALMS
AND FINGERS INTO
YOUR BACK

STRETCH THE SOLES
OF YOUR FEET

LIFT YOUR
INNER KNEES

PUSH YOUR HIPS
INTO YOUR BODY

TUCK IN YOUR
TAILBONE

KEEP YOUR ELBOWS
CLOSE TOGETHER

BRING YOUR CHEST
TO YOUR CHIN

हलासन
Halasana

- Plough posture -

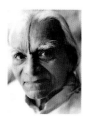

IN THIS ASANA, your body takes the shape of a plough. *Hala* is the Sanskrit word for "plough." Practicing Halasana regularly helps to increase your self-confidence and energy. The asana helps to restore calm and clarity of mind after a long illness. Halasana alleviates the effects of stress and strain by resting and relaxing your eyes and brain.

CAUTIONS
◆

Do not practice this asana if you have ischemia, cervical spondylosis, or diarrhea. Avoid this posture during menstruation. If you are prone to headaches, migraine, asthma, breathing difficulties, high blood pressure, physical and mental fatigue, or are overweight, practice Halasana with props (*see page* 214) and with your eyes closed.

REST YOUR HEAD ON THE FLOOR

1 Place 2 folded blankets, covered by a mat (*see page* 167), on the floor. Lie down with your back, neck, and shoulders resting on the blankets. Keep your legs stretched out and tightened at the knees. Focus on your inner legs and stretch from your thighs to your heels. Place your arms by your sides with your palms flat on the floor.

EXTEND THE ARCHES OF YOUR FEET UP

3 Raise your hips and buttocks toward the ceiling in a smooth, rolling action. Bring your knees close to your chin and raise your lower legs until your shins are perpendicular to the floor.

BEGINNERS Once you have raised your buttocks off the floor, ask a helper to hold your ankles and push your legs toward your head.

KEEP YOUR KNEES TOGETHER

2 Exhale, lift your buttocks off the floor, and bring your knees to your chest. Keep your arms straight and press your fingers firmly down onto the floor. Push your shoulders back and broaden your chest.

INTERLOCK YOUR FINGERS FIRMLY

STRAIGHTEN AND STRETCH YOUR ARMS

BENEFITS

◆

Relieves fatigue and boosts energy levels

◆

Controls hypertension

◆

Rejuvenates the abdominal organs and improves digestion

◆

Lengthens the spine and improves its alignment

◆

Helps to treat hernia and hemorrhoids if practiced with legs separated

◆

Relieves pain or cramps in the fingers, hands, wrists, elbows, and shoulders if practiced with arms and interlocked fingers extended toward the legs

4 Bend your elbows. Place your hands on the small of your back (*see inset*). Raise your hips and buttocks even further, until your torso is perpendicular to the floor and your thighs are positioned above your face. Bring your bent knees over your forehead before you lower your legs to the floor. Breathe evenly.

KEEP YOUR FEET, KNEES, AND THIGHS TOGETHER

RELAX YOUR FACIAL SKIN AND MUSCLES

5 Swing your hips and buttocks over your head until they are perpendicular to the floor and in line with your shoulders. Slowly straighten your legs and lower them until your toes rest onto the floor. Raise your chest, bringing your sternum to touch your chin. Stretch your arms out behind your back on the blankets. Then interlock your fingers firmly at the knuckles, rotating your wrists until your hands point toward the ceiling. Stay in the posture for 1-5 minutes. Breathe evenly.

BEGINNERS Initially, stretch your arms out toward your feet. Once you are comfortable in this posture, stretch your arms out behind your back.

TIGHTEN YOUR BUTTOCKS

OPEN BOTH SIDES OF THE CHEST

DO NOT BEND YOUR KNEES

PRESS YOUR TOES DOWN ONTO THE FLOOR

हलासन

Halasana

ADVANCED WORK IN THE POSTURE

When you hold this posture make sure that your brain is not tense. Consciously relax the skin and muscles of your face. Keep your gaze on your chest and do not look up. Drop your eyes down in their sockets since this helps relax the facial muscles. Your neck should be completely soft since this rests the brain. Remember that your throat is the site of the *Vishuddhi chakra* (*see page* 37). If it tightens, your brain will become tense. Lift your sternum and chest to relax your throat and ensure smooth and effortless breathing. Increase the space between your navel and diaphragm.

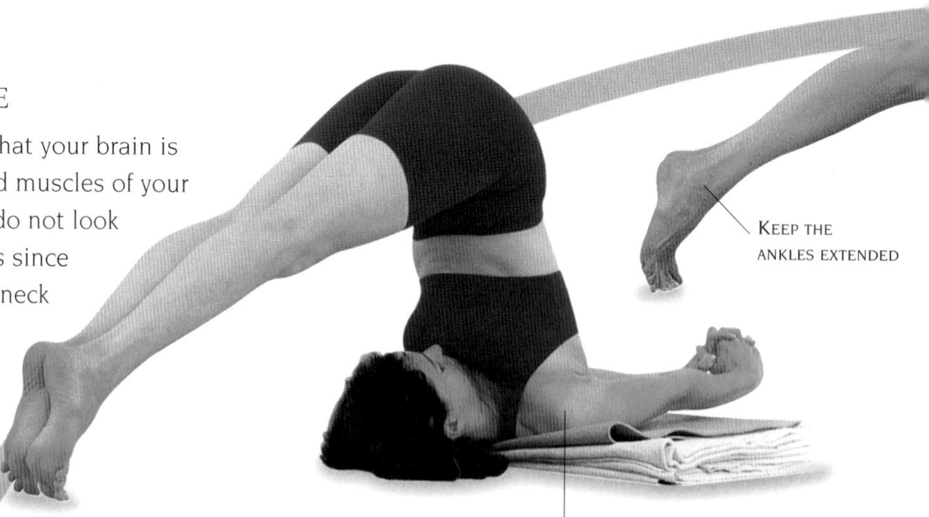

KEEP THE ANKLES EXTENDED

PUSH YOUR SHOULDERS INTO YOUR BODY

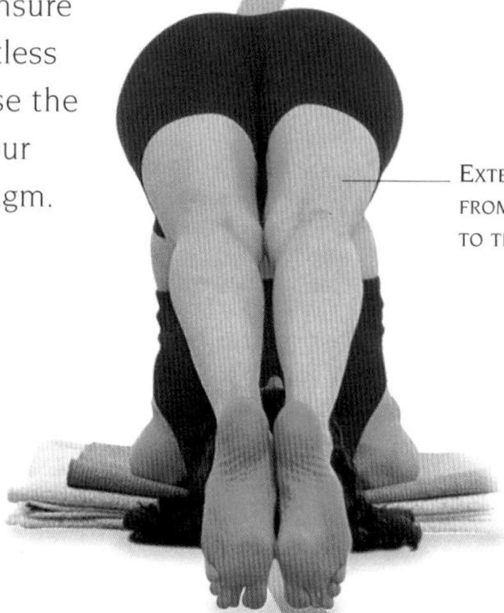

EXTEND YOUR LEGS FROM THE BUTTOCKS TO THE HEELS

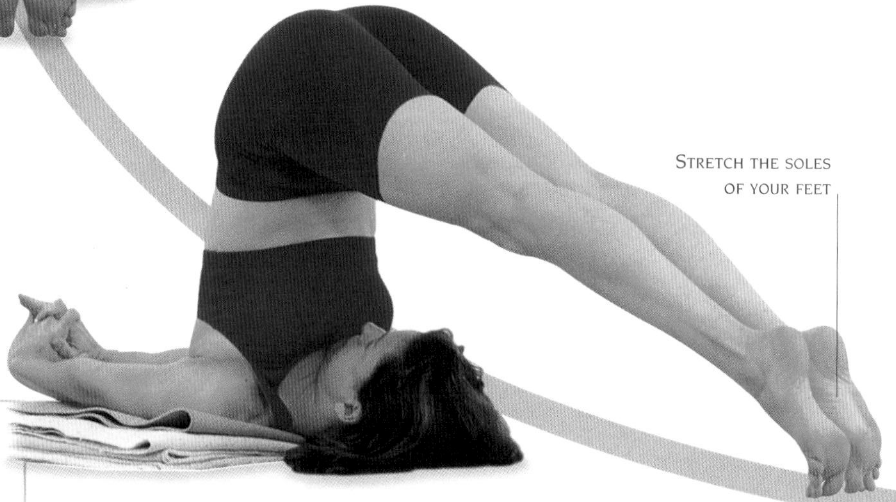

STRETCH THE SOLES OF YOUR FEET

COMING OUT OF THE POSTURE

◆

Slowly and with control lift your legs off the floor. Bring your thighs and knees toward your stomach. Push your buttocks back and lower them to the floor. Flatten your back and relax your entire body, breathing deeply.

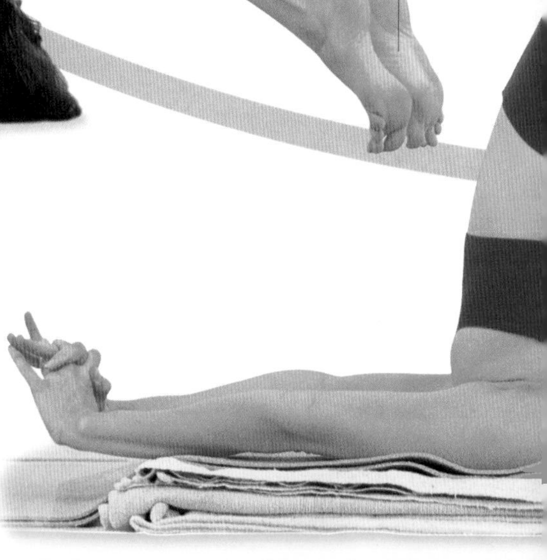

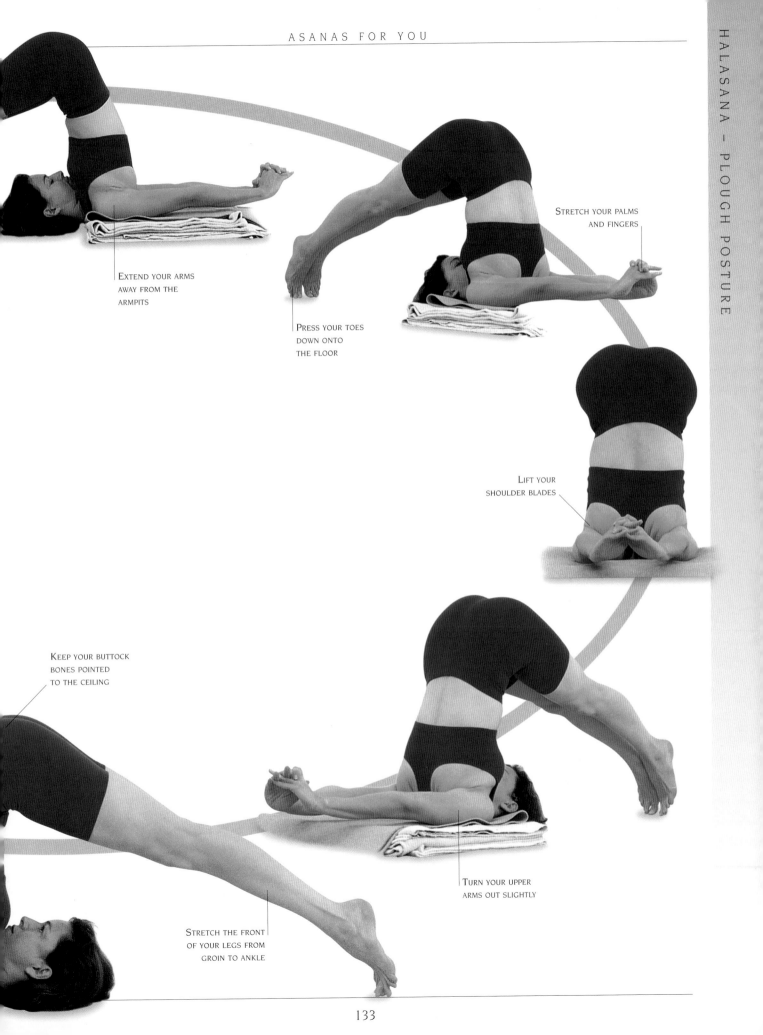

EXTEND YOUR ARMS
AWAY FROM THE
ARMPITS

STRETCH YOUR PALMS
AND FINGERS

PRESS YOUR TOES
DOWN ONTO
THE FLOOR

LIFT YOUR
SHOULDER BLADES

KEEP YOUR BUTTOCK
BONES POINTED
TO THE CEILING

TURN YOUR UPPER
ARMS OUT SLIGHTLY

STRETCH THE FRONT
OF YOUR LEGS FROM
GROIN TO ANKLE

Back Bends

"Asanas penetrate deep into each layer of the body and ultimately into the consciousness itself."

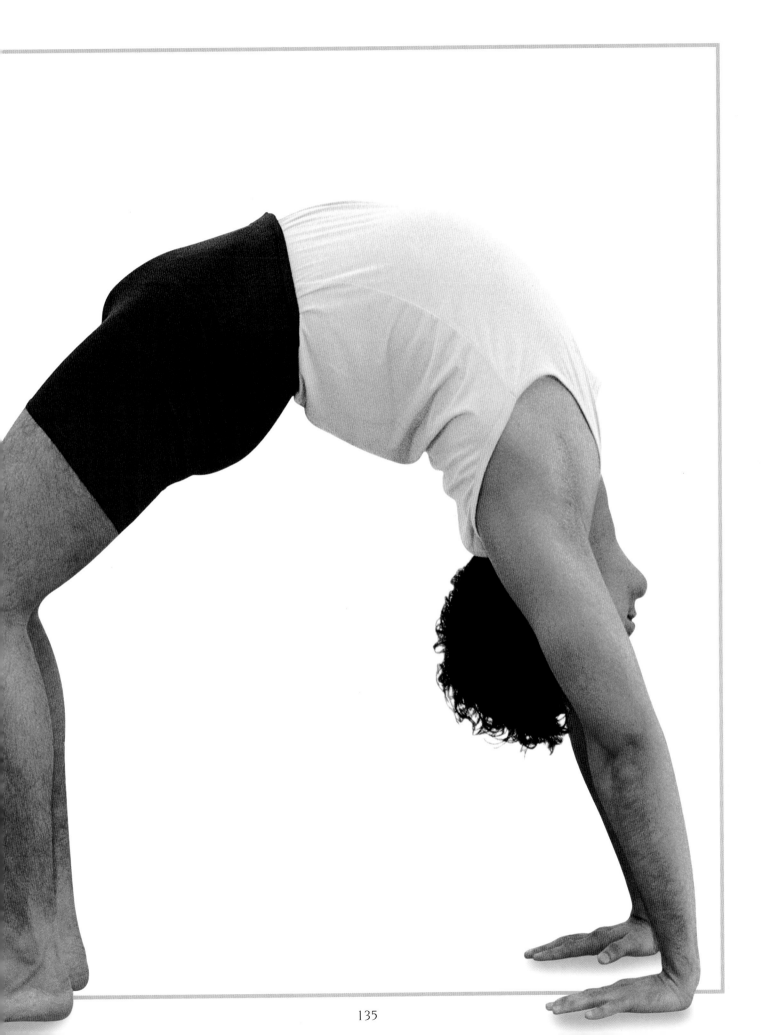

उष्ट्रासन

Ustrasana

- Camel posture -

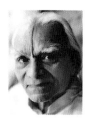

IN THIS ASANA, you bend back until the shape of your body resembles that of a camel. *Ustra* means "camel" in Sanskrit. Ustrasana is recommended for beginners as well as for the elderly because the balance of the final posture is relatively easy to attain. The asana also helps people in sedentary occupations whose work entails bending forward for long periods. Practicing the asana will relieve stiffness in the back, shoulders, and ankles.

CAUTIONS

◆

Do not practice this asana if you have severe constipation, diarrhea, headaches, migraine, or hypertension. If you are recovering from a heart attack, practice Ustrasana with props (*see page 222*).

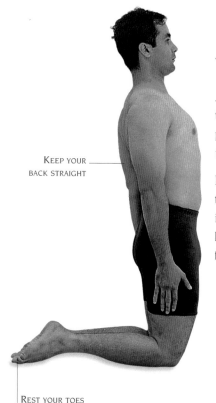

KEEP YOUR
BACK STRAIGHT

REST YOUR TOES
ON THE FLOOR

1 Kneel on the floor with your arms by your sides. Keep your thighs, knees, and feet together. Rest on the front of your feet, with the toes pointing to the back. Keep your torso upright and breathe evenly.

BEGINNERS If keeping your knees together leads to a feeling of strain in your thighs, practice with your knees slightly apart. This also allows for a freer movement of the spine.

KEEP YOUR
EYES OPEN

DO NOT TENSE
YOUR ARMS

2 Exhale and place your palms on your buttocks. Push your thighs forward slightly and then pull them up toward your groin. Push your spine into your body. Then gradually bend your back and lower it toward the floor. Simultaneously, extend your ribcage and broaden your chest. Continue to breathe evenly.

BENEFITS

◆

Helps to correct posture

◆

Increases lung capacity

◆

*Improves blood circulation
to all the organs of the body*

◆

*Tones the muscles of the back
and spine*

◆

*Removes stiffness in the shoulders,
back, and ankles*

◆

Relieves abdominal cramps

◆

Regulates menstrual flow

3 Push your shoulders back and stretch your arms from your shoulders toward your feet. Inhale, throw your head back, and hold both heels with your hands. Make sure that your thighs are perpendicular to the floor. Push your spine down toward your legs and breathe evenly.

BEGINNERS Initially hold one heel at a time by tilting each shoulder individually.

EXPAND YOUR CHEST

4 Push your feet down onto the floor. At the same time, press down on your soles with your palms. Your fingers should point toward your toes (*see inset*). Tighten your buttocks and tailbone. Push your shoulder blades back. Take your head as far back as possible, but take care not to strain your throat. Stay in the posture for 30 seconds.

LIFT YOUR STERNUM

DO NOT TILT YOUR
HEAD TOO FAR BACK

PULL YOUR
SPINE INTO
YOUR BODY

SLIDE YOUR HANDS OVER
THE HEELS TO COVER
YOUR SOLES FULLY

KEEP YOUR QUADRICEP
MUSCLES STRETCHED

उष्ट्रासन

Ustrasana

ADVANCED WORK IN THE POSTURE

Push your shins down on the floor and press your palms down onto your soles. Lift and stretch the length of your spine so that your body forms an arch. Your chest, armpits, and back should coil in since this will support the back of your chest. Consciously suck in your back ribs and feel your kidneys being drawn in and squeezed. Try to create a space between the dome of the diaphragm and the navel, and between the navel and the groin. By doing this, you will be extending your abdominal and pelvic organs as well as your intestines. Roll the inner sides of your upper arms to the front and the outer sides of your upper arms to the back. Keep your elbow joints locked. Breathe evenly.

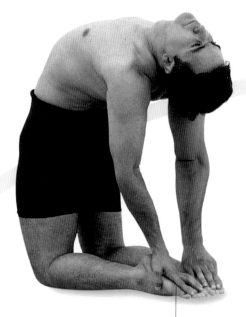

KEEP THE FRONT OF YOUR FEET ON THE FLOOR

LOCK YOUR ELBOWS

DO NOT STRAIN YOUR THROAT

EXTEND YOUR ARMS FROM YOUR SHOULDERS TO YOUR FEET

COMING OUT OF THE POSTURE

◆

Exhale and lessen the pressure of your palms on the feet. Raise your torso keeping your arms by your sides. The impetus for the upward movement should come from the thighs and chest. If you cannot raise both your arms together, lift them, one by one.

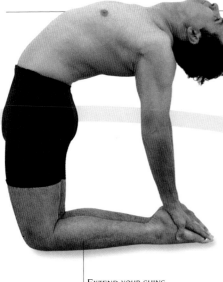

EXTEND YOUR SHINS

KEEP YOUR CHEST
RAISED AND EXPANDED

PUSH YOUR THIGHS
OUT AND UP

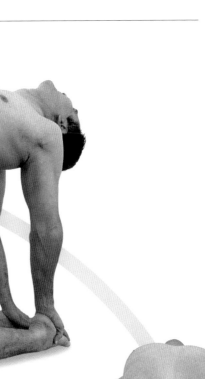

STRETCH THE
ABDOMINAL MUSCLES

CREATE SPACE BETWEEN
YOUR DIAPHRAGM
AND NAVEL

PUSH YOUR
COLLAR BONES BACK

ऊर्ध्व धनुरासन
Urdhva Dhanurasana

- Upward-facing bow posture -

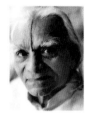

YOUR BODY ARCHES back to form an extended bow in this asana. *Urdhva* means "upward" in Sanskrit, while *dhanur* translates as "bow." Regular practice of Urdhva Dhanurasana keeps your body supple and creates a feeling of vitality and lightness. The asana stimulates the adrenal glands, strengthening your will power and increasing your capacity to bear stress.

CAUTIONS

◆

Do not practice this asana if your blood pressure is too high or too low. Avoid this posture if you have constipation or diarrhea, or when you are feeling tired. Do not practice during an attack of migraine or a severe headache. If you have a cardiac condition or ischemia, practice Viparita Dandasana (*see page* 220) instead of this posture.

PRESS YOUR THIGHS
AND CALVES TOGETHER

1 Lie on your back on the floor. Bend both knees and pull your heels to your buttocks. Spread your feet so that they align with your hips. Bend your elbows and bring them over your head. Place your palms on the floor on either side of your head. Your fingers should point toward your shoulders.

BEGINNERS At first, you may find it difficult to bring your heels close to your buttocks. Use your hands to pull the feet into position.

2 Focus on your palms and feet since you are going to use them to launch your posture. Push your shoulder blades back and pull the muscles of your back into your body. Exhale, then lift your torso and buttocks off the floor.

ENSURE THAT YOUR ELBOWS
ARE SHOULDER-WIDTH APART

KEEP YOUR SHOULDERS
ON THE FLOOR

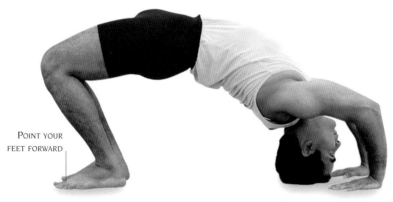

POINT YOUR
FEET FORWARD

3 Lift your chest and place the crown of your head on the floor. Take two breaths. Exhale sharply, and suck in your back and buttocks. Shift your weight from your palms to the front of your feet, and push up your torso in one single movement. Adjust your posture until your weight is equally distributed on your hands and feet.

BENEFITS

◆

Prevents the arteries of the heart from thickening and ensures healthy blood circulation throughout the body

◆

Tones the spine

◆

Strengthens the abdominal and pelvic organs

◆

Stimulates the pituitary, pineal, and thyroid glands

◆

Prevents prolapse of the uterus

◆

Helps to prevent excess menstrual flow and eases menstrual cramps

THE GURU'S ADVICE

"Do not merely push your chest forward, as this alone will not prevent the arch of the torso from collapsing. Look at how I am lifting the sides of my student's lower ribcage. You must lift both sides of your chest up toward the ceiling."

4 Push your body further up. Press both palms and soles down onto the floor and lift your head off the floor. Exhale, then pull your spine into your body. Straighten your arms and lock your elbows, sucking in the outer arms at the elbows. Now take your head back without straining your throat. Hold the posture for 5-10 seconds.

INTERMEDIATES For a more effective stretch, exhale, pull the muscles of your thighs up, and lift your heels off the floor (*see inset*). Extend your chest and push up your lower spine until your abdomen is as taut as a drum. Maintain the height of your body and stretch all your joints. Then bring your heels back onto the floor.

DO NOT TAKE YOUR HEAD TOO FAR BACK

SPREAD YOUR FINGERS AND STRETCH YOUR PALMS

KEEP YOUR WRISTS FIRM AND STEADY

ऊर्ध्व धनुरासन

Urdhva Dhanurasana

ADVANCED WORK IN THE POSTURE

In the final posture your body stretches in two directions: one from the palms, and the other from the feet. The meeting point is at the base of the spine. Try to raise this point higher and higher. Open up the spaces between the ribs, especially at the bottom of your chest. Broaden your diaphragm. Suck in your shoulder blades and back ribs. Imagine you are squeezing your kidneys. Make sure your weight is evenly distributed on your hands and feet. Initially, hold the posture for 5-10 seconds breathing evenly. With practice, repeat the asana 3 to 5 times. This will bring greater freedom of movement to your body and improve the effectiveness of your stretch.

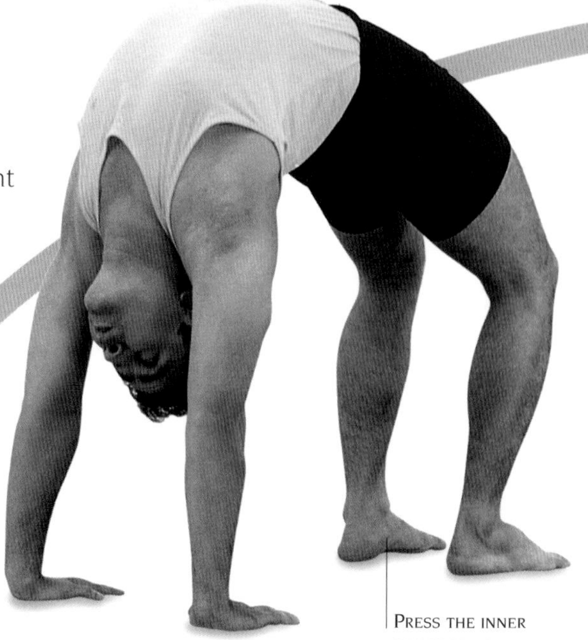

PRESS THE INNER EDGES OF YOUR FEET DOWN ONTO THE FLOOR

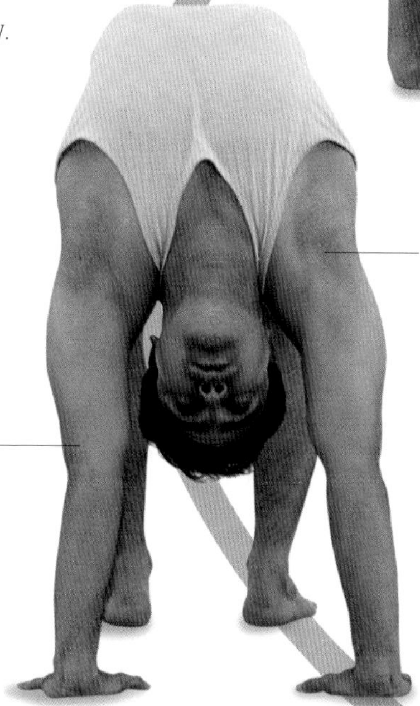

OPEN OUT YOUR ARMPITS

STRETCH YOUR ARMS FROM THE WRISTS TO THE ARMPITS

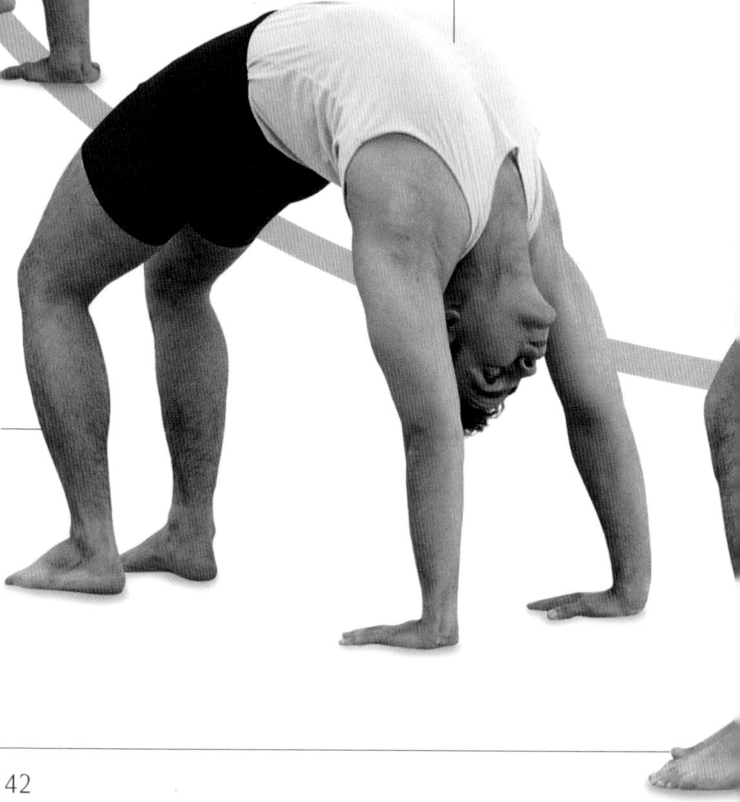

MOVE YOUR CHEST TOWARD YOUR HEAD

PULL YOUR SHINS UP TOWARD YOUR THIGHS

COMING OUT OF THE POSTURE

◆

Exhale and bend your elbows and knees. Lower your torso, then bring the crown of your head down to the floor. Lower your back and buttocks to the floor. Lie on your back and take a few breaths.

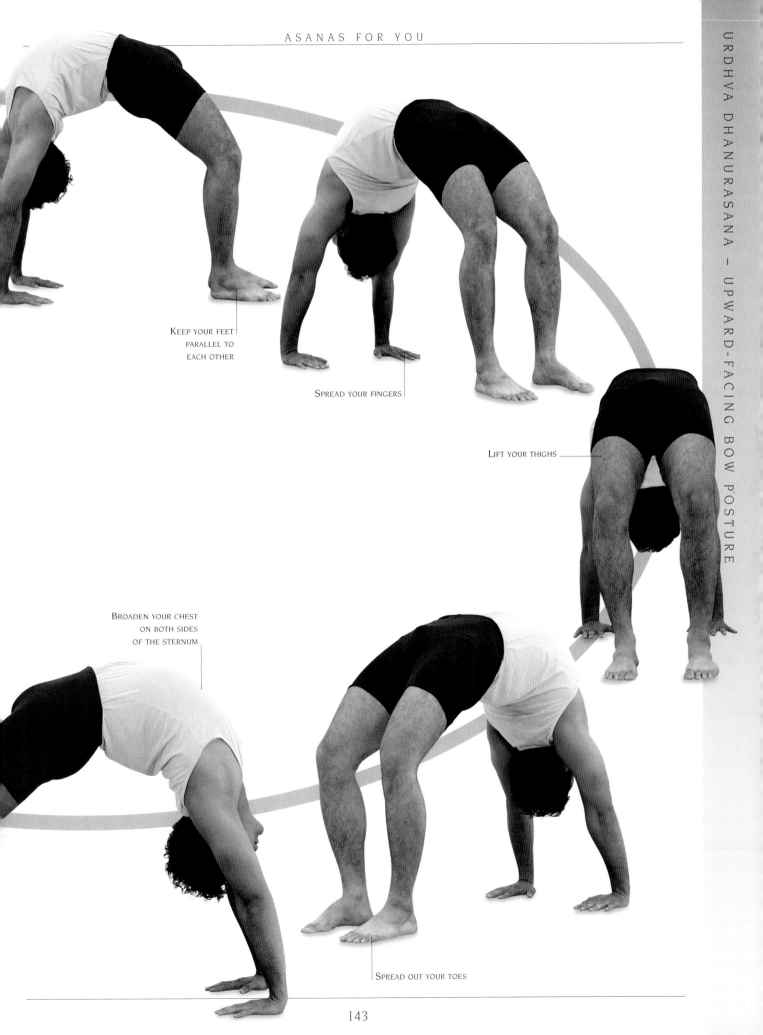

KEEP YOUR FEET
PARALLEL TO
EACH OTHER

SPREAD YOUR FINGERS

LIFT YOUR THIGHS

BROADEN YOUR CHEST
ON BOTH SIDES
OF THE STERNUM

SPREAD OUT YOUR TOES

Reclining Asanas

"Feel the inner mind touching your entire body – even the remotest parts where the mind does not normally reach."

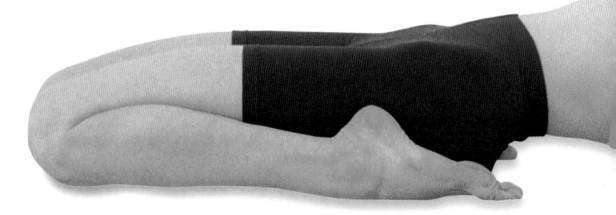

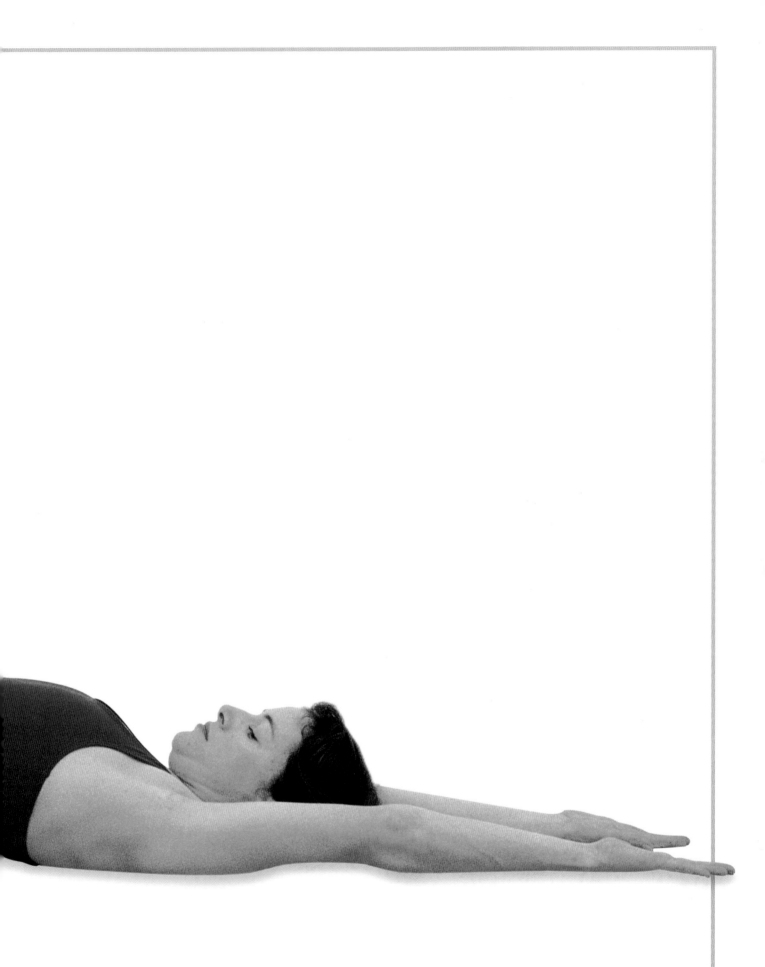

सुप्त वीरासन
Supta Virasana

- Reclining hero posture -

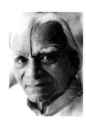

THIS IS A VARIATION OF the sitting posture, Virasana (*see page* 84). In this asana, you rest your torso on the floor. *Supta* means "lying down" in Sanskrit, while *vira* translates as "hero" or "champion." Athletes, and all those who are on their feet for long periods, will find this asana helpful since the legs receive an intense and invigorating stretch. If you practice this posture last thing at night, your legs will feel rested and rejuvenated in the morning.

CAUTIONS
◆

Do not practice this asana if you have a cardiac condition, lower backache, or osteoarthritis of the knees. Those with gout, arthritis of the ankles, or spinal disc disorders should practice with props (*see page* 228). Women should place a bolster under the back during menstruation (*see page* 228).

PUSH OUT YOUR ARMS SLIGHTLY

ENSURE THAT YOUR KNEES REMAIN TOGETHER

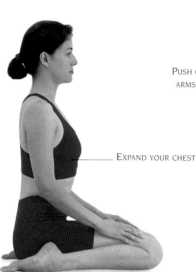

EXPAND YOUR CHEST

2 Hold your toes. Adjust your legs by slightly turning in your thighs and turning out your calves. Exhale and lower your back gradually toward the floor. Rest your elbows one by one onto the floor. Breathe evenly.

1 Sit in Virasana (*see page 84*). Keep both knees together and spread your feet about 18in (0.5m) apart until they rest beside your hips. To avoid strain, ensure that the inner side of each calf touches the outer side of each thigh. Turn your soles toward the ceiling. Each of your toes should rest on the floor. Stretch your ankles fully and extend the soles toward the toes. Let the energy flow in both directions through your feet.

KEEP YOUR THIGHS SLIGHTLY APART

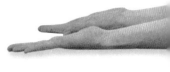

3 Place the crown of your head on the floor. Lower your shoulders and upper torso to rest your head, and then your back, onto the floor. Stretch your arms along your sides. Press your wrists against your soles.

BENEFITS

◆

Helps to reduce cardiac disorders

◆

Stretches the abdomen, back, and waist

◆

Relieves rheumatism and pain in the upper and middle back

◆

Aids digestion after a heavy meal

◆

Soothes acidity and stomach ulcers

◆

Relieves the symptoms of asthma

◆

Reduces menstrual pain and helps treat disorders of the ovaries

THE GURU'S ADVICE

"Do not push your buttocks toward the spine, since this causes your lumbar spine to arch. Look at how I am pushing my student's waist and buttocks toward her knees. You must lengthen your buttock muscles and allow the lumbar spine to extend. Then rest the spine on the floor."

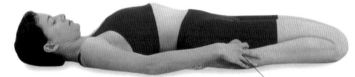

4 Move your elbows out to the sides and lie flat on the floor until the spine is fully extended. Bring your head down and spread your shoulders away from your neck. Rest your shoulder blades and knees on the floor.

PRESS YOUR HEELS DOWN WITH YOUR FINGERS

5 Take your arms over your head and stretch them out behind you on the floor with your palms facing the ceiling. Ensure that both shoulder blades remain flat on the floor and do not let your buttocks or knees lift off the floor. Release your back and allow it to descend completely to the floor. If your back arches, it causes stress to the lower back. Press your thighs together, taking care not to jerk your knees. Breathe evenly and stay in the posture for 30-60 seconds.

EXPAND YOUR CHEST EVENLY ON EITHER SIDE OF THE STERNUM

STRAIGHTEN YOUR ARMS AND KEEP THEM FLAT ON THE FLOOR

THE INNER SIDES OF YOUR FEET MUST TOUCH YOUR HIPS

सुप्त वीरासन

Supta Virasana

ADVANCED WORK IN THE POSTURE

In the final posture, the stretch of your arms pulls your thighs and abdomen toward your chest, massaging them in the process. Move both shoulder blades in and open your chest fully. Press your shoulders down ensuring that your knees and buttocks remain on the floor. The front and the back of your body should be evenly elongated and your armpits fully stretched. Push your pelvis toward the knees and press it down on the floor. Focus on your back ribs. Consciously extend them toward your head. Gradually, increase the time spent in the posture to 5-7 minutes.

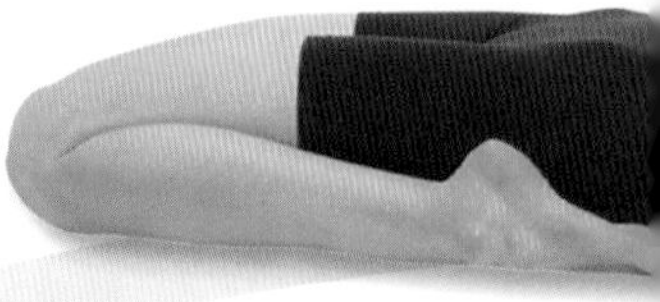

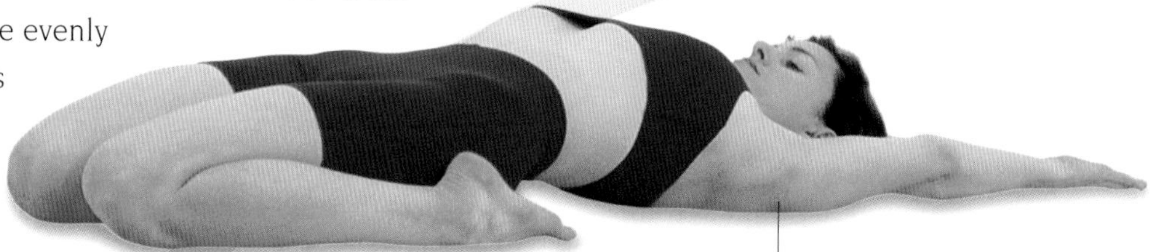

TUCK IN YOUR
SHOULDER BLADES

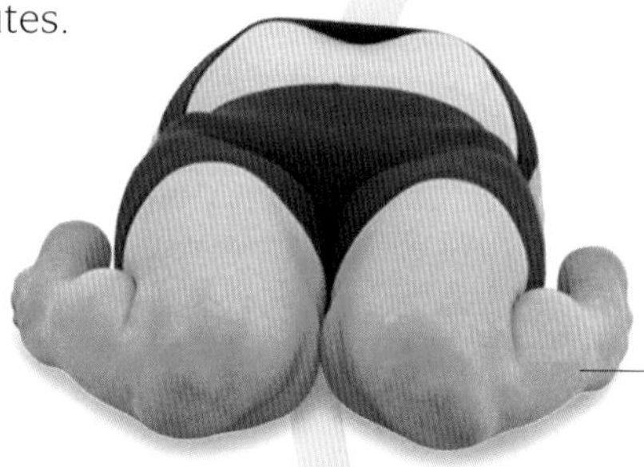

PRESS YOUR SHINS DOWN
ONTO THE FLOOR

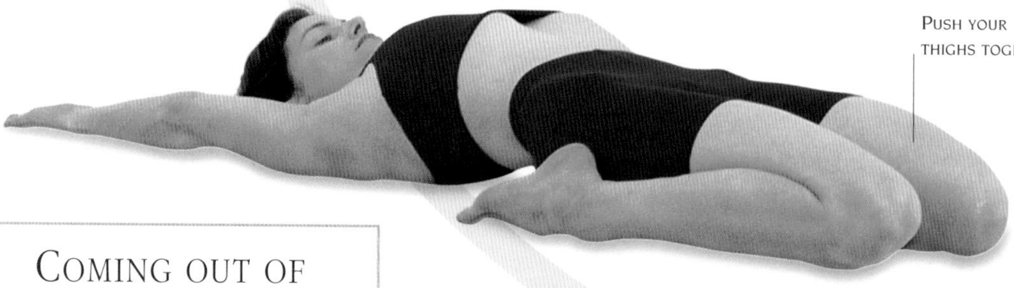

"When the
and still, what

PUSH YOUR
THIGHS TOGETHER

COMING OUT OF THE POSTURE
◆

Bring your hands over your head and hold your ankles. Lift your head and torso off the floor, supporting yourself on your elbows. Sit up in Virasana. Exhale and straighten your legs one at a time. Sit in Dandasana.

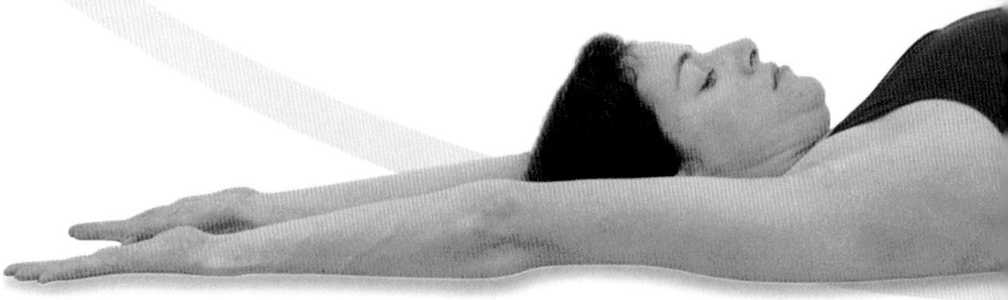

FIX YOUR GAZE ON
YOUR CHEST

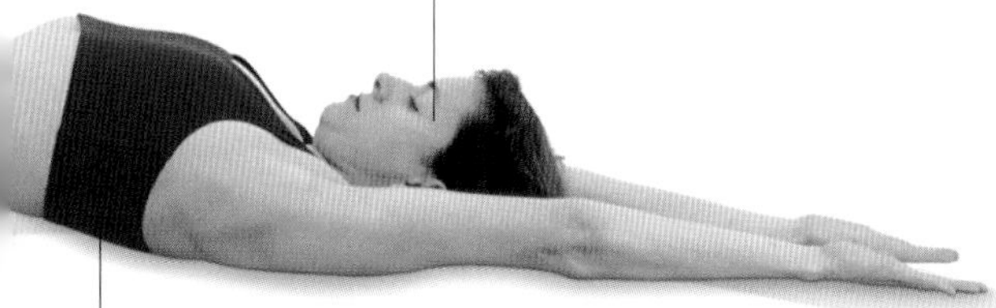

PUSH YOUR BACK TOWARD
YOUR HEAD – DO NOT
ALLOW IT TO ARCH

DO NOT ALLOW YOUR
ELBOWS TO TURN OUT

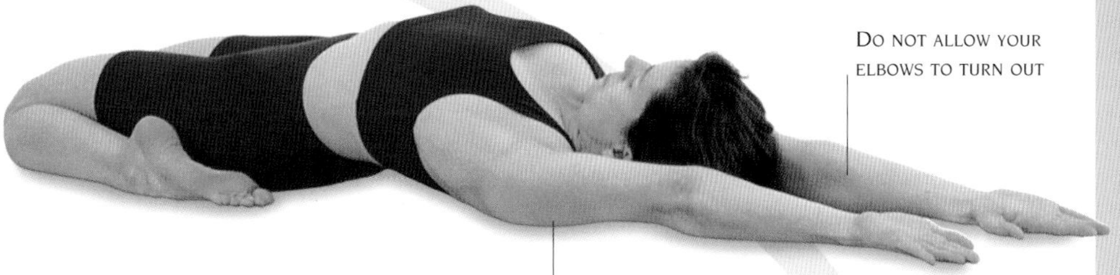

KEEP BOTH SHOULDERS IN
CONTACT WITH THE FLOOR

mind is controlled

remains is the soul."

MAKE SURE
YOUR CHEST
REMAINS EXPANDED

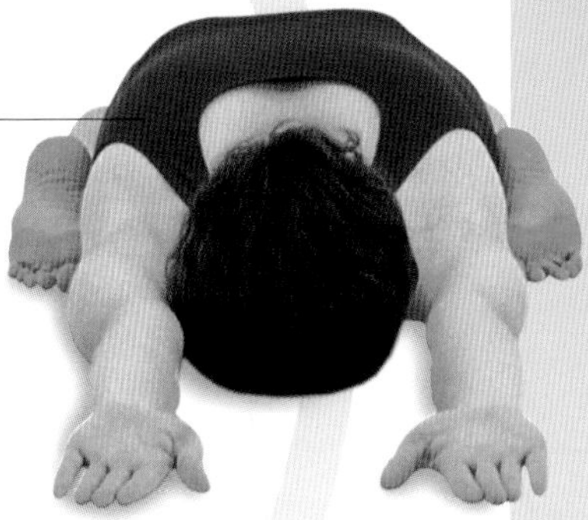

ENSURE THAT YOUR
PALMS ARE OPEN AND FLAT

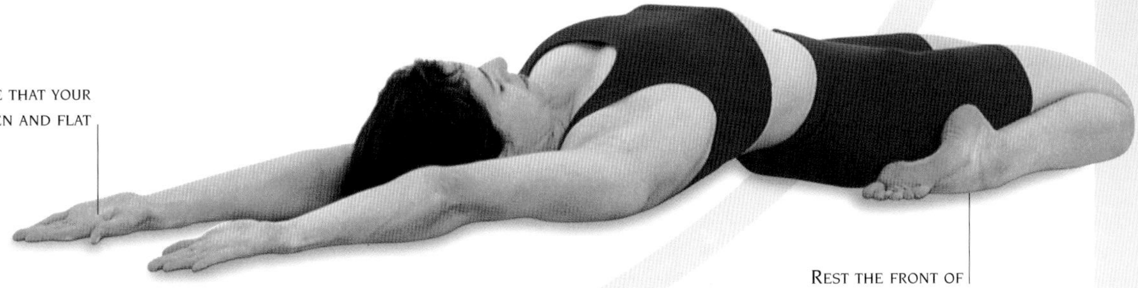

REST THE FRONT OF
YOUR FEET ON THE FLOOR

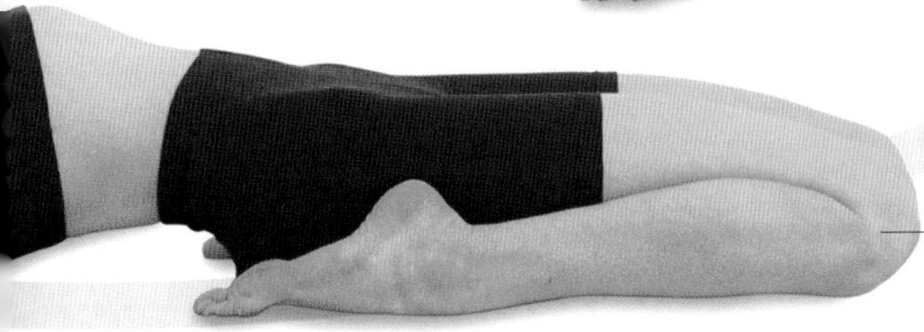

KEEP YOUR KNEES
PRESSED DOWN

शवासन

Savasana

- Corpse posture -

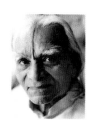

I N THIS ASANA, the body is kept as motionless as a corpse and the mind is alert, yet calm. The word *sava* means "corpse" in Sanskrit. Savasana removes fatigue and soothes the mind. Each part of the body is positioned properly to achieve total relaxation. When you practice this asana, your organs of perception, the eyes, ears, and tongue, withdraw from the outside world. The body and the mind become one, and you experience inner silence. This asana is the first step in the practice of meditation.

CAUTIONS
◆

If you are pregnant, have a respiratory ailment, or experience anxiety, practice Savasana with your head and chest raised on a bolster (*see page* 234). If you have a backache, lie with your back on the floor, and rest your calves on the seat of a chair, with your thighs perpendicular to the floor. Do not practice Savasana between other asanas.

PRESS THE BACKS OF YOUR KNEES TO THE FLOOR

SPREAD THE COLLAR BONES OUT TO THE SIDES

KEEP THE HEAD STRAIGHT – DO NOT TILT IT TO ONE SIDE

1 Sit in Dandasana (*see page* 82). Push the flesh of your buttocks out to the sides, distributing your weight equally on both buttock bones. Breathe evenly.

ENSURE THAT YOUR BACK IS STRAIGHT

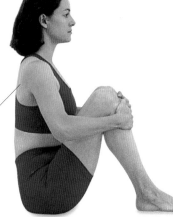

2 Bend your knees and bring your heels closer to the buttocks. Hold the tops of your shins and press your buttock bones down onto the floor. Check that your back is straight.

3 To lower your torso toward the floor, place your forearms and palms on the floor and lean back on your elbows. Do not move your feet, knees, or buttocks.

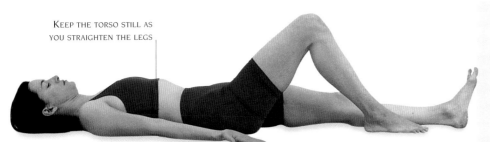

KEEP THE TORSO STILL AS
YOU STRAIGHTEN THE LEGS

BENEFITS

◆

*Helps to alleviate
nervous tension, migraine, insomnia,
and chronic fatigue syndrome*

◆

Relaxes the body and eases breathing

◆

*Soothes the nervous system and
brings peace of mind*

◆

*Enhances recovery from all long-term
or serious illnesses*

4 Lower your torso to the floor, vertebra by vertebra, until the back of your head rests on the floor. Turn your palms to face the ceiling. Close your eyes, then straighten your legs one by one.

INTERMEDIATES Stretch your torso away from your hips to straighten the spine. Extend the spine fully and keep it flat on the floor. Make sure that the stretch along the legs and the torso is equal on both sides of the body.

RELAX THE TOPS
OF YOUR THIGHS

TILT BOTH LEGS TO
THE SIDES EQUALLY

5 Relax your legs, allowing them to drop gently to the sides. Ensure that your kneecaps drop to the sides equally. Move your arms away from your torso without raising your shoulders off the floor. Push your collar bones out to the sides. Keep your eyes closed and focus on your breathing. Stay in this posture for 5-7 minutes.

INTERMEDIATES Visualize your spine. Rest the outer edge of your spine comfortably on the floor. Expand your chest out to the sides and relax your sternum. Focus on your diaphragm. It should be absolutely free of tension. As you push your collar bones out to the sides, allow your neck to dip to the floor. Relax the muscles of your neck.

RELAX THE FINGERS
AND THE CENTERS
OF THE PALMS

श्वासन

Savasana

ADVANCED WORK IN THE POSTURE

As your neck dips to the floor (*see Step 5, page* 151), you will feel a soothing sensation in the back of your brain. When this area of the brain relaxes, move onto the front of the brain. From the crown of the head, the energy should descend in a spiral action toward the bridge of the nose, and down to a point located at the sternum. When the energy reaches this point, the three layers and five sheaths that comprise your body (*see page* 24) come together and are integrated into a single, harmonious whole. This is the ultimate aim of Savasana.

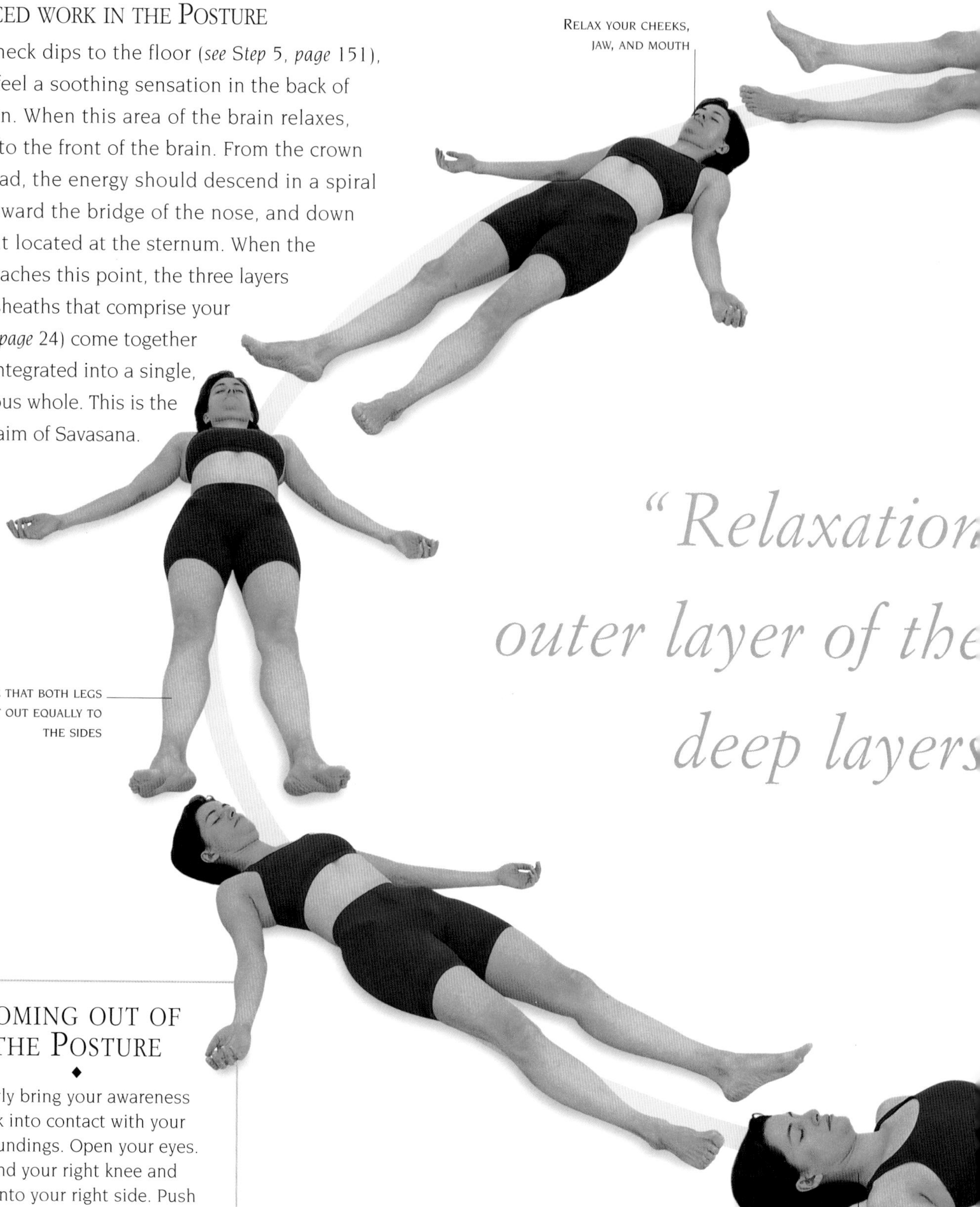

RELAX YOUR CHEEKS, JAW, AND MOUTH

"*Relaxation*

outer layer of the

deep layers

ENSURE THAT BOTH LEGS TILT OUT EQUALLY TO THE SIDES

COMING OUT OF THE POSTURE

◆

Slowly bring your awareness back into contact with your surroundings. Open your eyes. Bend your right knee and roll onto your right side. Push yourself up on your right arm and come to a cross-legged sitting position.

KEEP THE BACK OF THE NECK ON THE FLOOR

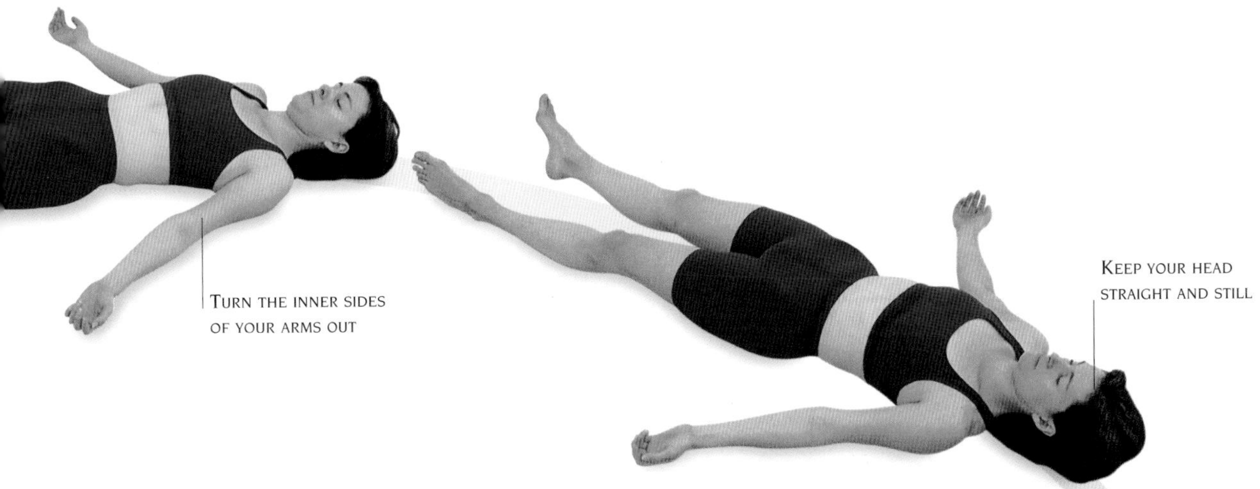

TURN THE INNER SIDES
OF YOUR ARMS OUT

KEEP YOUR HEAD
STRAIGHT AND STILL

begins from the body and penetrates the of our existence."

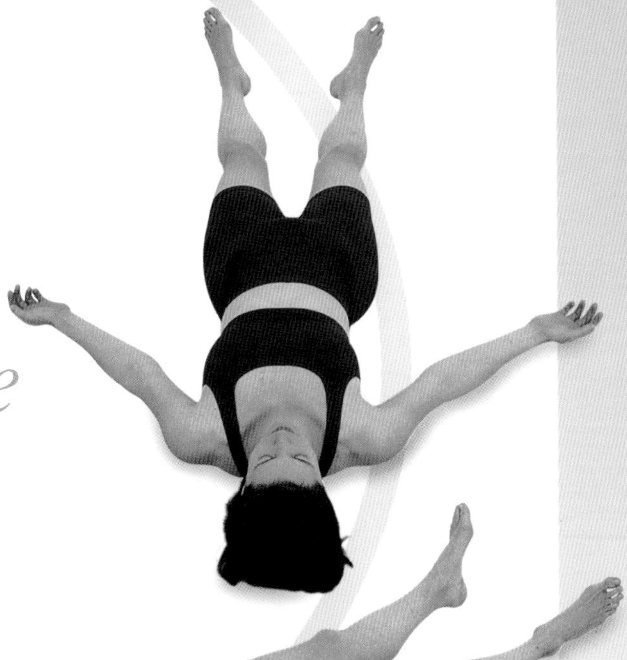

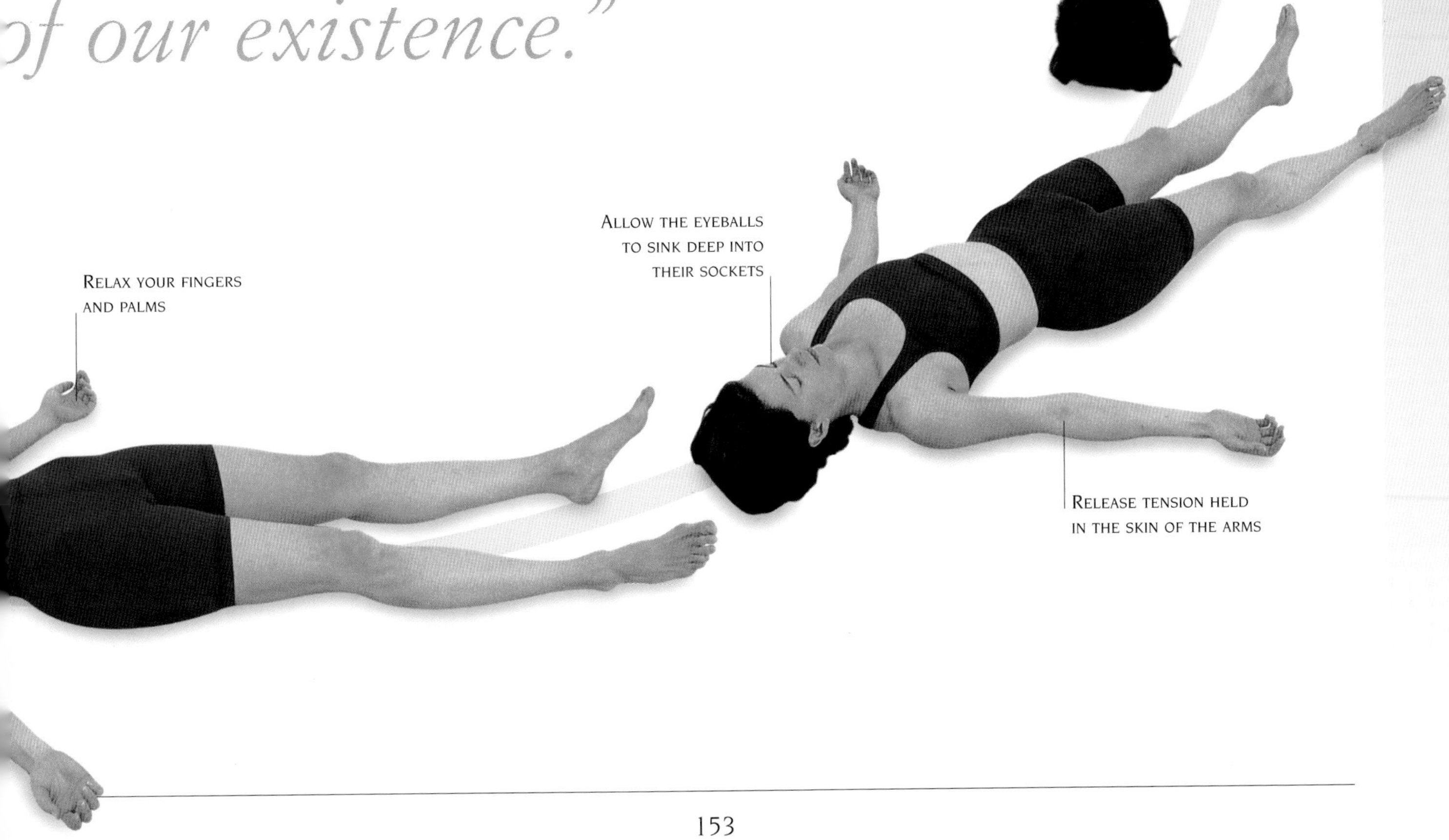

ALLOW THE EYEBALLS
TO SINK DEEP INTO
THEIR SOCKETS

RELAX YOUR FINGERS
AND PALMS

RELEASE TENSION HELD
IN THE SKIN OF THE ARMS

CHAPTER 4

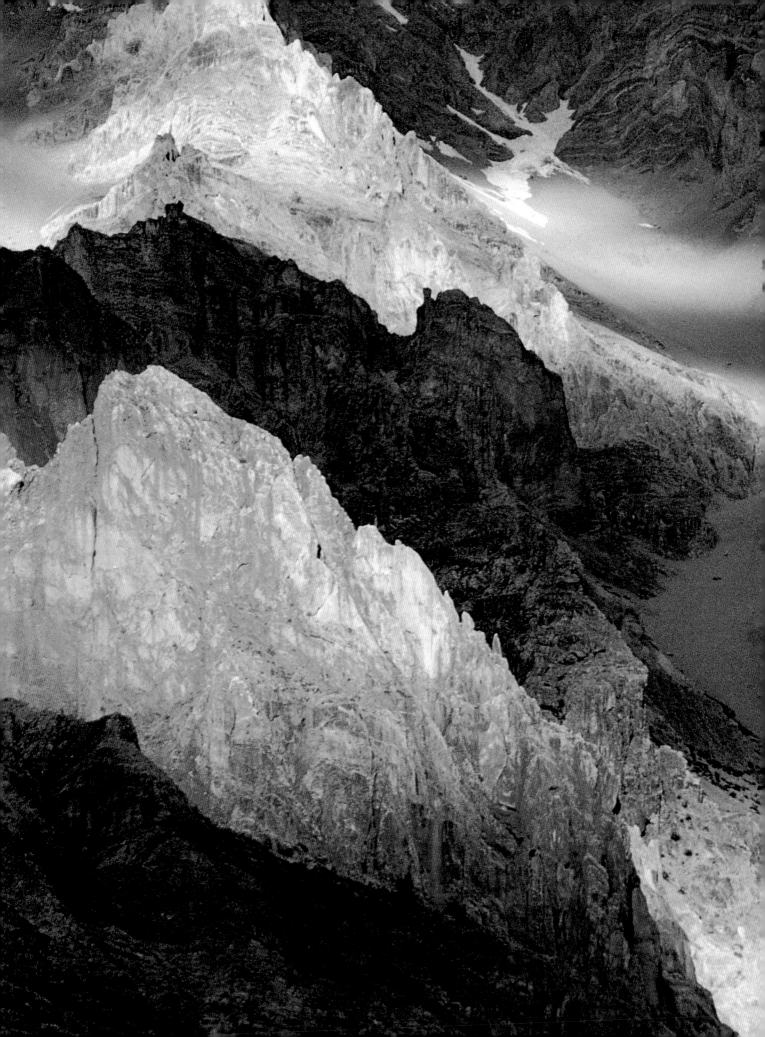

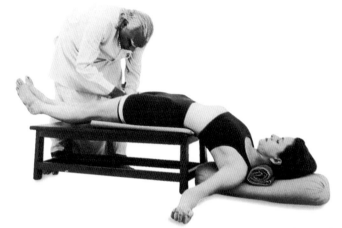

"An intellectual mind that is unconnected to the heart is an uncultivated mind."

Yoga for Stress

The practice of asanas and pranayama is not only the most effective, but also the most natural therapy for stress. Practiced together, they generate enormous amounts of energy in the body, stimulating the cells and relaxing tense muscles. The effect on the mind takes longer to register because yoga deals with the causes, and not just the symptoms of stress. With regular practice, the senses that divert the mind to the external environment are drawn inward, calming the restless mind. When your stress levels are high, it is sometimes hard to achieve the final posture effectively. In this case, practicing with the recommended props helps you to attain the benefits of the asanas in a relaxed manner.

Understanding Stress

Stress is as old as civilization itself. The ancient sages understood the impact on the mind and body of the turmoil of daily life. Yoga helps detach the mind from this turmoil and allows you to face the effects of stress with equilibrium.

We experience stress from the moment of birth, and spend our lives adjusting to it. Some of us manage better than others for a variety of reasons. It could be because of one's personality, environment, or one's physical condition. However, everyone has to deal with the effects of stress at some time, and in order to do so, he or she has to cultivate and discipline the mind, the physical body, psychological body, and spiritual body. We all evolve ways of coping with stress, checking and minimizing its effects with varying degrees of success. Yoga provides one of the most effective and comprehensive solutions to this problem.

Stress is not a modern phenomenon. It has always been with us. Our ancestors may not have had to deal with the same pressures that those of us who live in modern, technologically advanced cultures do, but even the ordinary events of daily life can cause inner turmoil. People have sought solutions for stress ever since civilization began.

Patanjali's understanding of stress led him to begin the *Yoga Sutras* with the phrase, "*Chittavritti niruddha.*" This translates as "controlling the thought waves or mental fluctuations which bring about stress." He goes on to describe how the path of yoga can help to cope with stressful situations.

THE CAUSES OF STRESS

All of us seek refuge in momentary and transient pleasures. Our desires, needs, or demands are ceaseless. We are often pulled in two opposite directions. On the one hand, our mind is attracted by the external world and our attention irresistibly drawn toward it. On the other, we yearn to look inward, to

STRESS IN DAILY LIFE
The external world exerts pressures that are hard to withstand

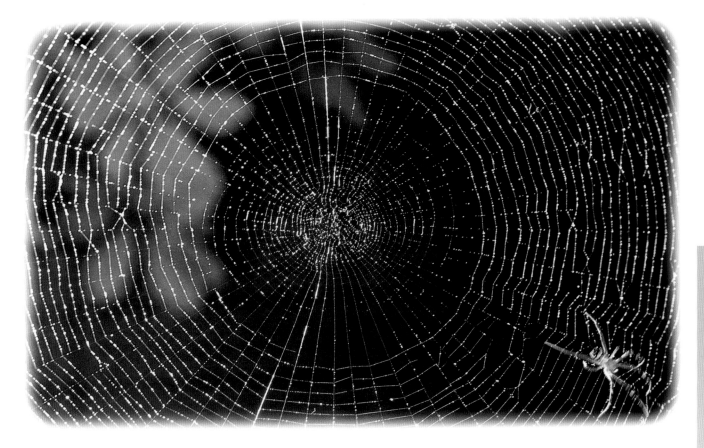

STRESS CONFUSES THE MIND
Our senses often betray us, trapping us in a web of avarice and discontent, from which it is difficult to escape

discover the core of our being and our inner self. This conflict entangles us in a web of desire, dissatisfaction, and anger, and manifests itself in feelings of anguish, exhaustion, and breathlessness.

CONTROLLING THE SENSES

The senses are directly controlled by the mind. Therefore, to control the senses, you must control the mind. By relaxing our senses and turning them inward, we can detach them from the mind. When a person is calm, his or her state of mind is meditative, and the senses are under control. At this point, external events cease to cause stress. It is only then that one can reflect on the emotional forces controlling one's life and analyse what should be discarded, and what should change. The practice of yoga harmonizes your body and mind. The steady rhythm of breath relaxes the body and detaches the mind from the worries of the external world. This healing effect can then be felt in your daily life when routine activities are performed efficiently and well.

A relaxed person possesses dynamic energy that does not dissipate. In this state of being, none of the common symptoms of stress, such as migraine, fatigue, or hypertension occur. Whatever the external environment may be, the mind remains cool and collected, and the body remains free from disease.

"We can rise above our limitations, only once we recognize them."

The Modern World

The technological and scientific advances of the modern world do not automatically bring happiness. If anything, modern life has led to greater levels of stress, since people are caught up in the pursuit of wealth, success, and worldly pleasures.

The information explosion has allowed access to more knowledge than ever before. Paradoxically, such scientific and technological advances have increased, rather than reduced stress levels. The pressures of financial security, the need for recognition and success, and the desire for worldly pleasures, all push us into a spiral of anxiety and haste. Inevitably, our spiritual life, peace of mind, and our health suffer.

If you are caught up in the maelstrom of constant challenge and competition, you lose your ability to perceive reality clearly. You may unknowingly twist the truth to suit your own personal goals and fail to recognize friendliness, honesty, and compassion, and instead see deceit, dishonesty, or pride.

An intellectual mind, if unconnected with the heart, is an uncultivated mind. The intelligence of the head must be controlled to allow the emotional center to awaken. It is only when the head and the heart are in harmony, that peace of mind, stability, and happiness can be achieved.

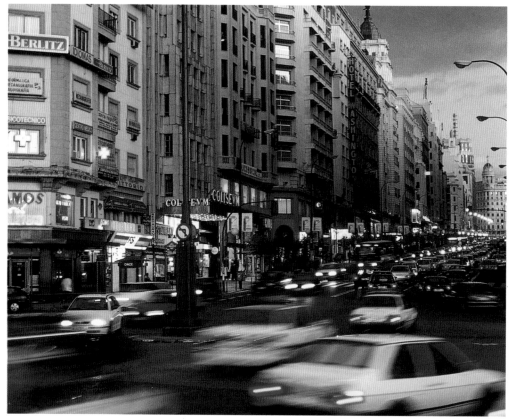

IN FRANTIC HASTE
The speed of modern life causes stress

Egoism and pride cause an individual to lose contact with his or her emotional center. In order to achieve a fully integrated personality, you must develop emotionally as well as intellectually. Only then will you be able to control the stresses and strains which knock you off balance from time to time. As long as your heart and your mind remain separate, stress will manifest itself physically and emotionally through contracted body muscles, tense facial expressions, and undesirable behavioral patterns.

Food & Nourishment

The food we eat and the surroundings we inhabit must be conducive to stress-free living. If we increase our intake of fruit and vegetables, and nourish our senses with calming scents, sounds, and sights, we will be on the way to a healthier lifestyle.

The *Upanishads*, ancient Indian scriptures compiled between 300 and 400 BC, divide food into 16 categories. Ten parts are classified as wastage, 5 parts affect the energy of the mind, and one part is vital for the intelligence. In this scheme, food can have positive or negative effects, depending on the immediate environment, the geographical and climatic conditions, and a person's constitution. Yogic science recognizes three different qualities of food: *sattva*, *rajas*, and *tamas*. *Sattva* means "pure essence," and represents the well-balanced and meditative aspect; *rajas* is the energy which seeks to accomplish, achieve, or create; and *tamas* indicates inertia and decay.

Sattvic food, which includes fruit and vegetables, is pure, wholesome, and fresh. *Rajasic* foods, such as onions, garlic, and pungent spices, are stimulants. *Tamasic* substances, such as alcohol and meats, are considered to be heavy and enervating. Junk food is a relatively new term, but its properties would certainly be categorized as *tamasic*.

Every activity in our modern world is fast, and this includes activities related to food and the way we eat it. Junk food and canned and packaged food have a tremendously negative impact on the body. The mind is as alert after a meal of *sattvic* food as it was before the food was eaten, but after meals which are largely *rajasic* or *tamasic* in nature, it becomes dull and sluggish. It is equally important to keep the mind healthy and the body well nourished.

The five organs of perception, the eyes, ears, nose, tongue, and skin, are the gateways to the mind. For better control of the mind, the senses need appropriate nourishment. Soothing music for the ears, soft, natural light, beautiful, peaceful scenery for the eyes, and fresh pure air with the scent of flowers for the nose, all help nourish the mind. The tongue needs nutritious, delicately flavored foods. The skin should be kept clean, soft, and supple. Finally, the mind must be nurtured by developing clarity of thought.

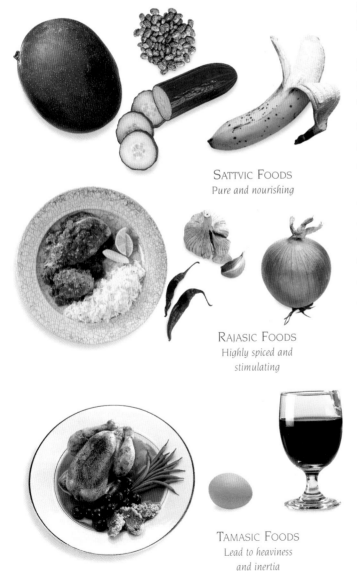

SATTVIC FOODS
Pure and nourishing

RAJASIC FOODS
Highly spiced and stimulating

TAMASIC FOODS
Lead to heaviness and inertia

Positive & Negative Stress

Stress can motivate an individual to develop creativity and achievement. This is positive stress. Negative stress can lead to illness, depression, and inertia. Yoga teaches you to transform negative stress into positive stress.

The cumulative effects of stress can damage your health and undermine your emotional stability. Stress can paralyze, and make you feel fragmented and off balance. There is a growing awareness today that stress is a health hazard. However, we should not forget that stress can also trigger the motivation to create and achieve. This type of stress can be positive, constructive, and healthy.

TYPES OF STRESS

We must distinguish clearly between positive stress and negative stress. Negative stress leads to the inability to adjust or react to illness, to feelings of uncertainty, or to certain harmful addictions. Negative stress, like some diseases, can remain dormant. It can be passive, but can also be active. The physical symptoms of negative stress include tremors or difficulty breathing.

Though positive and negative stress are two sides of the same coin, one type of stress usually predominates. Every person must find a way to transform negative stress into positive energy, so that it can be harnessed to build a healthy mind and body. The mind, body, and emotions are affected by physical, physiological, intellectual, emotional, and spiritual stress. The result may be tense or stiff muscles and joints, atrophying of skeletal bones, slowing down of body systems, or sluggishness in the vital organs. Emotional tension and muscular tension are closely related. Continuous stress causes habitual muscular contraction, severe muscle and joint pain, and tightness in the jaw or facial muscles. If you suffer from stress, you may experience severe indigestion or irritable bowel syndrome, headaches, migraine, a feeling of constriction in the diaphragm, breathlessness, or insomnia.

REACTIONS TO STRESS

Different people respond to the same stressful situation with different levels of intensity. Some may become irritable or angry, others may become confused or depressed. Regardless of how stress manifests itself, and how one responds to it, ultimately stress leads to disease, premature ageing, or in extreme cases, fatal illness. Turbulent emotions and physical ailments are directly connected. The science of psycho-neuroimmunology has established the connection between the body, mind, and emotions, a connection the ancient yogis recognized a millennium ago. According to yogic science, the health of the psyche is reflected in, and partly created by, the health of the body. Affliction and sorrow are often physiologically manifested as physical pain. Psychological pressures bring stress to bear on the anatomical body, the bodily organs, and on the nervous system.

POSITIVE ACTION
Stress can be harnessed to have a positive effect

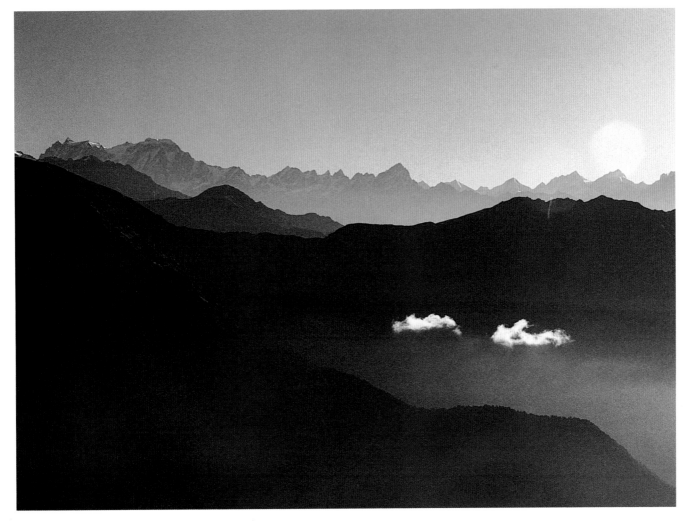

HORIZONS OF PEACE AND CALM
Yoga helps you see beyond the tension and strain of daily life

ALLEVIATING STRESS

To reduce stress, the body and mind cannot be treated as separate components. The tension associated with stress is stored mainly in the muscles, the diaphragm, and the nervous system. If these areas are relaxed, stress is reduced. Similarly, the organs of perception and the central nervous system react physically to stress. Yogic methods of deep relaxation have a profound effect on the central nervous system, as well as the circulatory, respiratory, and digestive systems. When a part of the body is tense, circulation to that area is decreased, reducing immunity. Yoga works on that area to relieve tension and increase circulation. Blood flow to all parts of the body improves and stabilizes the heart rate and blood pressure. Rapid, shallow breathing becomes deep and slow, allowing a higher intake of oxygen, and removing stress from the body and the mind.

"Words cannot convey the value of yoga. It has to be experienced."

Asanas & Stress

The practice of asanas and pranayama is the most natural therapy for stress. Practicing asanas with props builds your stamina and allows you to benefit from the posture without unnecessary strain.

Many people respond to stress by resorting to tranquillizers, alcohol, nicotine, or comfort eating. These may bring momentary relief, but as we all know, they are only temporary solutions and are, in fact, counterproductive. They also have dangerous side effects that actually increase stress levels. Simple relaxation techniques can alleviate stress levels for a short time, but cannot tackle the causes of stress comprehensively.

The yogis and sages of the past have emphasized that emotional turmoil or anxiety have to be faced with calmness and stability. Yoga can help you internalize those positive attitudes which allow you to face stressful situations with equanimity.

INTERNALIZING
POSITIVE ATTITUDES
Practicing Marichyasana helps relax your diaphragm and reduce stress

LEARNING TO DEAL WITH STRESS

Every individual has the power to discriminate between good habits and bad, and to develop his or her sense of ethical behavior. By adopting good habits, such as regular yoga practice, you can check the stress that depletes the body's bioenergy. The practice of asanas and pranayama is not just the most effective, but also the most natural therapy for stress, and unlike many other therapies, there is no danger of harmful side effects. Mere relaxation is not sufficient in itself to counter the negative effects of stress. The regular practice of yoga, along with a healthy diet and lifestyle, helps generate enormous amounts of energy in the body, stimulating the cells and relaxing tensed muscles.

While the effect of asanas and pranayama on the mind takes longer to be felt, with patience and dedication, you will soon discover a feeling of mental poise and well-being during and after your practice. While practicing asanas and pranayama, the five senses of perception that divert the mind to the external environment are drawn inward. When the restlessness of the mind is stilled, your entire being becomes calm and steady. The impact of negative stress is reduced, while the benefits of positive stress are enhanced, building the resilience and flexibility of the nerves, organs, senses, mind, and intelligence to create a healthy mind and body. Clarity, firmness of purpose, self-discipline, and ethical and moral sensibility follow naturally, enabling you to live a tranquil life, free of stress, and in harmony with your environment.

MINIMIZING STRAIN
Using simple props lessens strain and enables you to hold the posture for a longer period

individual, and even from season to season. Reclining asanas, inversions, and resting asanas, for example, are particularly beneficial on a hot day. These asanas slow the metabolism, and conserve energy. During the winter months, standing, back bends, and inverted asanas stimulate the body's systems, and help fight off common ailments such as colds, coughs, congestion in the chest, and sinusitis.

SEQUENCING AND TIMING

Sequencing is the method of practicing asanas in a particular order to maximize their effectiveness. Too much active practice may result in egoism and exhaust the body's systems. On the other hand, too much

ACTIVE AND PASSIVE PRACTICE

There are many different types of stress which we deal with every day, physical, psychological, and physiological. The only way to effectively combat the negative effects of these is through a balanced combination of active and passive practice. I use the term "passive practice" when talking of yoga with props, since this helps promote calmness of the mind, patience, and endurance. "Active practice," as the term suggests, is more vigorous, and generally refers to classical postures without the use of props. These postures, especially the standing postures and those involving back bends, help build stamina, vitality, and flexibility. The balance between active and passive postures will vary from individual to

passive practice may lead to depression, lethargy, and feelings of restlessness and irritability. As you gradually discover more and more about yoga and about your own body, you will be able to adjust the sequences of your practice, to achieve the ideal blend of active and passive postures. As your stamina and flexibility increase, you will also be able to hold postures for longer periods. The effect of an asana cannot take place in seconds, and timing is dependent on energy, intelligence, and awareness.

ASANAS WITH PROPS

If you are experiencing high levels of stress, or if you have a minor injury, or are fatigued in any way, it is best for you to practice yoga using props.

"The brain must be calm, and the body active."

Asanas with Props

The ancient yogis used logs of wood, stones, and ropes to help them practice asanas effectively. Extending this principle, Yogacharya Iyengar invented props which allow asanas to be held easily and for a longer duration, without strain.

Yoga asanas involve extension, exertion, as well as relaxation of the body. More importantly, the aim of the movements is to align the body correctly. This also includes mental alignment, in which the mind touches each and every part of the body evenly.

The practice of yoga requires you to be in good mental and physical condition. Yet, during my long years of teaching yoga, I have found that even those

whether they are weak or strong, young or old, beginners or advanced students, or those who wish to conserve their energy because of fatigue or injury.

HOW PROPS HELP

A yoga prop is any object that helps stretch, strengthen, relax, or improve the alignment of the body. It helps sustain the practice of asanas for a longer duration, and conserves energy. These props

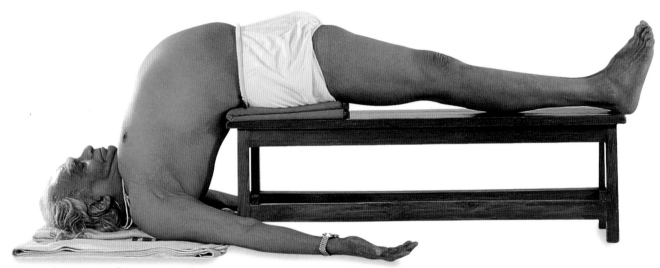

YOGACHARYA IYENGAR IN SETUBANDHA SARVANGASANA
This version of the posture requires considerable strength in the neck, shoulders, and back, requiring years of practice to achieve. It should not be attempted without supervision

in good condition occasionally find some postures difficult to sustain for the required length of time. Some asanas, too, entail body movements that are initially too complicated for even the healthiest students to attempt without help. It is for this reason that I developed the use of props in yoga. With these props, the practice of asanas has never been easier, less tiring, or more enjoyable, making each asana equally accessible to all yoga students,

allow asanas to be practiced in a relaxed way, and balance the body and mind actively as well as passively. At first, I would use my own body to support my students during their practice, but found that this exhausted my own reserves of energy. I then began experimenting with ordinary, everyday objects such as walls, chairs, stools, blocks, bolsters, blankets, and belts to help my students achieve the final posture. As I worked with people who were

affected by illness or disease, I realized the value of props. I discovered that props helped retain key movements and subtle adjustments of the body by providing more height, weight, or support.
I also found that the use of props improved blood circulation and breathing capacity. This inspired me to create props adjusted to suit individual needs.

The yoga asana practiced with props is unique in that it is the only form of exercise which allows both action and relaxation simultaneously. It activates the muscles, tones the body's organs, and relieves undue mental and physical stress or strain. Props help increase flexibility and stamina and, at the same time, relax slack and tired muscles. They help to rejuvenate the entire body, without increasing physical fatigue.

Students of yoga find the practice of asanas with props an encouraging exercise. It gives them the confidence to attempt difficult asanas, and ensures correct practice. Props provide a sense of direction and alignment, and help increase and enhance the understanding of each asana. They serve as silent instructors.

PROPS AND THERAPY

When the body is lethargic, sluggish, and fatigued, practice with props works wonders. The nervous system relaxes, the brain is calmed, and the mind soothed. Asanas with props build up emotional stability and will power. As stress is reduced, anxiety, fears, and depression also disappear, helping those under emotional strain cope better with all aspects of their lives. Blood circulation increases, and the heart, as well as the respiratory, abdominal, and pelvic organs are rested and rejuvenated. For instance, Setubandha Sarvangasana (*see page* 218) practiced on a broad wooden bench increases coronary blood supply and rests and energizes the heart without any bodily strain. This makes it ideal for cardiac patients.

Asanas practiced with the help of bolsters, blocks, stools, or chairs help relieve many common ailments. They regulate blood pressure, ease breathlessness and asthma, and remove stiffness in the back, hips, knees, and feet, alleviating rheumatism and arthritis. Yoga with props frees you from attachment to the body and liberates the spirit. It helps improve posture and maintain balance, allowing you to stretch, and experience a state of relaxation during practice.

Ultimately, yoga with props creates a feeling of peace and tranquillity, and culminates in a fresh perspective and renewed strength. Some of the props shown on the following pages have been specifically developed for your practice. Others are objects that you will find in your home.

PRACTICE AGAINST A WALL

The support of a wall helps maintain balance and a sense of alignment, particularly in standing and inverted asanas. It gives you the confidence to practice without fear of injury or strain. The wall is invaluable in the practice of Tadasana (*see page* 168). Make sure that you practice standing asanas on an even, smooth surface. To avoid slipping, do not practice on a mat or blanket, and do not wear socks. Always practice Tadasana and its variations with bare feet, since shoes restrict movement, cramp the toes, and reduce sensitivity in the soles, impairing your ability to sense all the adjustments in the posture.

A WALL GIVES YOU ALIGNMENT
Yogacharya Iyengar adjusts the position of the student's arms in Tadasana Urdhva Hastasana

Props

The props shown on these pages can be found in your home or can be bought at the addresses listed on page 416. When you practice with props, use them in a way that is the most suitable for you. I have provided some basic guidelines, but the most important point is that you should feel comfortable and relaxed when practicing an asana.

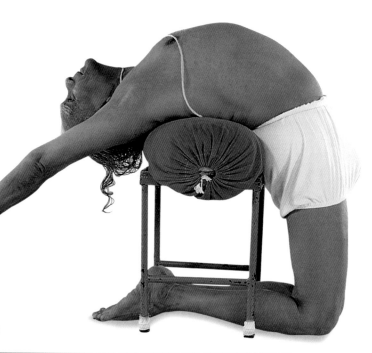

INVALUABLE SUPPORT
Yogacharya Iyengar in Ustrasana with one stool

The props shown below support the entire body when you practice the asana, give you the height to coordinate your movements more effectively, and allow better balance in the posture.

CHAIR

This folding metal chair has an open back rest which allows you to place your legs through it. This makes for an easier, yet still effective rotation of the torso in seated twists, such as Bharadvajasana. Holding the sides of the back rest steadies you when getting into the posture in Salamba Sarvangasana and Halasana. It provides support to the torso in back bends, such as Viparita Dandasana. Make sure that the chair is completely stable and rests firmly on the ground.

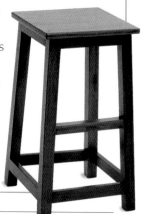

WOODEN BENCH

This bench should be broad enough to support your torso comfortably, and should be approximately 2ft (60cm) high. It must rest firmly on the ground. Cardiac patients or those with migraine or respiratory disorders will benefit from the use of this bench in their practice of Setubandha Sarvangasana.

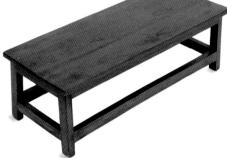

HALF-HALASANA STOOL

This stool should be approximately 1-1.5ft (30-45cm) high to support the back and feet in Paripurna Navasana, and the back in Ustrasana. It helps in the practice of asanas that require flexibility and strength in the back, abdomen, arms, and legs.

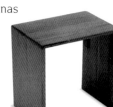

LOW, OPEN STOOL

A stool with open sides helps support the body in back bends, such as Ustrasana, and helps lift and arch the torso easily. The stool should not be more than 1.5ft (45cm) high, and should rest firmly on the ground.

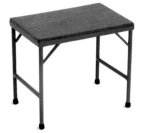

HIGH STOOL

This stool, of mid-thigh height, helps in the practice of standing twists, such as Utthita Marichyasana. The stool allows you to rotate the spine and torso effectively without strain. Make sure that the stool rests firmly on the ground and that it has a top wide enough for your whole foot to rest comfortably.

The props below support specific parts of the body and allow asanas to be held without strain and for a longer duration. Beginners, people with stiff joints or muscles, or those who have high blood pressure and need support for the head in forward bends, will find these useful.

BOLSTER

Bolsters support your body while enabling you to relax and stretch effectively without strain. The bolster should weigh about 7lbs (3kg) and be stuffed with dense cotton. The bolster should be about 2ft (60cm) long, with a diameter of 9in (23cm). It should preferably have a removable cotton cover.

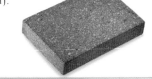

FOAM BLOCK

A foam block is placed under stacked wooden blocks to support the head in forward bends and the back in pranayama. Its dimensions are about 1ft (30cm) x 7in (18cm) x 2in x (5cm).

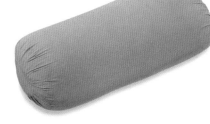

WOODEN BLOCK

The support of wooden blocks is used in all types of asanas. In sitting and standing asanas they support the legs, knees, or palms, and give height to seated twists. In Ujjayi Pranayama, a block supports the back and helps open the chest. In forward bends, such as Uttanasana, blocks provide support to the head and to the hands. The measurements of the block should be 9in (23cm) x 4.5in (12cm) x 3in (7cm). It can be placed on its short side (a); on its long side (b); and on its broad side (c); according to your requirement. While a height has been suggested for many asanas in this chapter, you should place the block at the height you find most comfortable.

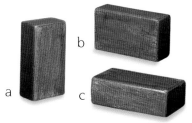

ROUNDED WOODEN BLOCK

A small block is used to give added height in the standing twist, Utthita Marichyasana. It helps you rotate your body more effectively and without strain. It is about 2in (5cm) high and 4in (10cm) long.

FOLDED BLANKET

Folded blankets are used to support the back, open the chest in reclining asanas and pranayama, and support the head and shoulders in inversions, such as Salamba Sarvangasana. They provide height in seated asanas, help keep the torso and spine erect, and also correct poor structural posture. Cotton blankets, measuring about 6.5ft (2m) x 4ft (1.2m), are most suitable. Fold one in half 3 times when using it to cushion the impact of a chair or a bench on the body. Fold in half 4 or 5 times to give added height for sitting asanas and seated twists.

ROLLED BLANKET

This is used to support the neck in reclining asanas and back bends, and the small of the back in back bends, such as Viparita Dandasana. It helps relieve strain on the chest and on the thighs and ankles in Virasana and Adhomukha Virasana. Fold a cotton blanket in half 4 times, and then tightly roll it up (see above).

These two props increase the effectiveness of some asanas. The belt prevents muscle or joint strain, and enhances the stretch. The bandage helps you relax completely by making it easier to turn your thoughts inward.

YOGA BELT

The belt helps to provide the required tension without strain in the final stretch of Supta Padangusthasana, Urdhvamukha Janu Sirsasana, and Paripurna Navasana. The belt is about 2ft (60cm) long, is made of strong woven material, and has a buckle at either end.

CREPE BANDAGE

The blindfold, 8-10ft (2.5-3m) long and 4in (10cm) broad, helps the eyes recede into their sockets. This cools the brain, and relaxes the facial muscles and the nervous system in Savasana and pranayama.

Tadasana Samasthithi

- Steady and firm mountain posture -

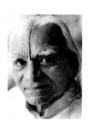

THIS POSTURE, THE starting point of all standing asanas, lifts the sternum, which is the site of the *anahata* or "heart" *chakra* (*see page* 37). This helps reduce stress and boost self-confidence, while the perfect balance of the final posture increases your alertness. In Sanskrit, *tadasana* means "mountain posture" while *samasthithi* indicates an "upright and steady state."

PROPS (*See page* 164) THE WALL helps you align your body correctly, makes adjustments in the posture easier, and gives stability to the final posture.

CAUTIONS
◆

Do not practice this asana if you have stress-related headaches, migraine, eye strain, low blood pressure, osteoarthritis of the knees, bulimia, diarrhea, insomnia, or leukorrhea. If you have had polio, or if you have a problem with balance, practice this asana with your feet about 10in (25cm) apart.

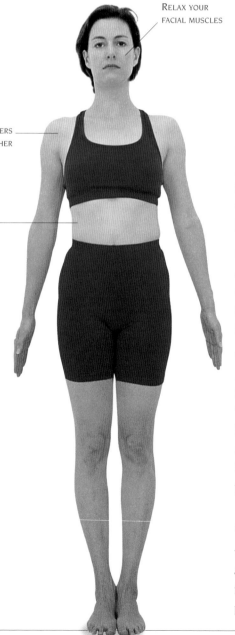

RELAX YOUR FACIAL MUSCLES

KEEP YOUR SHOULDERS LEVEL WITH EACH OTHER

LENGTHEN BOTH SIDES OF YOUR WAIST EVENLY

BENEFITS
◆
Helps treat depression
◆
Improves incorrect posture
◆
Strengthens the knee joints
◆
Revitalizes the feet and corrects flat feet
◆
Reduces sciatic pain
◆
Prevents hemorrhoids
◆
Improves bladder control
◆
Tones and lifts the pelvis and abdomen

1 With bare feet stand on a smooth, even surface. Keep your feet together, with your heels touching the wall. Beginners may find it easier to keep their feet (2in) 5cm apart.

2 Stretch your arms along your sides, with the palms facing your thighs, and your fingers pointing to the floor. Stretch your neck up, keeping the muscles soft and passive.

3 Distribute your weight evenly on the inner and outer edges of your feet, and on your toes and heels. Tighten your kneecaps and open the back of each knee. Turn in the front of your thighs. Tighten your buttocks. Pull in your lower abdomen, and lift your chest.

4 Keep your head erect and look straight ahead. Breathe evenly and with awareness. Experience your body and mind as an integrated whole and feel the surge of energy. Stay in the posture for 30-60 seconds.

Tadasana Urdhva Hastasana

- Mountain posture with arms stretched up -

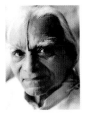

THIS IS A VARIATION of the mountain posture, with the arms extended up. *Urdhva* translates as "upward" in Sanskrit, while *hasta* means "hands." This is recommended for people in sedentary occupations, since it exercises the arms and the joints of the shoulders, wrists, knuckles, and fingers.

PROPS (*See page* 164) THE WALL helps you align your body correctly, makes adjustments in the posture easier, and gives stability to the final posture.

CAUTIONS
◆

Do not practice this asana if you have stress-related headaches, migraine, eye strain, low blood pressure, osteoarthritis of the knees, bulimia, diarrhea, insomnia, or leukorrhea. If you have high blood pressure, do not hold the posture for more than 15 seconds. If you have a slipped disc or a prolapsed uterus, keep your feet together, and your knees apart.

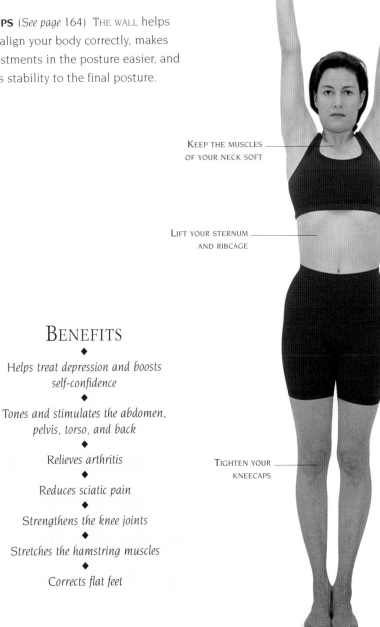

KEEP THE MUSCLES OF YOUR NECK SOFT

LIFT YOUR STERNUM AND RIBCAGE

TIGHTEN YOUR KNEECAPS

BENEFITS
◆

Helps treat depression and boosts self-confidence
◆
Tones and stimulates the abdomen, pelvis, torso, and back
◆
Relieves arthritis
◆
Reduces sciatic pain
◆
Strengthens the knee joints
◆
Stretches the hamstring muscles
◆
Corrects flat feet

1 With bare feet stand in Tadasana (*see page* 48) on an even, uncovered surface. Exhale, and stretching from your waist, lift up your arms in front of you to shoulder level. Keep your palms open and facing each other.

2 Raise your arms above your head, perpendicular to the floor. Stretch your arms and fingers. Push your shoulder blades into your body.

3 Stretch your arms further up from your shoulders keeping them parallel to each other. Extend your wrists, palms, and fingers toward the ceiling. Feel the stretch along both sides of your body.

4 Pull in your lower abdomen. Turn your wrists so that the palms face front. Hold the posture for 20-30 seconds. Breathe evenly.

Tadasana Urdhva Baddha Hastasana

- Mountain posture with bound hands -

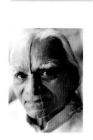

THIS IS A VARIATION of Tadasana, the "mountain posture." *Urdhva* means "upward" in Sanskrit, *baddha* indicates "caught" or "bound," while *hasta* translates as "hands." In this posture, the brain is relaxed but alert, and you are aware of the intense, whole-body stretch, from your feet to your interlocked fingers. Feel the energy flow from your feet up to your knuckles.

PROPS (*See page* 164) THE WALL helps you align your body correctly, makes adjustments in the posture easier, and gives stability to the final posture.

CAUTIONS
◆

Do not practice this asana if you have a cardiac condition, stress-related headaches, migraine, low blood pressure, insomnia, osteoarthritis of the knees, bulimia, diarrhea, or leukorrhea. If you have high blood pressure, do not hold the posture for more than 15 seconds. If you have had polio, are knock-kneed, or have a problem with your balance, keep your feet 8in (20cm) apart. If you are prone to backache, have a slipped disc, or a prolapsed uterus, keep your feet together and knees apart.

LIFT YOUR
STERNUM

BENEFITS
◆
Boosts confidence and helps treat depression
◆
Relieves arthritis
◆
Stretches the shoulders, arms, wrists, and fingers
◆
Helps treat spinal disorders
◆
Tones and activates the torso, back, abdomen, and pelvis
◆
Strengthens the knee joints
◆
Reduces sciatic pain
◆
Corrects flat feet

PULL UP YOUR
QUADRICEPS

EXTEND THE MOUNDS
OF YOUR TOES AWAY
FROM YOUR HEELS

1 With bare feet stand in Tadasana (*see page* 48) against a wall, on an even, uncovered surface. Bring your arms toward your chest, with your palms facing the chest. Interlock your fingers firmly, from the base of the knuckles, with the little finger of your left hand lower than the little finger of the right hand (*see inset above*).

2 Turn your interlocked palms inside out (*see inset below*). Exhale, and stretch your arms out in front of you at shoulder level. Then inhale, and raise your arms above your head until they are perpendicular to the floor. Extend your arms fully and lock your elbows. Feel the stretch in your palms. Hold the posture for 30-60 seconds.

Tadasana Paschima Baddha Namaskar

- Mountain posture with bound arms -

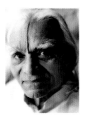

THE SANSKRIT WORDS *paschima baddha namaskar* mean "hands folded at the back in the salutation of *namaskar*." *Baddha* means "bound" or "caught." This asana is an easier version of Tadasana Paschima Namaskar (*see page* 172), and helps prepare you for the regular posture which calls for greater flexibility and extension of the back and arms.

(see page 172)

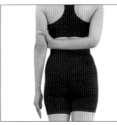
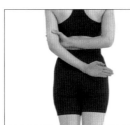

CAUTIONS
◆

Do not practice this asana if you have angina, stress-related headaches, migraine, eye strain, insomnia, low blood pressure, osteoarthritis of the knees, leukorrhea, or bulimia.
If you have a slipped disc, a displaced uterus, or painful wrist joints, keep your feet together and your knees apart. If you have had polio, or have any problems with your balance, keep your feet at least 10in (25cm) apart.

1 With bare feet stand in Tadasana (*see page* 48) on an even, uncovered surface. Take your right arm behind your back and hold your left arm just above the elbow. Bend your left arm and take it behind your back. Stretch both legs and imagine you are pulling the skin, muscles, and bones of your legs up to your waist.

(see page 48)

KEEP YOUR BACK ERECT

TIGHTEN YOUR BUTTOCK MUSCLES

BENEFITS
◆
Boosts confidence and helps reduce depression
◆
Helps in the treatment of cervical spondylosis
◆
Relieves arthritis of the shoulders, arms, wrists, and fingers
◆
Strengthens the knee joints and reduces sciatic pain
◆
Corrects flat feet

EXTEND YOUR HAMSTRINGS

2 Hold your right arm just above the elbow with your left hand. Your grip should be firm but not tight. Keep your forearms pressed to your back. Turn in your upper arms slightly. Push your elbows back, but do not allow them to lift. Initially, hold the posture for 20-30 seconds. With practice, increase the duration to 1 minute. Breathe evenly throughout.

REST YOUR WEIGHT EQUALLY ON BOTH FEET

Tadasana Paschima Namaskar

- Mountain posture with hands in prayer position -

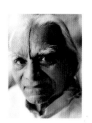

I N THIS STANDING ASANA, the hands are folded at the back in the Indian salutation of *namaskar* or "greeting." This stretch requires considerable flexibility in the upper body and arms. Practice Tadasana Paschima Baddha Namaskar (*see page* 171) until your shoulder, elbow, and wrist joints are sufficiently supple to perform this asana easily.

CAUTIONS
◆

Do not practice this asana if you have a cardiac condition, stress-related headaches, migraine, low blood pressure, insomnia, osteoarthritis of the knees, bulimia, diarrhea, or leukorrhea. If you have high blood pressure, do not hold the posture for more than 15 seconds. If you have had polio, or are knock-kneed, or have a problem with your balance, keep your feet 8in (20cm) apart. If you are prone to backache, have a slipped disc, or a prolapsed uterus, keep your feet together and knees apart.

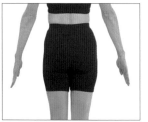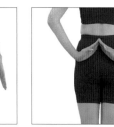

1 With bare feet stand in Tadasana (*see page* 48) on an even, uncovered surface. Gently turn your arms in and out a few times. Take them behind you and join your fingertips, pointing them to the floor. Rest your thumbs on your lower back. Move your elbows back and rotate your wrists, so that your fingertips turn and point first toward your back, and then up.

MOVE YOUR ELBOWS
BACK AND DOWN

BENEFITS
◆

Reduces depression
◆
Relieves cervical spondylosis
◆
Increases the flexibility of the upper body, arms, elbows, and wrists
◆
Strengthens the knee joints
◆
Reduces sciatic pain
◆
Corrects flat feet

OPEN OUT
THE BACKS OF
YOUR KNEES

2 Press your palms together, and move them up your back until they are in between your shoulder blades. Keep your palms joined from the base to the fingertips. Push your elbows down to stretch your upper arms and chest. Focus on keeping your chest and armpits open. Keep your neck and shoulders relaxed. Hold the posture for 30-60 seconds.

STRETCH YOUR
TOES AWAY
FROM YOUR HEELS

Tadasana Gomukhasana

- Mountain posture with hands held in the shape of a cow's face -

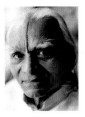

THE INTERLINKED HANDS in the final posture of this asana take the shape of *gomukha*, which means "a cow's face" in Sanskrit. The asana is a variation of Tadasana, the mountain posture. It activates the muscles of the shoulders and back. The stretch in the arms helps relieve arthritis in the shoulders, elbows, wrists, and fingers.

CAUTIONS
◆

Avoid this asana if you have a cardiac condition, stress-related headaches, migraine, eye strain, insomnia, low blood pressure, osteoarthritis of the knees, diarrhea, or leukorrhea. If you have had polio, or any congenital deformity of the legs, or are knock-kneed, keep your feet about 10in (25cm) apart. If you have backache, a slipped disc, a displaced uterus, or pain in the wrist joints, keep your feet together and your knees slightly apart.

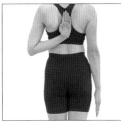

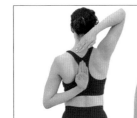

1 With bare feet stand in Tadasana (*see page* 48) on an even, uncovered surface. Take your left arm behind you and place the back of your left palm on the middle of your back. Raise your right arm. Bend your right elbow and move your hand down with your palm facing your body.

DO NOT ARCH YOUR BACK

PULL IN YOUR TAILBONE

BENEFITS
◆

Boosts confidence and helps treat depression
◆
Alleviates cervical spondylosis
◆
Improves breathing by opening up the chest
◆
Strengthens the knee joints
◆
Reduces sciatic pain
◆
Corrects flat feet

KEEP YOUR LEGS STRETCHED UP

2 Place your right palm on your left palm and interlink the fingers of both hands. If this proves difficult, touch the fingertips of both hands to each other. Do not force your arms to bend. Give yourself time to adjust to the action. Consciously relax your arms. Open your right armpit to create space between your chest and your upper right arm. Keep your right elbow pointed up and back, and your right forearm close to your head. Lower your left elbow further. Then place the back of your left wrist on your back. Hold the posture for 20-30 seconds. Repeat the posture on the other side.

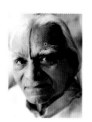

Utthita Trikonasana

- Extended triangle posture -

THIS ASANA IS A VARIATION of the classic posture (*see page* 50). Regular practice of this asana taps energy stored in the tailbone, an important source of vitality and strength. This helps those who require more energy to function efficiently under stress. The posture activates the spine, keeping it supple and well-aligned. It relieves backache and reduces stiffness in the neck, shoulders, and knees.

CAUTIONS
◆

Do not practice this asana if you have stress-related headaches, migraine, eye strain, diarrhea, low blood pressure, psoriasis, varicose veins, or if you are depressed or extremely fatigued. Patients of rheumatoid arthritis who have a fever should avoid this asana. Do not practice during menstruation. If you have high blood pressure, do not look up at the raised arm in the posture. If you have cervical spondylosis, do not look up for too long.

PROPS (*See page* 164) A WALL, A BLOCK, AND A MAT. Practice against a wall supports the body, reduces strain, and helps to align the body correctly. The mat prevents your feet from slipping,

helping to maintain the final balance in the posture. The block helps those with stiff backs reach the floor, and allows for greater extension of the spine, neck, and shoulders.

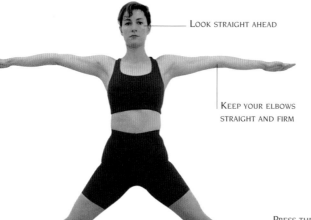

LOOK STRAIGHT AHEAD

KEEP YOUR ELBOWS STRAIGHT AND FIRM

PRESS THE INNER EDGES OF THE FEET TO THE FLOOR

PULL UP THE INNER SIDES OF YOUR LEGS

1 Spread a mat against a wall. Place a wooden block on its long side on the right edge of the mat. Stand in Tadasana (*see page* 48) on the center of the mat. Inhale, then spread your feet about 3.5ft (1m) apart. Your heels and buttocks should touch the wall. Raise your arms out to your sides until they are in line with your shoulders.

2 Turn out the right foot to the right until it is parallel to the wall. Turn in your left foot, slightly to the right. Your left heel and buttocks should touch the wall. Keep your left leg straight. Stretch your arms away from your body keeping them parallel to the floor, palms facing down.

BENEFITS

◆

Tones the abdominal organs

◆

Stimulates digestion, relieving
gastritis, acidity, and flatulence

◆

Tones the pelvic organs, correcting
the effects of a sedentary lifestyle
or faulty posture

◆

Alleviates backache

◆

Reduces stiffness in the neck,
shoulders, and knees

◆

Tones the ligaments of the
arms and legs

◆

Helps relieve menstrual
disorders

THE GURU'S ADVICE

*"You must keep your arms fully stretched out in this
asana. Look at how I am straightening and extending the
student's arm, wrist, and fingers."*

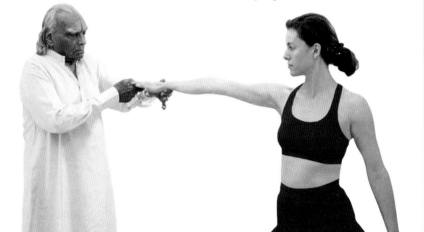

OPEN YOUR ARMPITS

DO NOT TILT
YOUR HEAD

PUSH YOUR RIGHT
SHOULDER INTO
YOUR BODY

LIFT YOUR KNEECAPS
BY CONTRACTING YOUR
QUADRICEP MUSCLES

EXTEND AND
RELAX THE TIPS
OF YOUR TOES

3 Bend to the right and extend your
right arm toward the floor. Place
your right palm on the block. Pull
the tailbone into your body, keeping
your left buttock and shoulders firmly
pressed to the wall. Raise up the left
arm toward the ceiling. Turn your head
and look at your left thumb. Rest
your weight on both heels, not on
your right palm. Breathe evenly,
not deeply. Hold the posture
for 20-30 seconds. Then
repeat the posture on the
other side.

Utthita Parsvakonasana

- Extended side angle stretch -

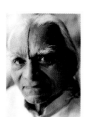

THIS ASANA IS A VARIATION of the classic posture (*see page* 60) and is practiced against a wall, with a block under the lowered hand. There is often a tendency to sink down on the bent leg in the final posture of this asana. Using the recommended props guards against this and gives greater freedom for adjustments in the posture without strain or injury.

PROPS (*See page* 164) A WALL AND A WOODEN BLOCK. The support of the wall reduces fatigue, helps you hold the posture longer, and aligns your neck and head correctly. A wooden block is placed at a suitable height under the lowered hand. This helps those who have a stiff spine or who find it difficult to reach the floor. It also helps maintain steadiness in the posture.

CAUTIONS
◆

Do not practice this asana if you have stress-related headaches, migraine, osteoarthritis of the knees, rheumatic fever, varicose veins, low blood pressure, chronic fatigue syndrome, diarrhea, psoriasis, insomnia, depression, or bulimia. Avoid the posture during menstruation, or if you have irregular or heavy periods, premenstrual stress, or leukorrhea. If you have cervical spondylosis, look up briefly in the final posture. Those with hypertension should look at the floor.

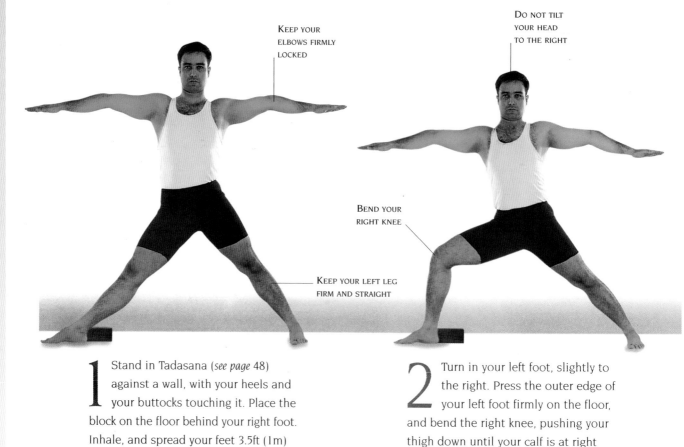

KEEP YOUR ELBOWS FIRMLY LOCKED

DO NOT TILT YOUR HEAD TO THE RIGHT

BEND YOUR RIGHT KNEE

KEEP YOUR LEFT LEG FIRM AND STRAIGHT

1 Stand in Tadasana (*see page* 48) against a wall, with your heels and your buttocks touching it. Place the block on the floor behind your right foot. Inhale, and spread your feet 3.5ft (1m) apart. Turn out your right foot to the right until it is parallel to the wall.

2 Turn in your left foot, slightly to the right. Press the outer edge of your left foot firmly on the floor, and bend the right knee, pushing your thigh down until your calf is at right angles to the floor. Stretch your left arm away from your left shoulder.

THE GURU'S ADVICE

"Look at how I am supporting the student's right side, in the region of his floating ribs. This support helps him to improve his balance by drawing in his left buttock and rotating the left side of his torso up toward the ceiling."

BENEFITS

◆

Corrects misalignment of the shoulders and shoulder blades

◆

Relieves backache and neck sprains

◆

Makes the hip joint and spinal column supple

◆

Strengthens the legs and knees, particularly the hamstring muscles

◆

Stretches and tones the abdominal and pelvic organs

◆

Stimulates digestion by relieving gastritis, acidity, and flatulence

◆

Helps relieve menstrual disorders

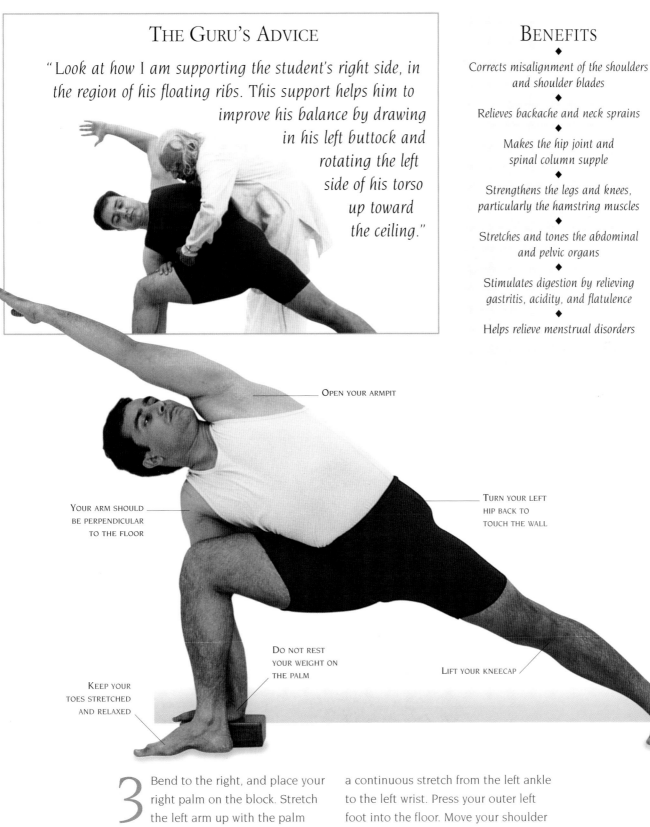

OPEN YOUR ARMPIT

YOUR ARM SHOULD BE PERPENDICULAR TO THE FLOOR

TURN YOUR LEFT HIP BACK TO TOUCH THE WALL

DO NOT REST YOUR WEIGHT ON THE PALM

LIFT YOUR KNEECAP

KEEP YOUR TOES STRETCHED AND RELAXED

3 Bend to the right, and place your right palm on the block. Stretch the left arm up with the palm facing forward. Now rotate the arm and bring it toward your left ear. Your left thumb should touch the wall. Turn your head and look at your left arm. Maintain a continuous stretch from the left ankle to the left wrist. Press your outer left foot into the floor. Move your shoulder blades into your body, and extend your spine toward your head. Stay in the position for 30 seconds. Then repeat the posture on the other side.

Ardha Chandrasana

- Half moon posture -

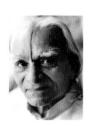

I N SANSKRIT, *ardha* means "half," while *chandra* translates as "moon." In this asana, your body takes the shape of a half moon. Regular practice enhances your span of concentration. It also improves coordination and motor reflexes. The intense stretch it gives to the spine, strengthens the paraspinal muscles, keeping the spine supple and well-aligned.

CAUTIONS

Do not practice this asana if you have stress-related headaches, migraine, eye strain, varicose veins, diarrhea, insomnia, or chronic fatigue syndrome. Avoid this posture if you are tired. If you have hypertension, do not look up at your raised arm. Look straight ahead.

PROPS (*See page* 164) A WALL AND A WOODEN BLOCK. The wall gives stability and helps align the head and neck. The wooden block makes the posture easier for those who have stiff backs and cannot reach the floor.

1 Stand in Tadasana (*see page* 48). Place a block on its short side against the wall. Inhale, spread your feet 3.5ft (1m) apart. Raise your arms to shoulder level.

2 Turn in your left foot, slightly to the right, and your right foot to the right, parallel to the wall. Bend your right knee, and place the right palm on the block. Raise your left arm.

POINT YOUR FINGERS TOWARD THE CEILING

EXTEND YOUR LEFT LEG AWAY FROM YOUR TORSO

BENEFITS

Rotates and flexes the vertebral joints, keeping the spinal muscles supple

Tones the lumbar and sacral spine, relieving backache

Corrects misalignment of the shoulders

Helps relieve sciatica

Improves circulation in the feet

Relieves gastritis and acidity

Corrects a prolapsed uterus

KEEP YOUR ARMS STRAIGHT

3 Straighten your right leg. Raise your left leg until it is parallel to the floor. Keep your left arm stretched up in line with the right arm. The back of your left hand should touch the wall.

4 Look up at your left thumb. Keep your weight on the right foot, thigh, and hip, not on your right palm. Hold the posture for 20 seconds. Repeat the posture on the other side.

Uttanasana

- Intense forward stretch posture -

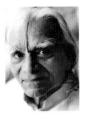

THIS IS A LESS STRENUOUS version of the classic posture (*see page* 72) that helps beginners and those with stiff backs achieve the final forward stretch. There are five variations of the final posture. Practice the one you find most comfortable and which suits your needs the best. This is both a calming and recuperative asana which rests and energizes the heart and lungs.

CAUTIONS
◆

Do not practice this asana if you have osteoarthritis of the knees, or diarrhea. Patients of rheumatoid arthritis who have fever should avoid this asana. Avoid the posture if you have excessive curvature of the lumbar spine or scoliosis. If you have low blood pressure, come out of the posture gradually to avoid dizziness.

PROPS (*See page* 164) A FOAM BLOCK AND FIVE WOODEN BLOCKS. Stack three wooden blocks on top of the foam block. Place a wooden block on either side of the stacked blocks.

SPECIFIC CAUTION Until your back muscles become more flexible, use props to support your head.

SPECIFIC BENEFIT Soothes and calms the body and brain.

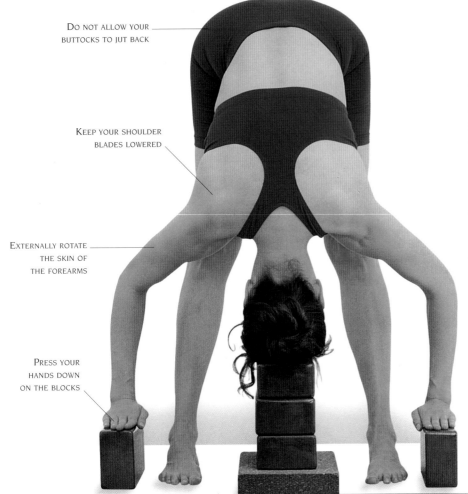

DO NOT ALLOW YOUR BUTTOCKS TO JUT BACK

KEEP YOUR SHOULDER BLADES LOWERED

EXTERNALLY ROTATE THE SKIN OF THE FOREARMS

PRESS YOUR HANDS DOWN ON THE BLOCKS

1 Stand in Tadasana (*see page* 48). Separate your legs to a distance of 1ft (30cm). Keep your feet parallel to each other, toes pointing forward. Pull up your kneecaps.

2 Inhale and raise your arms toward the ceiling, palms facing forward. Push your spine up.

3 Bend from the waist toward the floor. To increase the stretch of your spine, vital for correct practice, press your heels down on the floor.

4 Rest the crown of your head on the blocks in front of you, and place your palms on the blocks beside your feet. Pull in your kneecaps. Extend your hamstrings and pull your inner legs up. Feel one single stretch from the crown of your head to your heels. Hold the posture for 1 minute.

"*The regular, persevering, and alert practice of yoga is the foundation for stabilizing the consciousness.*"

BENEFITS

◆

*Reduces depression
if practiced regularly*

◆

Cures insomnia and relieves fatigue

◆

*Increases blood flow to the brain,
soothing the brain cells
and sympathetic nervous system*

◆

Regulates blood pressure

◆

*Relieves migraine and
stress-related headaches*

◆

Tones the abdominal organs

◆

*Relieves stomach ache by
neutralizing acidity*

◆

*Strengthens and stretches the
hamstring muscles*

◆

Increases the flexibility of the hip joint

◆

*Strengthens the knee joint and its
surrounding tissue and muscles*

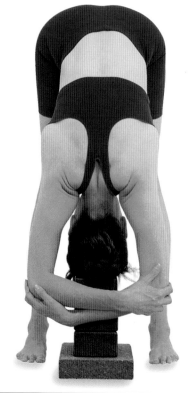

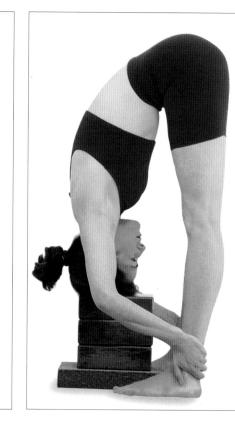

VARIATION 1 Hands on Elbows

PROPS (*See page* 164) A FOAM BLOCK AND THREE WOODEN BLOCKS. This variation is easier for beginners and for those who are too stiff to place their palms on the floor or on blocks.

GETTING INTO THE POSTURE Place the foam block on the floor and stack the 3 wooden blocks on it. Follow Steps 1, 2, and 3 of the main asana. Bend your right arm. Clasp your left elbow with your right hand. Hold the right elbow with your left hand. Place the crown of your head on the stacked blocks. Hold the posture for 1 minute.

VARIATION 2 Hands on Ankles

PROPS (*See page* 164) A FOAM BLOCK AND THREE WOODEN BLOCKS. The blocks support the head and make the forward bend easier.

GETTING INTO THE POSTURE Place the foam block on the floor and stack the 3 wooden blocks on it. Then follow Steps 1, 2, and 3 of the main asana. Exhale, and place the crown of your head on the blocks. Hold your right ankle with your right hand. At the same time, hold the left ankle with your left hand. Breathe evenly, and stay in the posture for 1 minute.

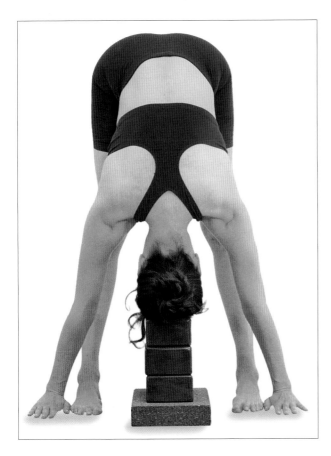

VARIATION 3 Palms on Floor

PROPS (*See page* 164) A FOAM BLOCK AND
THREE WOODEN BLOCKS. Once the muscles
of your back feel flexible enough, do
not use blocks to support your hands.
Instead, place your palms flat on the
floor in the final posture.

GETTING INTO THE POSTURE Place
the blocks, as given for Variation 2 on
page 180. Then follow Steps 1, 2, and 3
of the main asana. Ensure that both
your heels are pressed onto the floor,
and stretch the hamstring muscles at

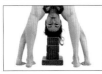 the back of your
thighs. Then place
your palms flat on
the floor just
beyond your feet (*see inset*). The thumb
of each hand should touch the little
toe of each foot. Distribute your body
weight equally on the toes and heels
of both your feet. Breathe evenly, and
hold the posture for 1 minute.

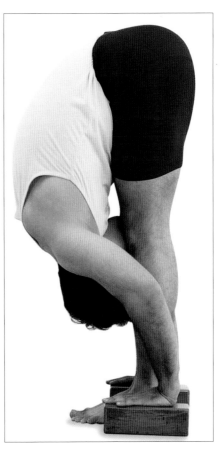

VARIATION 4 Palms on Blocks

PROPS (*See page* 164) TWO WOODEN
BLOCKS. Practice this variation only
when you feel your back muscles are
sufficiently flexible to hold the forward
bend without the support of blocks for
your head.

SPECIFIC CAUTIONS This variation
is not recommended for beginners.
Do not practice this posture if you are
prone to hypertension, headaches,
cervical spondylosis, insomnia,
migraine, or prolapsed discs.

GETTING INTO THE POSTURE Stand
with your feet together. Place a block
on its broad side on either side of your
feet, long edges parallel to your feet.
Follow Steps 1, 2, and 3 of the main
asana. When you bend from the waist,
place your palms on the blocks. Press
your chin to your knees. Hold the
posture for 1 minute.

Prasarita Padottanasana

- Expanded leg intense stretch -

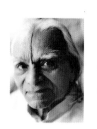

IN SANSKRIT, *prasarita* means "stretched out" or "spread out," while *pada* means "leg" or "foot." This asana gives an intense stretch to your legs. The torso is inverted in the posture, and your head rests on the floor, on a block, or on a bolster. This restful and recuperative asana is usually practiced toward the end of the standing posture cycle, just before Salamba Sirsasana (*see page* 118). Practicing the asana cools the body and brain, and gives you a feeling of tranquillity and repose.

CAUTIONS
♦

Do not hold this asana for more than 1 minute, especially if you are a beginner. If you have low blood pressure, come out of the posture gradually to avoid dizziness. Do not tilt your head or compress your neck while practicing this posture.

FLEX YOUR ELBOWS

PULL UP THE INNER SIDES OF YOUR LEGS

KEEP YOUR BACK CONCAVE AND PULL IN YOUR TAILBONE

1 Stand in Tadasana (*see page* 48). Place your hands on your hips with your thumbs on your back and your fingers on the front of the hips. Inhale, and spread your feet 4ft (1.2m) apart. Your feet should be parallel, toes pointing forward. Press the outer edges of your feet to the floor. Ensure that you keep your back erect.

2 Exhale, and lift both kneecaps. Bend forward, extend your spine, and bring your torso down toward the floor. Look up as you bend to ensure that your back is concave. Take both hands off your hips, and lower them to the floor. Place your palms flat on the floor with your fingers spread out.

3 Widen your elbows, keeping your palms flat on the floor. Place the crown of your head on the floor between your palms. Push your sternum forward and draw in the abdomen. Move back the thighbones and groin to reduce the pressure on your head. Stay in the posture for 1 minute.

STRETCH YOUR HAMSTRING MUSCLES

ENSURE THAT YOUR HANDS AND HEAD ARE IN LINE

KEEP YOUR HEAD AND NECK PASSIVE

BENEFITS

◆

Reduces depression, boosts confidence

◆

Soothes the brain and the sympathetic nervous system

◆

Energizes the heart and lungs

◆

Reduces blood pressure

◆

Relieves stress-related headaches, migraine, and fatigue

◆

Tones the abdominal organs

◆

Relieves stomach ache by neutralizing acidity

◆

Relieves lower backache

◆

Strengthens the knee joint and makes the hip joint supple

◆

Regulates menstrual flow

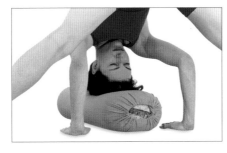

VARIATION 1 Head on Bolster

PROPS (*See page* 164) A BOLSTER helps those with stiff lower backs achieve the final posture more effectively and without strain.

GETTING INTO THE POSTURE Place a bolster on the floor, flat end between your feet. Follow Steps 1, 2, and 3 of the main asana. When you bend toward the floor, place your crown on the center of the bolster. Keep your head and neck relaxed. Shift your weight onto your heels and hold the posture for 1 minute.

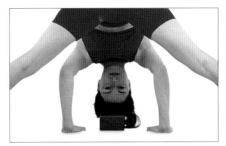

VARIATION 2 Head on Block

PROPS (*See page* 164) A WOODEN BLOCK will help you if you have a stiff spine and find it difficult to place your head on the floor. Use the block until your spine and the muscles of your back become more flexible.

GETTING INTO THE POSTURE Place a wooden block on its broad side, on the floor, and in front of your feet. Then follow Steps 1, 2, and 3 of the main asana and bend forward. Place the crown of your head on the center of the block. Hold the posture for 1 minute.

Adhomukha Svanasana

- Downward-facing dog posture -

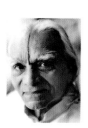

THIS INVERTED STRETCH brings fresh blood to the heart and the lungs, increasing the fitness of the entire body. *Adhomukha* means "facing down" in Sanskrit, while *svan* translates as "dog." This posture and its variations are less strenuous versions of the classic posture (*see page* 68), and allow a better stretch of the limbs while calming and soothing the mind.

PROPS (*See page* 164) A WALL AND THREE WOODEN BLOCKS. Two blocks against the wall support the hands, stretch the arms, and reduce strain on the shoulder joints. The third block helps those with a stiff back achieve the final posture.

SPECIFIC BENEFITS Helps increase self-confidence. Relieves headaches and hypertension. Helps rest and rejuvenate the heart. Reduces the "heavy-headed" feeling associated with menopause.

CAUTIONS
◆

Do not practice this asana if you have diarrhea or varicose veins. Patients of rheumatoid arthritis who have fever should avoid this asana. If you have a stiff spine or high blood pressure, or are prone to recurrent headaches, always practice all these variations with your head supported by a block. Beginners should not hold the final posture for more than 30 seconds. Gradually increase the duration to 1 minute.

LOWER YOUR HEAD TOWARD THE FLOOR

PUSH YOUR HEELS BACK AND PULL YOUR INNER ANKLES UP

1 Stand in Tadasana (*see page* 48) facing a wall, about 3.5ft (1m) away from it. Place 2 of the blocks on their broad sides, shoulder-width apart, against the wall. Place the third block on its long side, 18in (45cm) away from the wall. Separate your feet to a distance of 18in (45cm). Kneel, and place your palms on the 2 blocks against the wall.

BEND THE BACKS OF YOUR KNEES

2 Press your palms down on the blocks and walk your feet back until they are 4ft (1.2m) away from your hands. Make sure that your feet are in line with your hands and the same distance apart. Raise both heels, stretch your legs, and then lower your heels to the floor. Stretch your arms fully.

STRETCH YOUR
BUTTOCKS TOWARD
THE CEILING

3 Consciously stretch each leg from
heel to buttock, and from the
front of the ankle to the top of
the thigh. Raise your buttocks, stretch
your chest, and push your sternum
toward your hands. Exhale, then rest
your head on the third block. Press your
hands down on the blocks, extending
your arms fully. Stretch your spine and
expand your chest. Keep your throat
soft and elongated. Relax your eyes
and keep your brain passive.

PULL UP YOUR
KNEECAPS

EXTEND YOUR ARMS
FROM THE ELBOWS
TO THE SHOULDERS

PRESS YOUR FEET
DOWN ONTO
THE FLOOR

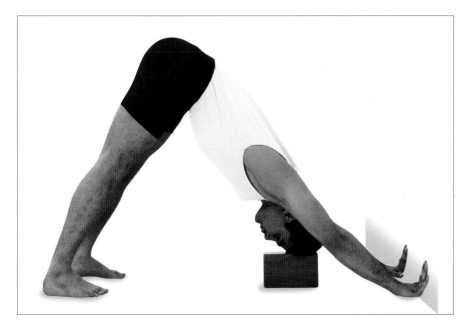

VARIATION 1
Hands against a Wall

PROPS (*See page* 164) A WALL AND A
WOODEN BLOCK. Placing the fingers
against the wall supports the shoulders
and reduces strain in the shoulder joints.

SPECIFIC BENEFITS Helps relieve
arthritis of the shoulders, elbows,
wrists, and fingers.

GETTING INTO THE POSTURE Follow
Steps 1 and 2 of the main asana,
omitting the blocks for the hands. Place
your fingers on the wall, ensuring that
both palms rest firmly on the floor.
Then follow Step 3 of the main asana.

ADHOMUKHA SVANASANA

BENEFITS

◆

Tones and relaxes the nervous system, helping relieve depression and anxiety

◆

Cures breathlessness, palpitation, extreme fatigue, and sunstroke

◆

Stabilizes blood pressure and heart rate

◆

Helps relieve chronic constipation, indigestion, and excess bile formation

◆

Relieves arthritis in the shoulders, wrists, and fingers

◆

Reduces lower backache

◆

Increases the flexibility of the hip, knee, and ankle joints, and strengthens the ligaments and tendons of the legs

◆

Counters the damage to the cartilage of the knee or hamstring muscles, caused by jogging, walking, and other sports

◆

Strengthens the arches of the feet and prevents calcaneal spurs

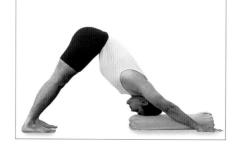

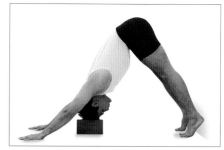

VARIATION 2
Head on Bolster

PROPS (*See page* 164) A BOLSTER AND A MAT. The bolster supports the head, helping those with stiff backs achieve the forward bend easily and without strain. The mat prevents you from slipping when you stretch out.

GETTING INTO THE POSTURE Place a mat on the floor. Place a bolster on the mat, its long sides parallel to the long sides of the mat. Follow Steps 1, 2, and 3 of the main asana and place your head on the near end of the bolster. In this variation, you should place your palms directly on the floor, omitting the blocks as support for the hands.

VARIATION 3
Heels against a Wall

PROPS (*See page* 164) A WALL AND A WOODEN BLOCK. Placing the heels against the wall reduces strain in the knee and hip joints.

SPECIFIC BENEFITS Strengthens the calf muscles, Achilles tendons, and the arches of the feet. Reduces cramps in the calf muscles. Stretches the back.

GETTING INTO THE POSTURE Stand in Tadasana with your back 4ft (1.2m) away from the wall. Kneel, then place your hands on the floor. Walk your feet back and place your heels against the wall. Lock your elbows, then follow Step 3 of the main asana.

"The ethical discipline of the asana comes when you extend your body correctly, evenly, and to the maximum."

Dandasana

- Staff posture -

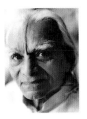

THIS ASANA IS the starting point of all the seated forward bends and twists. It has many positive effects, the most important being the improvement of posture. Dandasana teaches you to sit up straight with an absolutely erect spine, and is helpful to those in sedentary professions. Regular practice of this posture massages and stimulates the abdominal and pelvic organs.

CAUTIONS

◆

If you have asthma, bronchitis, breathlessness, rheumatoid arthritis, ulcers, or bulimia, or are experiencing premenstrual stress, practice the asana with your back supported by a wall. Also practice against a wall during menstruation.

PROPS (See page 164) A MAT, TWO WOODEN BLOCKS, AND A FOLDED BLANKET. The folded blanket placed under the buttocks helps stretch the legs, while the two blocks under the hands, help extend the torso.

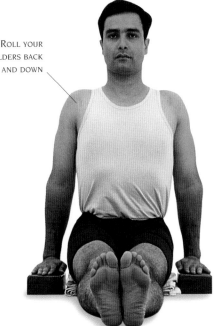

ROLL YOUR SHOULDERS BACK AND DOWN

1 Sit on a folded blanket, with your spine erect and your knees bent. Position the blocks on their broad sides on either side of your hips. Place your palms on the blocks and sit on your buttock bones.

2 One at a time, straighten each leg and join the inner sides of your legs and feet. Lengthen the calf muscles, and stretch your knees and toes. Keep your knees straight. Press your palms down onto the blocks and stretch your elbows and arms.

3 Lift your abdomen, freeing the diaphragm of tension. Hold the posture for 1 minute. Beginners may find it easier to separate their feet slightly, and should hold the posture for just 30 seconds.

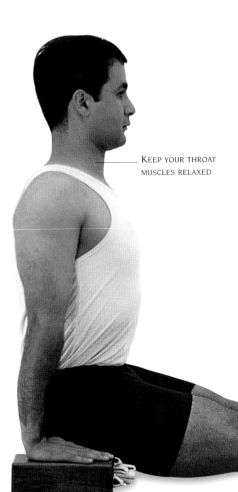

KEEP YOUR THROAT MUSCLES RELAXED

BENEFITS

◆

Improves digestion

◆

Tones the kidneys

◆

Helps prevent sciatic pain

◆

Stretches and activates the muscles of the legs

◆

Prevents tiredness in the feet by stretching the muscles of the feet

Virasana

- Hero posture -

THESE VERSIONS OF THE classic asana, Virasana (*see page* 84), are designed to make the posture easier for those with stiff hips, knees, or ankle joints by using rolled or folded blankets and a block or bolsters. In addition, the extension of the spine enhances the functioning of the heart, and helps improve blood circulation to all parts of the body.

PROPS (*See page* 164) TWO BOLSTERS AND TWO BLANKETS. The bolsters support the legs and give the torso an upward extension. The blankets, one folded to sit on, the other rolled and placed between the calves and thighs, relieve pressure on the knees and ankles, and distribute body weight evenly.

STRETCH YOUR SPINE UP

BENEFITS
◆

Reduces stiffness in the hip joints
◆
Reduces inflammation in the blood vessels of the legs caused by standing for long periods
◆
Alleviates pain or inflammation in the knees and tones knee cartilage
◆
Relieves gout and rheumatic pain
◆
Tones the hamstring muscles
◆
Strengthens the arches of the feet, and relieves pain in the calves, ankles, and heels
◆
Helps correct calcaneal spurs and flat feet

CAUTIONS
◆

If you experience leg cramps while practicing this asana, stretch out your legs in Dandasana (*see page* 82). Avoid practicing this asana if you have a headache, migraine, or diarrhea.

1 Place 2 bolsters parallel to each other on the floor. Kneel on the bolsters, keeping your knees together. Place the rolled blanket on your shins, and the folded blanket under your buttocks. Sit with your back upright.

2 Keep your chest stretched out. Imagine you are squeezing your kidneys and drawing them into the body. Place your palms on your knees. Look straight ahead. Stay in the posture for 30-60 seconds.

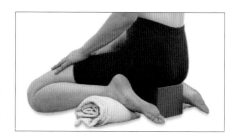

VARIATION 1 Sitting on a Block

PROPS (*See page* 164) A BLANKET AND A BLOCK. The blanket eases strain on the knees. The block supports the buttocks.

GETTING INTO THE POSTURE Kneel on the floor. Separate your feet and place the block between them. Sit on the block. As you become more supple, replace the block with a folded blanket. Position the rolled blanket in front of the block and place it under both your ankles. Your feet should point back and your toes should rest on the floor. Stretch the soles of your feet. Follow Step 2 of the main asana. Hold the posture for 30-60 seconds.

Urdhvamukha Janu Sirsasana

- Upward-facing single leg forward bent knee posture -

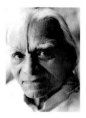

THIS ASANA IS A creative adaptation of the classic posture (*see page* 94). In this version, the back is erect and the head is tilted back. In Sanskrit, the word *urdhvamukha* means "looking up." In this posture, the action of the eyes looking up, synchronized with the upward movement of the head, stimulates the pineal and pituitary glands. This movement also helps refresh the mind.

CAUTIONS

◆

Avoid this asana if you are tired, have low blood pressure, blocked arteries, stress-related headaches, migraine, eye strain, insomnia, or diarrhea. If you have osteoarthritis of the knees, place a block under your bent knee.

PROPS (*See page* 164) A MAT, A BLANKET, AND A YOGA BELT. The blanket supports the buttocks. The belt helps those who are overweight or have stiff backs and find it hard to reach their feet. It also intensifies the stretch.

RELAX THE EYES
AND FACIAL MUSCLES

DO NOT TILT YOUR
HEAD TOO FAR BACK

BENEFITS

◆

Relieves lower and middle backache

◆

Reduces stiffness in the neck

◆

Tones the kidneys and the abdominal organs

◆

Relieves hemorrhoids

◆

Massages the reproductive and pelvic organs, improving their functioning

◆

Prevents prostate gland enlargement

◆

Regulates menstrual flow and relieves menstrual disorders

◆

Corrects a prolapsed uterus

1 Spread a mat on the floor and place a folded blanket on it. Then sit in Dandasana (*see page* 82) on the blanket. Bend your right knee, so that the sole of your right foot touches your left thigh. The right heel should rest against the groin. Loop the belt around your left upper heel. Pull strongly on the belt and lift the torso.

2 Straighten and stretch both arms. Press both thighs and the bent knee down on the floor. Tighten your grip on the belt, and stretch your spine up. Tilt your head back, breathing evenly. Hold the posture for 20-30 seconds. Repeat the posture on the other side.

Baddhakonasana

- Bound angle posture -

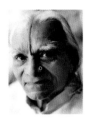

IN THIS SITTING ASANA, the knees are bent and the feet are joined to form a fixed angle. *Baddha* means "fixed" or "bound" in Sanskrit, and *kona* translates into "angle." The use of the props makes this version easier and more comfortable than the classic posture (*see page* 88). Regular practice of this asana helps relieve stiffness in the hips, groin, and in the hamstring muscles.

PROPS (*see page* 164) A BOLSTER AND TWO WOODEN BLOCKS.
The bolster below the buttocks lifts the abdomen and relaxes the groin, allowing the knees to descend easily. A block under each knee relieves stiffness in the hips.

CAUTIONS

◆

Practice this asana sitting against a wall if you have asthma, bronchitis, breathlessness, rheumatoid arthritis, peptic ulcers, or premenstrual stress. Make sure that your lower spine does not become concave, since this will strain your waist and hips.

1 Sit on a bolster placed at right angles to your body (*see inset below*). Place a block on either side of your hips. Sit in

Dandasana (*see page* 82). Bend your knees and join both soles together. Pull your heels closer to the bolster.

Beginners may find it easier to use a bolster positioned parallel to the hips (*see inset above*).

BENEFITS

◆

Stimulates the heart and improves circulation in the entire body

◆

Tones the spine, and the abdominal and pelvic organs

◆

Prevents hernia

◆

Alleviates sciatica and varicose veins

◆

Reduces menstrual pain, irregular periods, and leukorrhea

DO NOT TILT YOUR HEAD

RELAX YOUR EYES

KEEP YOUR NECK ERECT

LIFT YOUR DIAPHRAGM

2 Push your knees away from each other and lower them gradually onto the blocks. Place your hands behind your back and press your fingertips to the bolster. Open up your chest and draw in the abdomen. Initially, hold the posture for 1 minute. Gradually increase the duration of the asana to 5 minutes.

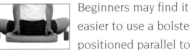

Swastikasana

- Cross-legged posture -

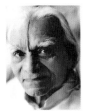

IN SANSKRIT, *swastika* means "crossed legs." This asana is one of the basic postures of yoga and symbolizes its meditative spirituality and physical rigor. Regular practice improves blood circulation in the legs. This asana is recommended for those who are on their feet for long periods. The posture also calms and rejuvenates the mind.

CAUTIONS
◆
If your feet ache while performing the asana, place a folded blanket under them. Beginners should hold the posture for only 20-30 seconds.

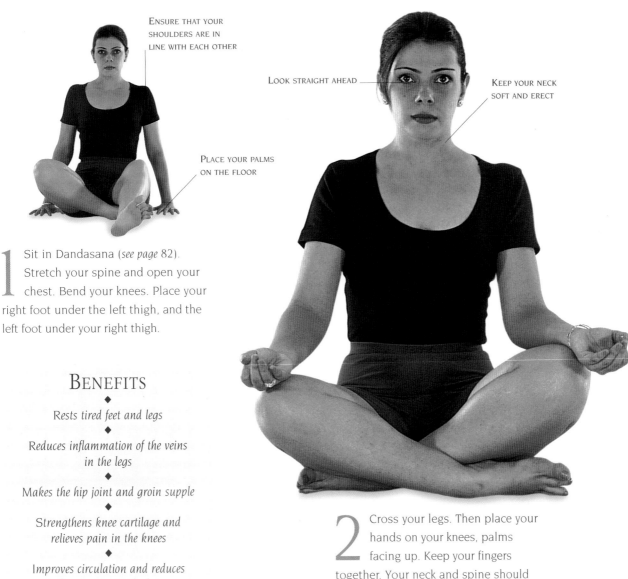

ENSURE THAT YOUR SHOULDERS ARE IN LINE WITH EACH OTHER

LOOK STRAIGHT AHEAD

KEEP YOUR NECK SOFT AND ERECT

PLACE YOUR PALMS ON THE FLOOR

1 Sit in Dandasana (*see page* 82). Stretch your spine and open your chest. Bend your knees. Place your right foot under the left thigh, and the left foot under your right thigh.

BENEFITS
◆
Rests tired feet and legs
◆
Reduces inflammation of the veins in the legs
◆
Makes the hip joint and groin supple
◆
Strengthens knee cartilage and relieves pain in the knees
◆
Improves circulation and reduces inflammation in the knees

2 Cross your legs. Then place your hands on your knees, palms facing up. Keep your fingers together. Your neck and spine should be straight and erect, but not tensed. Hold the posture for 30-60 seconds.

Paripurna Navasana

- Full boat posture -

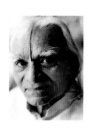

IN THIS ASANA, the body takes the shape of a boat. The word *paripurna* means "complete" or "full" in Sanskrit, while *nava* means "boat." The use of props in this asana allows the posture to be held without straining your stomach and back muscles. Regular practice of this asana tones the muscles and abdominal organs. It also exercises the neck and stimulates the thyroid gland.

CAUTIONS
◆

Do not practice this asana if you have a cardiac condition or low blood pressure. Avoid it if you have breathlessness, asthma, bronchitis, a cold and congestion, migraine, chronic fatigue syndrome; or insomnia, cervical spondylosis, severe backache, diarrhea, or menstrual disorders.

PROPS (*See page* 164) A WALL, TWO HALF-HALASANA STOOLS, TWO BLANKETS, A MAT. The stools support the legs and back, freeing the abdomen of tension. The mat is spread on the floor, and the two blankets cushion the back and legs.

SPECIFIC CAUTIONS The stools are essential until your stomach muscles, arms, legs, and back are strong enough to allow you to hold the posture on your own. Ensure that your neck and head are not strained during practice.

REST YOUR UPPER BACK
AGAINST THE STOOL

KEEP THE
MUSCLES OF YOUR
NECK RELAXED

KEEP YOUR
FEET RELAXED

1 Spread a mat on the floor, its short side against a wall. Place a stool against the wall. Place the other stool about 4ft (1.2m) away from the first stool, in line with it. Place a folded blanket on each stool. Sit between both stools, resting your back against the stool touching the wall. Place your palms behind your buttocks, fingers pointing forward. Bend your knees.

2 Sit on your buttock bones and press your palms down on the mat. Raise your right leg and place your calf on the stool in front of you. Your heel should rest on the stool. Breathe evenly.

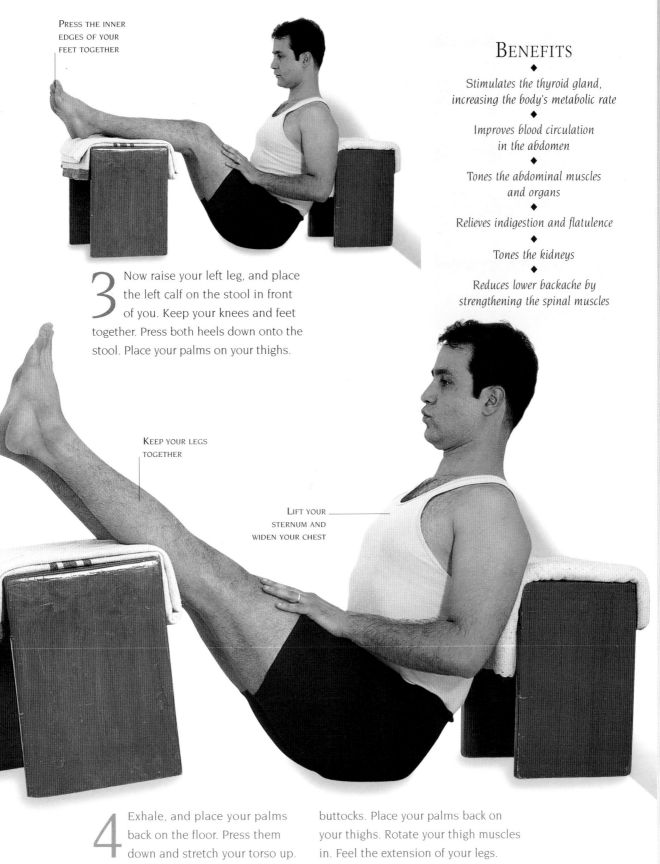

PRESS THE INNER EDGES OF YOUR FEET TOGETHER

BENEFITS

◆

Stimulates the thyroid gland, increasing the body's metabolic rate

◆

Improves blood circulation in the abdomen

◆

Tones the abdominal muscles and organs

◆

Relieves indigestion and flatulence

◆

Tones the kidneys

◆

Reduces lower backache by strengthening the spinal muscles

3 Now raise your left leg, and place the left calf on the stool in front of you. Keep your knees and feet together. Press both heels down onto the stool. Place your palms on your thighs.

KEEP YOUR LEGS TOGETHER

LIFT YOUR STERNUM AND WIDEN YOUR CHEST

4 Exhale, and place your palms back on the floor. Press them down and stretch your torso up. Pull in your shoulder blades. Straighten your legs and lift your calves off the stool, tilting the stool away from your buttocks. Place your palms back on your thighs. Rotate your thigh muscles in. Feel the extension of your legs. Keep your abdomen soft. Hold the posture for 1 minute, increasing the duration to 5 minutes with practice.

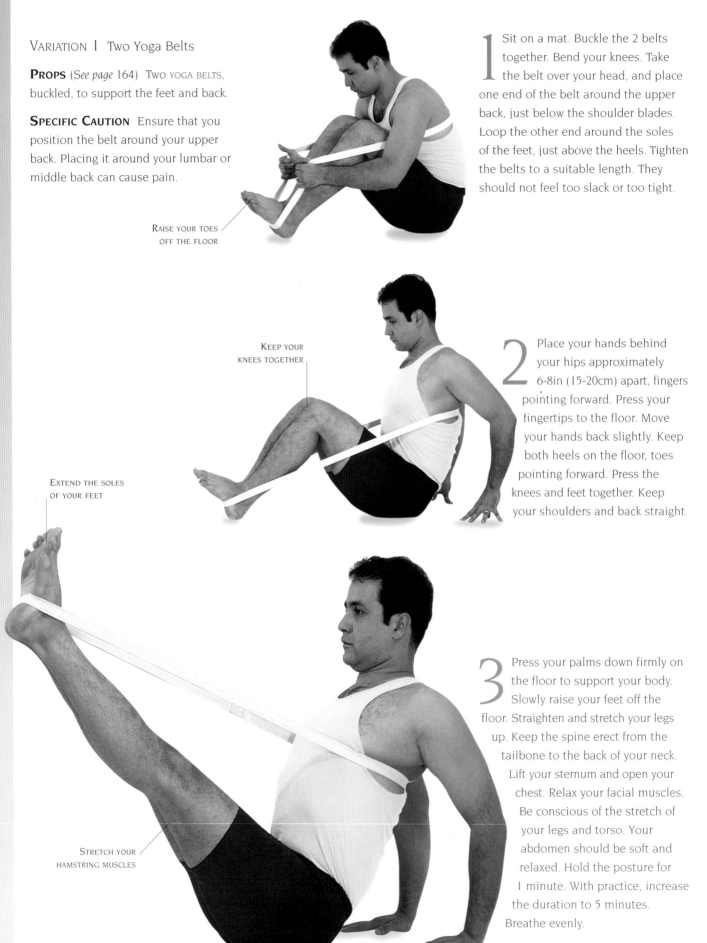

VARIATION 1 Two Yoga Belts

PROPS (*See page* 164) TWO YOGA BELTS, buckled, to support the feet and back.

SPECIFIC CAUTION Ensure that you position the belt around your upper back. Placing it around your lumbar or middle back can cause pain.

RAISE YOUR TOES
OFF THE FLOOR

1 Sit on a mat. Buckle the 2 belts together. Bend your knees. Take the belt over your head, and place one end of the belt around the upper back, just below the shoulder blades. Loop the other end around the soles of the feet, just above the heels. Tighten the belts to a suitable length. They should not feel too slack or too tight.

KEEP YOUR
KNEES TOGETHER

2 Place your hands behind your hips approximately 6-8in (15-20cm) apart, fingers pointing forward. Press your fingertips to the floor. Move your hands back slightly. Keep both heels on the floor, toes pointing forward. Press the knees and feet together. Keep your shoulders and back straight.

EXTEND THE SOLES
OF YOUR FEET

STRETCH YOUR
HAMSTRING MUSCLES

3 Press your palms down firmly on the floor to support your body. Slowly raise your feet off the floor. Straighten and stretch your legs up. Keep the spine erect from the tailbone to the back of your neck. Lift your sternum and open your chest. Relax your facial muscles. Be conscious of the stretch of your legs and torso. Your abdomen should be soft and relaxed. Hold the posture for 1 minute. With practice, increase the duration to 5 minutes. Breathe evenly.

Upavista Konasana

- Seated wide-angle posture -

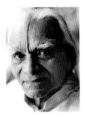

BY OMITTING THE forward bend of the original asana, this version of Upavista Konasana is adapted to help beginners and those with stiff backs stretch their legs out to the sides. The posture gets its name from the Sanskrit words *upavista*, which means "seated," and *kona*, which translates into "angle." This asana relaxes stress-related tension in the abdominal muscles.

CAUTIONS
◆
If you have asthma, you must practice this asana sitting on a folded blanket. The wall and blanket lift and open the chest, allowing for easy breathing. Avoid practicing this asana during menstruation.

PROPS (*See page* 164) A WALL supports the back and eases breathing.

1 Sit against a wall. Then sit in Dandasana (*see page* 82) with your shoulders and back touching the wall. Keep your back erect. Sit on your buttock bones. Place your palms on the floor, beside your hips, fingers pointing forward. Look straight ahead.

2 Press your palms down onto the floor and push your torso up. Exhale, and spread your legs as far apart as possible. Use your hands, one by one, to help you push your legs even further out to the sides.

POINT YOUR TOES TO THE CEILING

BENEFITS
◆
Helps treat arthritis of the hips
◆
Relieves sciatic pain
◆
Helps prevent and relieve hernia
◆
Massages the organs of the reproductive system
◆
Stimulates the ovaries, regulates menstrual flow, and relieves menstrual disorders
◆
Corrects a prolapsed uterus or bladder

3 Move your hands behind your buttocks and place both palms on the floor. Press your heels and thighs down onto the floor. Lift your waist and the sides of your torso. Rotate your thighs to the front. Shift your weight from the buttocks to the pelvic bone. Stretch each leg from thigh to heel. Hold the posture for 30-40 seconds.

KEEP YOUR NECK STRETCHED BUT NOT TENSE

PUSH YOUR HAMSTRING MUSCLES DOWN ON THE FLOOR

Paschimottanasana

- Intense west stretch posture -

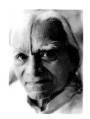

THIS VERSION OF Paschimottanasana uses five combinations of props that make the posture less strenuous than the classic asana (*see page* 102). These variations, which give an intense stretch to the back, relieve lower backache and make the spine more supple. When practiced, this asana cools the brain, calms the mind, and rejuvenates the entire body.

CAUTIONS
◆

Do not practice this asana if you have asthma, bronchitis, or diarrhea. Do not practice this posture if you have cervical spondylosis.

PROPS (*See page* 164) Two BOLSTERS support the head and allow people with stiff backs hold the posture more easily.

SPECIFIC BENEFITS Prevents sciatica and varicose veins. Relieves arthritis of the shoulders and elbows. Improves the circulation of blood in the arms, strengthening the elbow and wrist joints. Rests tired feet and legs. Helps treat incontinence.

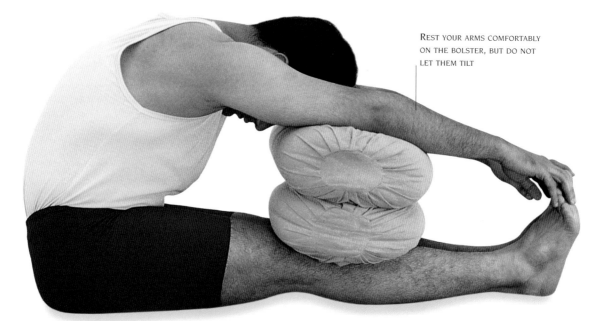

REST YOUR ARMS COMFORTABLY ON THE BOLSTER, BUT DO NOT LET THEM TILT

1 Sit in Dandasana (*see page* 82). Place 2 bolsters across your knees, one on top of the other. Make sure that your ankles, heels, and big toes are close together. Stretch your arms over the bolsters and bend forward. Hold your feet just below the toes, keeping both legs straight. Press your thighs and your knees together.

2 Bend from the base of your spine and push your waist forward. Elongate your torso toward your feet, stretching it from the groin to the navel. Make sure that your abdominal muscles do not contract. Rest your elbows and forehead on the bolsters. Keep the muscles of your thighs and calves fully stretched.

3 Stretch your neck. Push both your shoulders down and back, moving them away from your ears. Rest your forehead evenly on the bolsters, and do not tilt your head to one side. Your arms should be straight, but not tensed. Consciously relax your neck, face, eyes, and ears. Breathe evenly, and stay in this posture for 5 minutes.

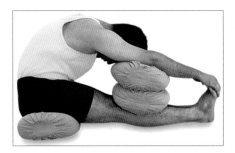

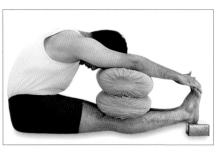

VARIATION 1
Three Bolsters

PROPS (*See page* 164) THREE BOLSTERS. Sitting on a bolster gives the torso height, making the forward bend easier.

SPECIFIC CAUTION Avoid this variation if you have varicose veins.

SPECIFIC BENEFITS Reduces acidity and prevents ulcers. Relieves menstrual pain and premenstrual stress. Helps treat stress-related disorders of the reproductive system. Prevents fibroid formation. Regulates menstrual flow by relaxing the uterine muscles. Relieves vaginal dryness and itching.

GETTING INTO THE POSTURE Place a bolster behind you, so that the center of the long side touches the back of the buttocks. Bend your knees. Press your palms down on the bolster and place your buttocks on it. Now follow Steps 1, 2, and 3 of the main asana.

VARIATION 2
Two Bolsters and a Block

PROPS (*See page* 164) TWO BOLSTERS AND A WOODEN BLOCK. The block under the heels gives the legs an intense stretch.

SPECIFIC BENEFITS Relieves arthritis of the shoulders and elbows. Alleviates osteoarthritis of the knees and ankles. Prevents varicose veins and sciatic pain. Reinvigorates tired feet.

GETTING INTO THE POSTURE Position the block near your feet with its long side facing you. Place your heels, one after the other, on the block, supporting the backs of your knees with your hands. Now follow Steps 1, 2, and 3 of the main asana. Make sure that you do not contract your leg muscles. Extend your thigh muscles and keep your knees firmly down on the floor.

BENEFITS
◆
Sharpens memory
◆
Soothes the sympathetic nervous system
◆
Prevents fatigue
◆
Rests the heart, normalizes blood pressure and the pulse rate
◆
Reduces angina pain
◆
Relieves chronic headaches, migraine, and eye strain.
◆
Reduces stress in the facial muscles
◆
Alleviates stress-related compression or a feeling of tightness in the throat and diaphragm
◆
Improves blood circulation in the pelvic area, toning the pelvic organs
◆
Regulates blood supply to the endocrine glands, activating the adrenal glands and relaxing the thyroid gland
◆
Cools the temperature of the skin
◆
Strengthens the vertebral joints and stretches the ligaments of the spine

"It is while practicing yoga asanas that you learn the art of adjustment."

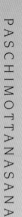

PASCHIMOTTANASANA

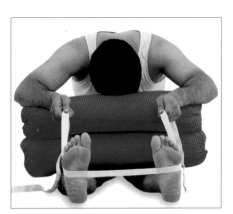

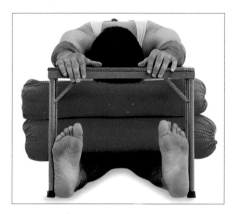

VARIATION 3
Two Bolsters and a Belt

PROPS (*See page* 164) A BELT AND TWO BOLSTERS. The belt helps those who are too stiff to hold their feet.

SPECIFIC BENEFITS Rests tired feet. Relieves osteoarthritis of the ankles. Prevents sciatica and varicose veins.

GETTING INTO THE POSTURE Follow Step 1 of the main asana, but separate your legs to a distance of 1ft (30cm). Point your toes toward the ceiling. Hold one end of the belt in each hand and loop it over your feet. Keep shortening the length of the belt until the pull feels intense. Then follow Steps 2 and 3 of the main asana. Widen your elbows and keep the belt taut.

VARIATION 4
Two Bolsters and a Stool

PROPS (*See page* 164) A LOW, OPEN STOOL AND TWO BOLSTERS. The stool helps you stretch your arms and spine. It relaxes the back of the head, throat, diaphragm, chest, and back.

SPECIFIC BENEFITS Helps relieve depression. Stimulates the liver and kidneys. Reduces ulcers, flatulence, constipation, and indigestion. Prevents varicose veins and sciatic pain. Relieves osteoarthritis of the hips. Prevents fibroids. Relieves vaginal itching. If practiced during menstruation, it regulates menstrual flow and reduces menstrual pain. Relieves stress-related headaches and migraine, if practiced with a crepe bandage around the eyes.

GETTING INTO THE POSTURE Place the stool on the floor. Sit in Dandasana and stretch your legs through the stool. Separate your legs until they touch the inner sides of the stool. Then follow Steps 1, 2, and 3 of the main asana, but do not hold your toes. Stretch your arms over the bolsters, and hold the further edge of the stool. Rest your forehead on the top

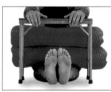

bolster and close your eyes. Breathe evenly. This variation, if practiced with the feet together (*see inset*) relaxes the neck, diaphragm, and back.

"Focus on keeping your spine straight. It is the job of the spine to keep the brain alert."

Adhomukha Paschimottanasana

- Downward-facing intense west stretch -

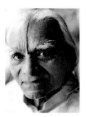

I N SANSKRIT, *paschim* literally means "west." In yogic terms, this refers to the back of the whole body, from the heels to the head. Although this asana intensely stretches this region, the props enable you to hold the posture comfortably, without strain. Regular practice of the asana tones the liver and kidneys. The stretch also alleviates lower backache.

PROPS (*see page* 164) A LOW, OPEN STOOL AND TWO BOLSTERS. The stool gives the torso height and helps those with stiff backs to bend forward easily. The bolsters support the torso and help make the posture restful and relaxing.

1 Sit on the front edge of the stool and place 2 bolsters beside it. Hold the stool and straighten your legs, keeping your legs and feet together. Place a bolster on your legs, parallel to them. Place the second bolster on top of the first, but about 2-3in (5cm) closer to your toes. Straighten your back and stretch your torso up. Take several breaths.

2 Look down and push your torso toward your legs. Stretch your arms out over the bolsters. Ensure that you stretch from the base of the spine. Keep your abdomen soft and breathe normally. Stretch your hands beyond the bolsters and hold the upper soles of your feet.

3 Rest your chest comfortably on the bolsters and place your forehead on the top bolster. Now, holding on to your feet, extend your torso down even further. If you cannot reach your toes, rest your hands as far down on the top bolster as possible. Hold the posture for 1 minute. With practice, increase the duration to 5 minutes.

PUSH YOUR
SPINE FORWARD

SIT ON THE FRONT
EDGE OF THE STOOL

BENEFITS
◆

Relieves stress-related appetite loss
◆

Helps in the treatment of acidity, ulcers, anorexia, bulimia, and alcoholism
◆

Tones the liver and kidneys
◆

Relieves lower backache

KEEP YOUR LEGS
FULLY EXTENDED

Janu Sirsasana

- Head on knee posture -

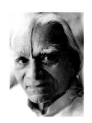

THIS ASANA CALMS the brain and the sympathetic nervous system. The mind detaches from the senses and feelings of restlessness and irritability are soothed. This adapted version of the classic posture (*see page* 94) is supported by props. It rests the heart and activates the *anahata* or "heart" *chakra* (*see page* 37), helping treat depression and alleviate insomnia.

CAUTIONS

Do not practice this asana if you have asthma or bronchitis. Avoid the posture if you have diarrhea as it will aggravate the condition. If your knees are stiff, or if you have osteoarthritis of the knees, practice with a wooden block under the bent knee. If you have a stress-related headache or migraine, practice the asana with a crepe bandage over your eyes.

PROPS (*See page* 164) A BOLSTER, A BLANKET, AND A LOW, OPEN STOOL. The bolster and blanket support the head and help those with stiff backs bend forward easily. The low, open stool facilitates the arm extension from the shoulders to the fingers. It also relaxes and stretches the back of the head and neck, creating a traction-like extension of the spine.

1 Place a low stool on the floor. Sit in Dandasana (*see page* 82) with your feet through it. Sit on your buttock bones. Press your palms to the floor beside your hips and straighten your back. Bend your left leg and bring the heel to your groin. Your toes should touch your right thigh and your legs should be at an obtuse angle. Push the bent knee as far back as you can. Keep your right leg absolutely straight. Place the bolster across your right calf, and place a folded blanket on top of it for added height.

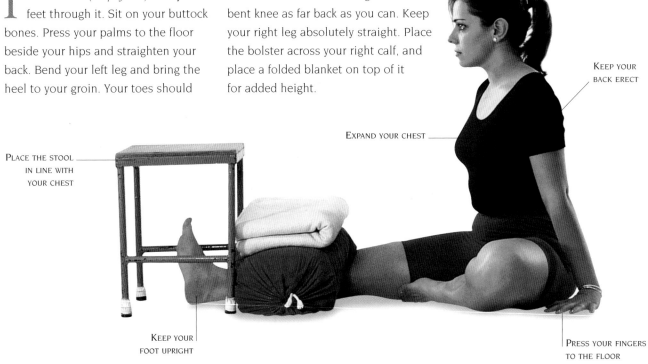

KEEP YOUR BACK ERECT

EXPAND YOUR CHEST

PLACE THE STOOL IN LINE WITH YOUR CHEST

KEEP YOUR FOOT UPRIGHT

PRESS YOUR FINGERS TO THE FLOOR

2 Exhale, and bend forward from the base of your spine, not from the shoulder blades. Stretch your arms over the bolster and rest your palms on the stool. Keep your left knee pressed to the floor.

PUSH YOUR
TORSO FORWARD

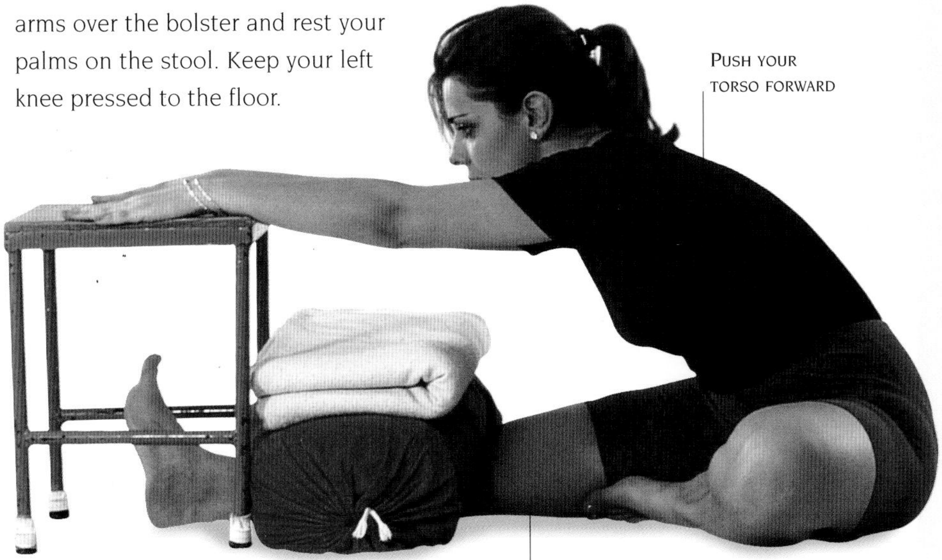

STRETCH THE RIGHT
LEG FROM THIGH
TO HEEL

BENEFITS

◆

Sharpens the memory

◆

Relieves chronic headaches, migraine,
or eye strain

◆

Helps normalize blood pressure

◆

Reduces angina pain

◆

Reduces stress-related appetite loss

◆

Vitalizes the adrenal gland and
relaxes the thyroid gland

◆

Improves bladder control

◆

Prevents enlargement of the
prostate gland

◆

Reduces menstrual cramps and
relieves dryness and itching
in the vagina

◆

Prevents fibroids and regulates
menstrual flow

3 Push your torso forward and hold the far edge of the stool. Stretch from the groin to the navel. Do not allow your abdomen to contract as you bend forward. Rest your forehead on the blanket and close your eyes. Exhale slowly to release the tension in your neck and head. Stay in this position for approximately 1 minute. Repeat the posture on the other side.

KEEP YOUR HEAD
AND NECK RELAXED

EXTEND YOUR
SPINE FORWARD

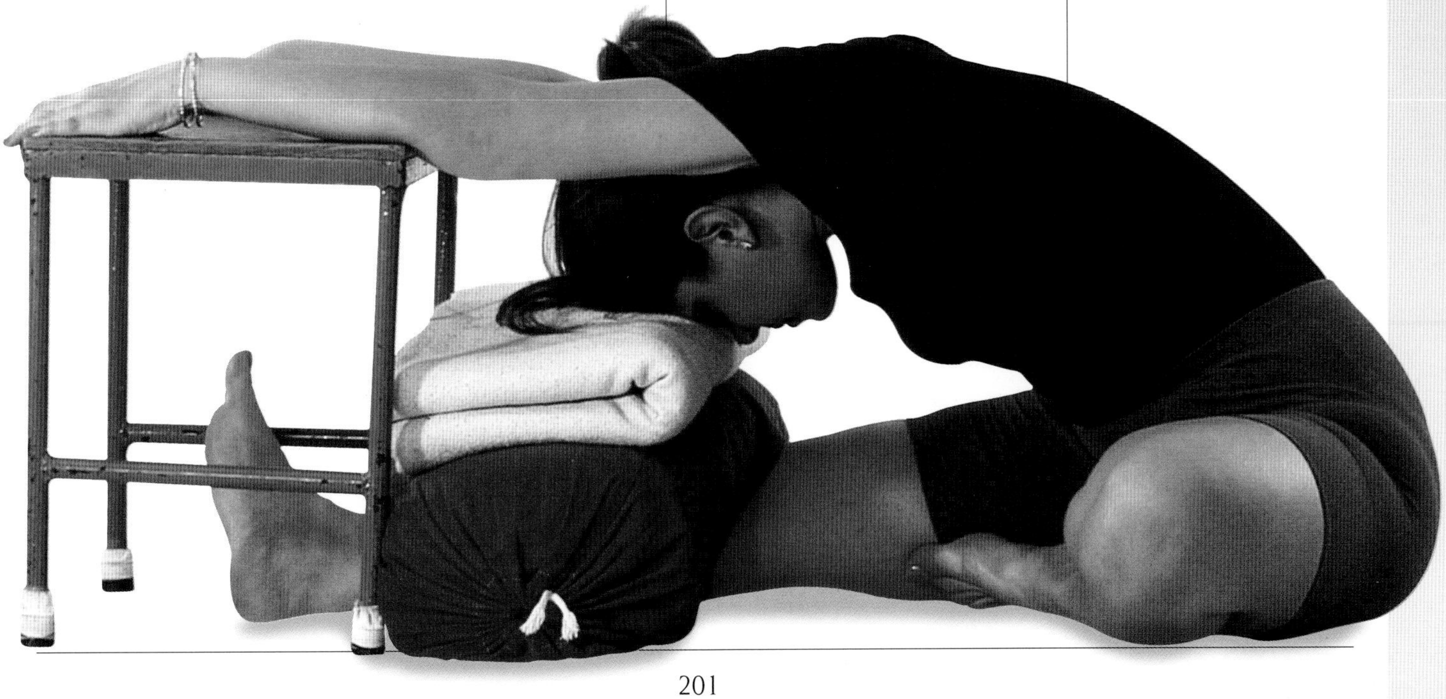

Adhomukha Virasana

- Downward-facing hero posture -

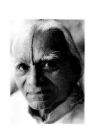

THIS ASANA IS A VARIATION of the classic posture, Virasana (*see page* 84). *Vira* means "hero" or "warrior" in Sanskrit, *adho* indicates "downward," and *mukha* means "face." This is a very restful asana to practice as it pacifies the frontal brain by reducing stress, soothing the eyes and nerves, and calming the mind. It also helps you rejuvenate after a tiring day.

CAUTIONS
◆
Do not practice this asana if you have osteoarthritis of the knees, breathlessness, bronchitis, diarrhea, or if you are incontinent.

PROPS (*See page* 164) A BOLSTER AND TWO BLANKETS. The bolster supports the head and eases stiffness in the back. A blanket supports the chest, while the second blanket under the thighs relieves painful ankles. If you have migraine, or a stress-related headache, wrap a crepe bandage around your eyes.

RELAX YOUR NECK

KEEP YOUR BACK ERECT

PLACE YOUR PALMS ON YOUR KNEES

EXTEND YOUR TORSO FORWARD

1 Place a bolster on the floor and put a rolled blanket on it. Kneel with the bolster between your knees. Place the second blanket across your calves and heels. Lower your buttocks onto the blanket. Place both palms on your knees and your feet close together. Imagine you are pulling your kidneys into your body. Pause for 30 seconds.

2 Move the bolster toward you. The front end should be in between your knees. Draw the bolster closer to your body so that it is just below your abdomen. Position the rolled blanket on the bolster so that you can rest your face on it. Now exhale, and move your torso forward. Fully stretch your arms out and place your hands on the floor on either side of the far end of the bolster.

3 Lower your chest to the bolster. Stretch your arms forward, extend the nape of your neck, and rest your forehead and face on the blanket. Push your thighs down, and lower your buttocks to the floor. Keep your abdomen soft. Open your armpits and extend your sternum. Push your chest forward, broadening your ribs. In order to relax your body, increase the forward stretch of your torso and spine on the bolster. Make sure your buttocks rest on the other blanket. Stay in the posture for 30-60 seconds.

THE GURU'S ADVICE

"The pressure of my hands on the student's sacro-lumbar area is like a fulcrum. In this posture, do not lift the buttocks. Extend the torso and hands forward. Keep the lower back firm and extend it forward."

STRETCH YOUR FINGERS AWAY FROM THE WRIST

REST ON THE FRONT OF YOUR FEET

BENEFITS

♦

Relieves breathlessness, dizziness, fatigue, and headaches

♦

Reduces high blood pressure

♦

Stretches and tones the spine, relieving pain in the back and neck

♦

Reduces acidity and flatulence

♦

Alleviates menstrual pain and depression associated with menstruation

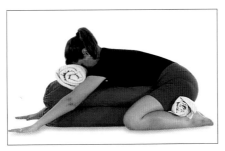

VARIATION 1 Two Bolsters

PROPS (*See page* 164) TWO BOLSTERS AND TWO BLANKETS. The bolsters help those with stiff backs hold the posture easily. The added height makes it easier to lower the chest.

GETTING INTO THE POSTURE Place 2 bolsters in front of you and follow Step 1 of the main asana. Now move the bolsters toward you. The front end of the lower bolster should be in between your knees. Then draw the 2 bolsters closer to your body so that the end of the top bolster touches your abdomen. Place the rolled blanket on the far edge of the top bolster. Now follow Steps 2 and 3 of the main asana.

Adhomukha Swastikasana

- Downward-facing cross-legged posture -

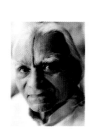

IN THIS ASANA, YOU sit cross-legged and rest your head, chest, and shoulders on a bench, bolster, and blanket. This is an extremely relaxing posture, relieving strain in your back, neck, and heart. It also alleviates the symptoms of premenstrual stress. Regular practice of the asana helps people who are prone to anxiety, tension, and frequent mood swings.

CAUTIONS
◆

If your feet ache while you practice this posture, place a folded blanket under them. If you have stress-related headaches or a migraine, wrap a crepe bandage around your eyes.

PROPS (*See page* 164) TWO BOLSTERS, A LONG BENCH, A MAT, AND A BLANKET. The bolster to sit on gives the torso height for the forward stretch. The bench, mat, bolster, and blanket between the chest and the bench, support the head and prevent neck strain.

REST YOUR UPPER TORSO ON THE BLANKET

STRETCH THE SOLES OF YOUR FEET

BENEFITS
◆

Soothes the sympathetic nervous system, relieving stress and fatigue
◆
Relieves migraine and stress-related headaches
◆
Relieves palpitation and breathlessness
◆
Helps prevent nausea and vomiting
◆
Relieves pain in the hip joints
◆
Rests tired legs and improves blood circulation in the knees

1 Place a bolster on the floor at right angles to the bench. Place a mat and a bolster along the length of the bench. Place a folded blanket between the front end of the bolster and the front edge of the bench.

2 Sit cross-legged as in Swastikasana (*see page* 191) on a bolster. Ensure that you are sitting on the inner sides of your buttock bones.

3 Exhale, bend forward, and rest your chest on the folded blanket. Place your forehead on the bolster. Bring your arms forward and bend your elbows. Place your right palm on your left forearm, and your left palm on your right forearm. Exhale slowly, and feel the tension in the head and neck dissipate. Keep your neck muscles soft and elongated. Hold the posture for 2 minutes. Breathe evenly.

Bharadvajasana on a chair

- Torso twist -

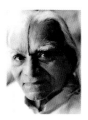

THE CLASSIC VERSION OF this posture (*see page* 108) is the basic seated twist, and can sometimes be difficult for beginners to perform. However, the asana can also be practiced seated on a chair. These adaptations of the classic posture are recommended if you are elderly, overweight, or recovering from a long illness.

PROPS (*See page* 164) A CHAIR supports you and allows for effective and safe rotation of the torso.

1 Sit sideways on the chair with the right side of your body against the chair back. Sit erect and exhale. Hold the outer sides of the chair back.

2 Widen your elbows. Push the right side of the chair back away from your body, exerting pressure, while pulling the left side toward you. Exhale as you rotate, but do not hold your breath. Look over your right shoulder. Hold the posture for 20-30 seconds. Repeat the posture on the other side.

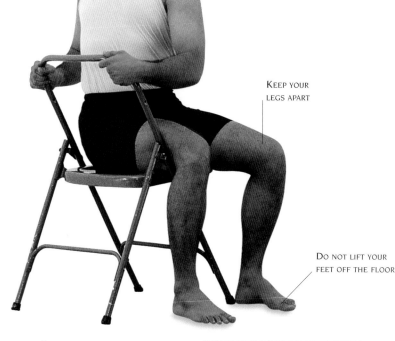

KEEP YOUR LEGS APART

DO NOT LIFT YOUR FEET OFF THE FLOOR

CAUTIONS
◆

Avoid this asana if you have blocked arteries, high or low blood pressure, bronchitis, headaches, migraine, eye strain, diarrhea, insomnia, fatigue, osteoarthritis of the knees, or during menstruation.

BENEFITS
◆

Makes the spinal muscles supple
◆
Relieves arthritis of the lower back
◆
Reduces stiffness in the neck and shoulders
◆
Alleviates rheumatism of the knees
◆
Exercises the abdominal muscles
◆
Improves digestion

VARIATION 1
Legs through the chair back

SPECIFIC CAUTION Avoid this posture if you have varicose veins.

GETTING INTO THE POSTURE Step your legs between the chair back and the seat. Hold the seat with your right hand and the chair back with your left hand. Rotate your torso to the right. Hold the posture for 20-30 seconds. Repeat the posture on the other side.

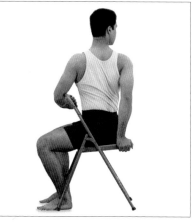

Bharadvajasana

- Torso stretch -

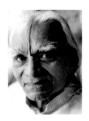

THIS ASANA IS A VARIATION of the classic seated twist (*see page* 108). It works on the dorsal and lumbar spine and improves blood circulation in the organs of the abdomen. Regular practice of this asana increases the flexibility of the entire body. It also helps in the treatment of arthritis, cervical spondylosis, and rheumatism of the heels, knees, hips, and shoulders.

PROPS (*See page* 164) A BLANKET AND TWO WOODEN BLOCKS. The folded blanket supports the buttocks and helps keep the body straight. The blocks placed under the hands keep the spine erect and improve its rotation.

CAUTIONS
◆
Do not practice this asana if you have a cardiac condition, high or low blood pressure, migraine, headaches, severe eye strain, a cold or chest congestion, diarrhea, chronic fatigue syndrome, depression, insomnia, or osteoarthritis of the knees. Do not practice during menstruation.

1 Sit in Dandasana (*see page* 82) on a folded blanket. Bend your knees and bring your feet next to your left buttock. Place your left ankle on the arch of your right foot (*see inset*). Press your knees together.

2 Place the blocks on their long sides, one behind the right buttock and the other beside your right knee. Then stretch your spine and inhale.

3 Exhale, and turn to the right. Move your right shoulder back. Place your right hand on the block behind you and your left hand on the block beside you. Press both hands down on the blocks. Raise your spine. Exhale and look over your right shoulder. Do not hold your breath. Hold the posture for 30 seconds. Repeat the posture on the other side.

KEEP YOUR BRAIN
AND EYES RELAXED

DRAW YOUR
SHOULDER BLADES
INTO YOUR BODY

BENEFITS
◆
Alleviates stiffness and pain in the lower back, neck, and shoulders
◆
Reduces pain in the hip joints, calves, heels, and ankles
◆
Relieves gout and rheumatism in the knees, and makes the hamstrings supple
◆
Helps treat disorders of the kidneys, liver, spleen, and gall bladder
◆
Relieves indigestion and flatulence
◆
Tones the muscles of the uterus

PRESS YOUR
HANDS DOWN
ON THE BLOCKS

Marichyasana

- Spinal twist -

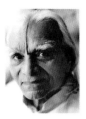

THIS ASANA ADAPTS and combines the two classic versions of Marichyasana, one a forward bend, and the other a twist (*see page* 112). The props help keep the torso centered and erect. They also enhance the rotation of the spine, working the dorsal and lumbar region. Practicing this asana helps reduce stiffness in the back, neck, and shoulders.

PROPS (*See page* 164) A BLANKET AND A WOODEN BLOCK. The blanket supports the buttocks and lifts the torso, increasing the spinal twist. It also prevents the bent leg from tilting to the side. The block, placed on its broad side under the hand, improves the spinal twist and keeps the torso erect.

CAUTIONS
◆
Do not practice if you have a cardiac condition, high or low blood pressure, migraine, headache, a cold or chest congestion, diarrhea, constipation, chronic fatigue syndrome, insomnia, depression, or osteoarthritis of the knees. Do not practice during menstruation.

1 Sit in Dandasana (*see page* 82) on a folded blanket. Place a block behind you. Bend your right leg at the knee. Make sure the shin is perpendicular to the floor and your right heel touches your groin. Keep your left leg straight.

2 Bend your right elbow and place your upper right arm against your inner right leg (*see inset*). Place your left hand on the block behind you, keeping your left arm straight. Press your right arm and your right knee against each other with equal pressure. Press your left hand down on the block.

3 Lift your torso, exhale, and turn to the left. Ensure that your bent leg does not tilt, and that there is no gap between your right arm and knee. Look over your left shoulder. Hold the posture for 20-30 seconds. Repeat the posture on the other side.

BENEFITS
◆
Alleviates lower backache and cervical spondylosis
◆
Increases blood circulation to the abdominal organs
◆
Aids digestion and reduces flatulence
◆
Helps in the treatment of hernia
◆
Tones the liver and kidneys

KEEP YOUR HEAD, EYES, AND NECK PASSIVE

KEEP YOUR PALM OPEN

REST YOUR FOOT ON THE CENTER OF YOUR HEEL

Utthita Marichyasana

- Standing spinal twist -

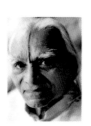

THIS VARIATION OF the classic posture (*see page* 112) is practiced against the wall with the help of a high stool. This asana works the paraspinal muscles and ligaments which rarely get exercised in our normal, day-to-day routine. The props allow the twist to be achieved without strain. Utthita Marichyasana is recommended for those with lower backache.

PROPS (*See page* 164) A WALL, A HIGH STOOL, AND A ROUNDED BLOCK. The stool makes the twisting action easier for those with stiff backs. The block placed under the left leg allows for a more effective rotation.

CAUTIONS

◆

Do not practice this asana if you have a serious cardiac condition, blocked arteries, high or low blood pressure, migraine, severe eye strain, a cold, bronchitis, breathlessness, chronic fatigue, depression, insomnia, diarrhea, constipation, or osteoarthritis of the knees. Women should avoid this asana during menstruation.

1 Place a stool against a wall. Stand facing the stool, with your left shoulder touching the wall. Put the block under your right heel. Place your left foot on the stool, and your left palm on the wall at waist level. Keep your right leg stretched.

ENSURE THAT THE STOOL IS AT MID-THIGH HEIGHT

KEEP YOUR FINGERS TOGETHER

2 Bend your right arm and rest its elbow on the outer side of your left knee. Place your right palm on the wall. Press your left palm against the wall and push your torso away from the wall. Ensure that your body is perpendicular to the floor.

MAKE SURE YOUR RIGHT LEG IS PARALLEL TO THE WALL

"*Total extension brings total relaxation.*"

BENEFITS

◆

Relieves stiffness in the neck and shoulders

◆

Improves the alignment of the spinal column and keeps it supple

◆

Alleviates pain in the lower back, hips, and tailbone

◆

Prevents the shortening of the leg muscles associated with ageing

◆

Prevents sciatica

◆

Cures indigestion

◆

Relieves flatulence

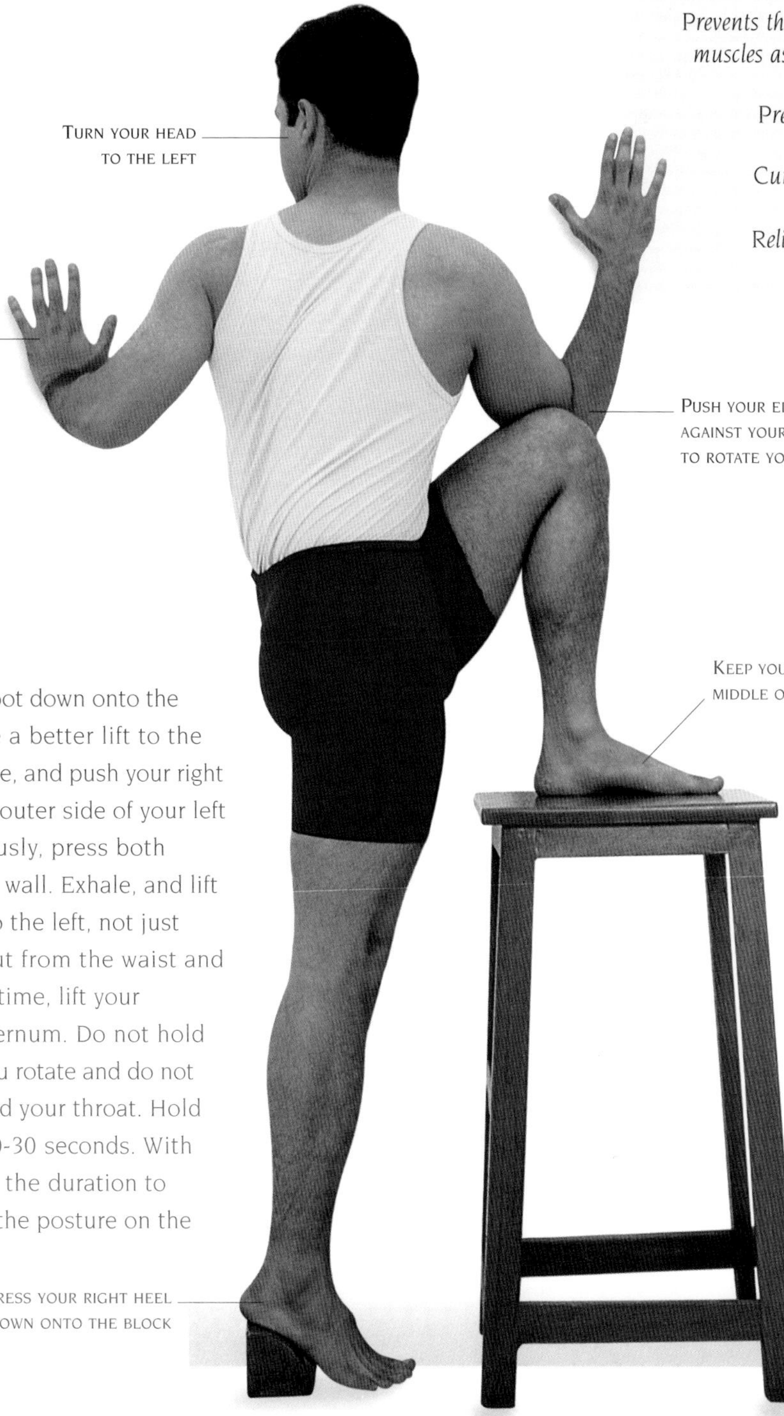

TURN YOUR HEAD
TO THE LEFT

PLACE YOUR
LEFT PALM FLAT
ON THE WALL

PUSH YOUR ELBOW
AGAINST YOUR THIGH
TO ROTATE YOUR SPINE

KEEP YOUR FOOT ON THE
MIDDLE OF THE STOOL

3 Press your foot down onto the stool to give a better lift to the spine. Exhale, and push your right elbow against the outer side of your left knee. Simultaneously, press both palms against the wall. Exhale, and lift your torso. Turn to the left, not just from the spine, but from the waist and ribs. At the same time, lift your diaphragm and sternum. Do not hold your breath as you rotate and do not tense your neck and your throat. Hold the posture for 20-30 seconds. With practice, increase the duration to 1 minute. Repeat the posture on the other side.

PRESS YOUR RIGHT HEEL
DOWN ONTO THE BLOCK

Parsva Virasana

- Spinal twist in hero posture -

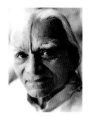

THIS ASANA VIGOROUSLY stretches the sides of your waist and back, improves blood circulation in the spinal area, and makes the shoulders and neck more flexible. *Parsva* means "side" or "flank" in Sanskrit, while *vira* translates as "hero." This asana rests and rejuvenates tired legs and is recommended for those who are on their feet for long periods.

CAUTIONS

◆

Avoid this asana if you have blocked arteries, cardiac disorders, high or low blood pressure, migraine, headaches, severe eye strain, bronchitis, a cold and congestion in the chest, or diarrhea. Do not practice during menstruation, or if you are prone to depression, extreme fatigue, or insomnia.

PROPS (*See page* 164) A BLANKET AND A WOODEN BLOCK. Sitting on the blanket reduces pressure on the knees and on the ankle joints. The wooden block, positioned on its long side and placed under your hand, makes it easier to rotate your torso and to lift and stretch your spine more effectively.

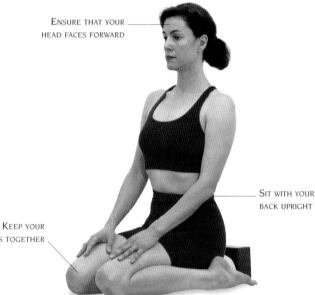

ENSURE THAT YOUR HEAD FACES FORWARD

SIT WITH YOUR BACK UPRIGHT

KEEP YOUR KNEES TOGETHER

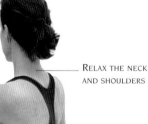

KEEP YOUR LEFT ARM EXTENDED

RELAX THE NECK AND SHOULDERS

1 Kneel on the mat with your knees close together. Gradually separate your feet. Fold the blanket, and place it between your feet. Lower your buttocks onto the blanket, making sure that you do not sit on your feet. Place the block on the floor behind your buttocks and parallel to them. Place your palms on your knees. Sit with your head, neck, and back erect. Pause for 30-60 seconds.

2 Exhale, then place your left hand on the outer side of your right thigh. Rest your right hand on your right hip. The inner sides of your calves should touch the outer sides of your thighs. Push the inner sides of both heels against your hips. Stretch your ankles and then your feet, from the toes to the heels. Feel the energy flow through your feet.

BENEFITS
◆

Improves digestion and cures flatulence by exercising the abdominal muscles

◆

Relieves lower backache

◆

Alleviates gout, rheumatism, and inflammation of the knees

◆

Lessens stiffness in the hip joints, and makes the hamstrings supple

◆

Reduces pain in the calves, ankles, and heels

◆

Strengthens the arches of the feet and corrects flat feet or calcaneal spurs

3 Open your chest and focus on your kidneys. Imagine you are pulling them into your body. Keep your spine upright by pulling up the inner portion of your buttocks. Press your knees firmly down onto the floor and stretch your torso up further. Exhale, then turn your chest and abdomen to the right. Move your right shoulder blade into your body, and increase the pressure of your left palm against the right thigh.

MOVE YOUR RIGHT
SHOULDER BACK

KEEP YOUR TOES
ON THE FLOOR

TUCK YOUR
SHOULDER BLADES
INTO YOUR BODY

KEEP YOUR NECK
STRAIGHT, BUT RELAXED

4 Turn, lifting your ribs and waist away from your hips, and twisting your torso further to the right. Straighten your left arm and pull in your left shoulder blade toward your spine. Place your right palm on the block and press it down firmly. Ensure that your buttocks rest on the folded blanket. Exhale, and twist your torso even further to the right. If you feel discomfort while rotating your torso, place a rolled towel under each ankle and sit on a wooden block (*see inset*). Hold the posture for 20-30 seconds. With practice, increase the duration to 1 minute. Repeat the posture on the other side.

211

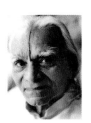

Salamba Sarvangasana

- Shoulderstand -

IN THE CLASSIC VERSION of this asana (*see page* 124), your hands and shoulders support your back, making the asana quite strenuous to practice. In this adaptation, a chair allows the posture to be held more easily and without strain. Regular practice brings benefits to the entire body. This asana is recommended during recuperation after a major illness.

CAUTIONS
◆

Do not practice if you have a migraine or a stress-related headache. Do not practice during menstruation. Ensure that your shoulders do not slide off the bolster onto the floor. This will compress the neck and might cause injury.

PROPS (*See page* 164) A CHAIR, A BOLSTER, AND A BLANKET. The chair supports the body, preventing strain, and helps you balance better in the posture. Holding the back legs of the chair keeps the chest expanded. The bolster supports the neck and shoulders, helping those with stiff necks. The blanket prevents the edge of the chair from cutting into your back.

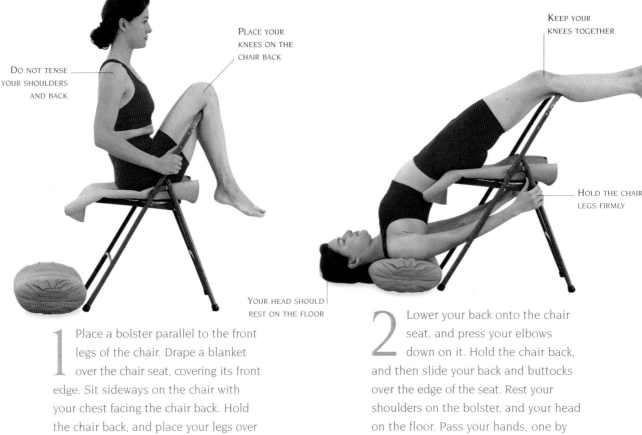

DO NOT TENSE YOUR SHOULDERS AND BACK

PLACE YOUR KNEES ON THE CHAIR BACK

KEEP YOUR KNEES TOGETHER

HOLD THE CHAIR LEGS FIRMLY

YOUR HEAD SHOULD REST ON THE FLOOR

1 Place a bolster parallel to the front legs of the chair. Drape a blanket over the chair seat, covering its front edge. Sit sideways on the chair with your chest facing the chair back. Hold the chair back, and place your legs over it, one by one. Slide your hands down the chair back and move your buttocks toward the back of the seat.

2 Lower your back onto the chair seat, and press your elbows down on it. Hold the chair back, and then slide your back and buttocks over the edge of the seat. Rest your shoulders on the bolster, and your head on the floor. Pass your hands, one by one, through the front legs of the chair and hold the back legs. Straighten your legs and pause for 1 minute.

KEEP YOUR INNER
THIGHS TOGETHER

PRESS YOUR SOLES
ON THE CHAIR BACK

BENEFITS

◆

Relieves stress and nervous disorders

◆

Alleviates hypertension and insomnia

◆

Reduces palpitation

◆

*Improves the functioning of the thyroid
and parathyroid glands*

◆

*Relieves cervical spondylosis and
shoulder pain*

◆

*Relieves bronchitis, asthma, sinusitis,
and congestion*

◆

Prevents varicose veins

◆

*Alleviates ulcers, colitis, chronic
constipation, and hemorrhoids*

3 Rest your head comfortably on the floor, and keep your neck and shoulders on the bolster. Hold the back edges of the chair seat. Bend your knees and place your feet on the top edge of the chair back. Make sure that your buttocks rest on the front edge of the chair.

SUCK IN YOUR
KNEECAPS

ROTATE YOUR
FRONT THIGHS IN

CONTRACT YOUR
BUTTOCKS

4 Maintain your grip on the chair seat and straighten your legs, one by one. Your buttocks, lower back, and waist should rest on the front edge of the chair seat. Lift your dorsal spine and shoulder blades. Intensify your grip on the chair seat. Extend your inner legs from the groin to the heels. Rotate your thighs in. Keep your neck soft. Do not hold your breath. Hold the posture for 5 minutes.

COMING OUT OF THE POSTURE

Exhale, and place your feet on the chair back. Push the chair away slightly. Slide your buttocks and back onto the bolster. Rest for a few minutes. Turn on your right, slide off the bolster and sit up.

Halasana

- Plough posture -

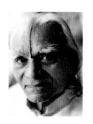

THIS VERSION OF Halasana (*see page* 130) uses a chair, a stool, and two bolsters to support the neck, spine, torso, and legs, allowing the posture to be held without strain. Practicing this asana helps alleviate the effects of anxiety and fatigue. The chinlock in this posture soothes the nerves and relaxes the brain. This asana is recommended for those with thyroid disorders.

CAUTIONS
◆

Do not practice this asana if you have blocked arteries or cervical spondylosis, or during menstruation. If you suffer from osteoarthritis of the hips, backache, peptic ulcers, or premenstrual stress; or if you are overweight, separate your legs in the final posture. If you feel choked or heavy headed in the final posture, separate your legs.

PROPS (*See page* 164) A CHAIR, A BLANKET, TWO BOLSTERS, AND A STOOL. The chair helps you go into and out of the posture with confidence, and allows the spine to be stretched comfortably. The blanket draped over the chair's edge cushions your back. The bolster placed beneath the shoulders prevents strain to the neck and head. The second bolster, placed on the stool, supports the thighs. The stool bears the weight of the body and supports the legs.

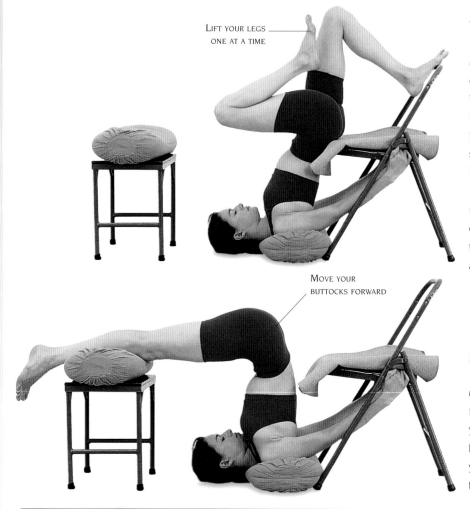

LIFT YOUR LEGS
ONE AT A TIME

MOVE YOUR
BUTTOCKS FORWARD

1 Place a folded blanket on the seat of the chair, ensuring that it covers the chair's front edge. Place a bolster on the floor, its long sides touching the front legs of the chair. Place a stool about 2ft (60cm) away from the bolster, and position the second bolster on top of the stool, in line with the first. Now follow Steps 1, 2, and 3 of Salamba Sarvangasana (*see page* 212). Then hold the back edge of the chair seat and bring both legs toward the stool. Keep your buttocks against the chair seat.

2 Place your legs, one at a time, on the bolster on the stool. Ensure that your neck is stretched and rests comfortably on the floor. Keep your shoulders on the bolster on the floor. Move your buttocks forward until your shins rest on the bolster and your torso is perpendicular to the floor.

BENEFITS

◆

Reduces fatigue, insomnia, and anxiety

◆

Relieves stress-related headaches, migraine, and hypertension

◆

Relieves palpitation and breathlessness

◆

Improves the functioning of the thyroid and parathyroid glands

◆

Alleviates throat ailments, asthma, bronchitis, colds, and congestion

◆

Relieves backache, lumbago, and arthritis of the back and spine

3 Bring your arms back through the chair legs. Shift your weight slightly to the back of your shoulders, and bring your arms over your head. Rest them, parallel to each other, on either side of your head, palms facing the floor. Bend your arms, and place your left hand just below your right elbow, and your right hand just below your left elbow. Keep your abdomen and pelvis soft. Stretch both legs from your heels to your thighs. Allow your eyes to recede into their sockets. Do not look up. Relax your facial muscles and your throat. It is vital to keep your throat stretched in the posture. You must bring your chest to your chin, and not the other way around. As your brain rests, your breathing will become deeper and longer. Close your eyes. Stay in this posture for 3 minutes. Breathe evenly.

EXTEND YOUR LEGS FROM THE THIGHS TO THE HEELS

LIFT YOUR BUTTOCKS

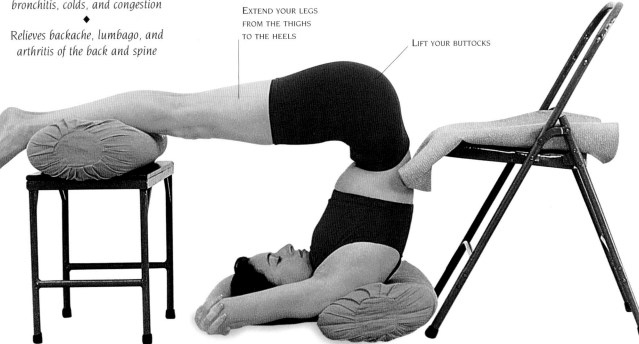

COMING OUT OF THE POSTURE

After you have held the final posture for the recommended duration, open your eyes slowly. Stretch your arms out on either side of your head. Then follow Steps I, II, and III carefully (*see right*). Make sure that your movements are not jerky, since this might strain your neck or back. Pause for a few seconds between each step.

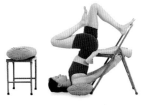

I *Hold the sides of the chair. Move your hips back until your buttocks rest on the front of the chair. Lift your legs, one by one, off the bolster and place your feet on the chair back.*

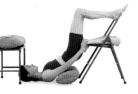

II *Hold the front of the chair. Move your buttocks off the chair. Push your shoulders off the bolster onto the floor. Slide your torso back until your head moves between the legs of the stool.*

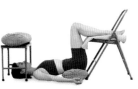

III *Rest your arms on the floor and your buttocks on the bolster. Rest your calves on the seat of the chair. Push the stool back. Bring your legs down. Roll onto your right side and sit up.*

Viparita Karani

- Inverted lake posture -

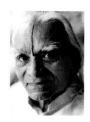

THIS IS A RESTORATIVE and relaxing asana, but the final posture is quite difficult for beginners and those with stiff backs. The use of props makes the posture easier and more restful. The name of this asana means "inverted lake" in Sanskrit, and is based on the belief that blood and hormones circulate better through the body when it is inverted. This asana alleviates nervous exhaustion, boosts confidence, and reduces depression.

CAUTIONS

◆

Do not practice during menstruation, although at other times this asana alleviates menstrual disorders. Make sure that you rest your neck and shoulders firmly on the floor. If necessary, use just 1 bolster.

PROPS (*See page* 164) A WALL, A WOODEN BLOCK, TWO BOLSTERS, AND A BLANKET. The wall supports the legs. The bolsters support the back and buttocks. A block placed between the wall and the bolsters creates the space to lower the buttocks slightly. The blanket makes the bolsters and block a single unit.

YOUR RIGHT KNEE SHOULD TOUCH THE WALL

PRESS YOUR HEELS AGAINST THE WALL

KEEP YOUR ELBOWS STRAIGHT

PRESS YOUR FINGERS DOWN ON THE FLOOR

1 Place the block on its long side against and parallel to the wall. Place the bolsters, one behind the other, parallel to the block. Drape the blanket over all 3 props. Then sit sideways in the middle of the bolsters, and place your fingers flat on the floor behind you.

2 Turn your torso toward the wall, simultaneously lifting your legs, one by one, onto the wall. Keep your knees slightly bent. Support your body on both palms, fingers pointing toward the bolsters. Push both palms down on the floor, and move your buttocks closer to the wall.

THE INNER EDGES
OF YOUR FEET SHOULD
TOUCH EACH OTHER

BENEFITS

◆

Regulates blood pressure

◆

Helps treat ear and eye ailments,
stress-related headaches, and migraine

◆

Relieves palpitation, breathlessness,
asthma, bronchitis, and throat
ailments

◆

Alleviates arthritis and
cervical spondylosis

◆

Relieves indigestion, diarrhea,
and nausea

◆

Helps treat kidney disorders

◆

Prevents varicose veins

DO NOT ALLOW
YOUR FEET TO TILT

3 Bend your elbows and lower your torso until your shoulders rest on the floor. Fully straighten your legs. If your buttocks have moved away from the wall, bend your knees and place both feet against the wall. Then press your palms down onto the floor, lift your hips, and move the buttocks closer to the wall. Straighten your legs.

4 Rest your head and neck on the floor. Lift your chest. Spread your arms out to the sides, palms facing the ceiling. Allow your chest, abdomen, and pelvis to expand and relax. Straighten and stretch your legs. Close your eyes and experience the serenity of the posture. Stay in the posture for 3-4 minutes. Gradually increase the duration to 5-8 minutes.

KEEP YOUR
ABDOMEN SOFT

EXTEND YOUR
ARMS AWAY FROM
YOUR TORSO

PRESS YOUR SHOULDERS
DOWN ONTO THE FLOOR

Setubandha Sarvangasana

- Full bridge posture -

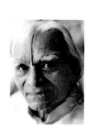

THE SANSKRIT WORD *setu* means "bridge," *bandha* translates as "formation," and *sarvanga* means "entire body." In this asana, the body arches to take the shape of a bridge. The chinlock in the asana calms the flow of thoughts and soothes the mind. The posture sends a fresh supply of blood to the brain, resting and revitalizing the mind and body.

CAUTIONS
◆

Make sure that your lower back touches the edge of the bench in the final posture. Your buttocks should not touch the edge of the bench, but should not be too far from it. Otherwise your shoulders will lift, causing neck strain. If you are recovering from a major illness, practice Variation 2.

PROPS (*See page* 164) A LONG BENCH, A BOLSTER, THREE BLANKETS, AND A YOGA BELT. The bench stretches the legs and buttocks and keeps the back arched. A bolster, with a folded blanket on top of it, supports the head and neck. Adjust the height and stability of the bolster by rolling a blanket around it, if required. The belt helps keep the legs together without strain.

SPECIFIC BENEFITS The reverse movement of the torso in the posture strengthens the back muscles, relieving neck strain and backache.

DO NOT ALLOW
THE BELT TO TWIST

1 Place a folded blanket on one end of the bench. Place a bolster on the floor in line with the bench, and touching one end of it. Place a folded blanket on the bolster. Then sit on the blanket on the bench with your legs stretched out. Place a yoga belt under your thighs and bind it around the middle of your thighs.

DO NOT TILT
YOUR HEAD

PRESS YOUR
THIGHS DOWN ONTO
THE BENCH

2 Exhale, and lower your back toward the bolster. Press each palm down onto the floor on either side of the bolster, fingers pointing forward. Both arms should support your upper back. Keep your thighs, knees, and feet close together, heels on the bench, and toes pointing up. Lower your arms to the floor.

3 Slide further down until the back of your head and your shoulders rest on the bolster. Straighten your legs, keeping your feet together. Stretch the heels and toes away from the torso to increase the stretch of the legs. Extend your arms to the sides, with the palms facing the ceiling. Hold the posture for 3 minutes. With practice, increase the time to 5-8 minutes.

RELAX YOUR FACIAL MUSCLES, NECK, AND SHOULDERS

BENEFITS

◆

Helps prevent arterial blockages or cardiac arrest by resting the heart muscles and increasing blood circulation to the arteries

◆

Combats fluctuating blood pressure, hypertension, and depression by soothing the brain and expanding the chest

◆

Relieves eye or ear ailments, migraine, stress-related headaches, nervous exhaustion, and insomnia

◆

Improves digestion and strengthens the abdominal organs

◆

Relieves backache, strengthens the spine, and relieves neck strain

◆

Helps rest tired legs and prevent varicose veins

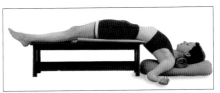

VARIATION 1 With a Rolled Blanket

PROPS (*See page* 164) A LONG BENCH, A MAT, A BLANKET, A YOGA BELT, AND A BOLSTER. The blanket supports the neck.

SPECIFIC BENEFIT Helps relieve cervical spondylosis.

GETTING INTO THE POSTURE Place a rolled blanket on the center of the bolster. Place a mat on the bench. Follow Steps 1, 2, and 3 of the main asana, bending your arms in the final posture. A bolster under the calves

 (*see inset*), stretches the legs, prevents varicose veins, and relieves

osteoarthritis of the hips and knees.

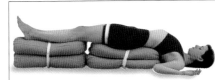

VARIATION 2 On 4 Bolsters

PROPS (*See page* 164) FOUR BOLSTERS, A MAT, AND THREE YOGA BELTS. This variation is easier for beginners, and if you are elderly, overweight, or convalescent.

SPECIFIC BENEFITS The bolsters help increase chest expansion, relieving breathlessness and chronic bronchitis.

GETTING INTO THE POSTURE Place 2 bolsters lengthwise on a mat. Place 2 more bolsters over these. Bind each set and your thighs with yoga belts. Lie on the bolsters. Slide down until your head and shoulders rest on the mat, your palms on either side of your head. Then follow Step 3 of the main asana.

Viparita Dandasana

- Inverted staff posture -

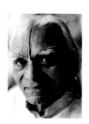

I N THE CLASSIC VERSION of this asana, the feet, hands, and head rest on the earth. The posture is believed to symbolize the yogi's salutation to the divine force. This adaptation with props makes the posture easier to practice, and helps soothe an emotional or restless mind. The word *viparita* means "inverted" in Sanskrit, while *danda* translates as "staff."

PROPS (*See page* 164) A CHAIR, A BOLSTER, A BLANKET, A MAT, AND A TOWEL. The chair supports your back and increases the flexibility of the neck and shoulders. Holding the chair's legs expands the chest, relieving respiratory and heart ailments. The bolster, with the blanket on top of it, supports the head. This soothes the nerves, and regulates blood pressure. The mat prevents the chair's edge from cutting into your back. The towel supports the lumbar spine.

CAUTIONS

◆

Do not practice this asana during an attack of migraine. Avoid the posture if you have stress-related headaches, eye strain, constipation, diarrhea, or insomnia. Discontinue the asana if you feel dizzy. If you suffer from backache, you must practice a few twists before and after this posture.

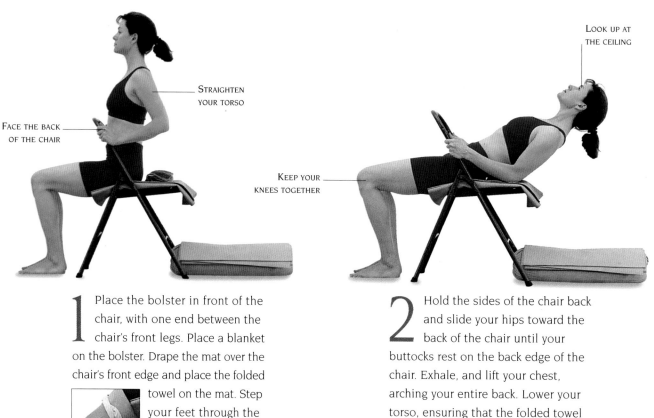

FACE THE BACK OF THE CHAIR

STRAIGHTEN YOUR TORSO

KEEP YOUR KNEES TOGETHER

LOOK UP AT THE CEILING

1 Place the bolster in front of the chair, with one end between the chair's front legs. Place a blanket on the bolster. Drape the mat over the chair's front edge and place the folded 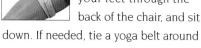 towel on the mat. Step your feet through the back of the chair, and sit down. If needed, tie a yoga belt around your legs to keep them together (*see inset*).

2 Hold the sides of the chair back and slide your hips toward the back of the chair until your buttocks rest on the back edge of the chair. Exhale, and lift your chest, arching your entire back. Lower your torso, ensuring that the folded towel supports your lumbar spine.

3 Place the crown of your head on the bolster. Ensure that your lower back rests on the front edge of the seat. Insert your hands, one at a time, through the chair to hold its back legs. Do not press your head down on the bolster. Keep it perpendicular to the floor since tilting the head too far back strains the neck and throat. Close your eyes. (Beginners should keep their eyes open to avoid disorientation.) Straighten your legs to increase the stretch of the back. Hold the posture for 30-60 seconds and, with practice, for 5 minutes.

KEEP YOUR STERNUM LIFTED

ROLL YOUR SHOULDERS BACK TO EXPAND YOUR CHEST

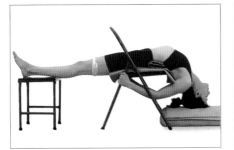

VARIATION 1 Feet on a Stool

PROPS (*See page* 164) A CHAIR, A LOW OPEN STOOL, A ROLLED TOWEL, A FOLDED BLANKET, A MAT, A BOLSTER, AND A YOGA BELT. The stool supports the feet. The belt keeps the legs together.

SPECIFIC BENEFITS Relieves diarrhea, abdominal cramps, and indigestion. Alleviates cervical spondylosis. Reduces pain in the back, shoulders, and neck.

GETTING INTO THE POSTURE Place a stool 2ft (60cm) from the chair. Follow Step 1 of the main asana. Place your legs on the stool, and follow Steps 2-3.

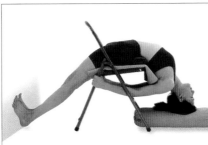

VARIATION 2 Feet against a Wall

PROPS (*See page* 164) A WALL, A CHAIR, A ROLLED TOWEL, A FOLDED BLANKET, AND A MAT. The wall supports the feet and intensifies the final stretch.

SPECIFIC BENEFITS Prevents varicose veins. Tones the hamstrings, ankles, and heels.

GETTING INTO THE POSTURE Place the chair about 2ft (60cm) from the wall. Follow Steps 1, 2, and 3 of the main asana, but press your soles against the wall. Stretch your legs, pushing the chair a little away from the wall, if necessary.

BENEFITS
◆
Soothes and relaxes the brain
◆
Builds up emotional stability and self-confidence
◆
Stimulates the adrenal, thyroid, pituitary, and pineal glands
◆
Gently massages and strengthens the heart, preventing arterial blockage
◆
Increases lung capacity
◆
Relieves indigestion and flatulence
◆
Increases the flexibility of the spine
◆
Alleviates lower backache
◆
Corrects a displaced bladder or prolapsed uterus
◆
Relieves menstrual pain and helps treat the symptoms of menopause

Ustrasana

- Camel posture -

THIS VERSION OF THE classic posture (*see page* 136), uses props to support the back, making the asana less strenuous to practice. The expansion of the chest in the posture alleviates stress by calming turbulent emotions. If you are feeling depressed or are prone to mood swings or anxiety, this will help to boost your self-confidence. The posture is especially beneficial to adolescents.

CAUTIONS
◆

Avoid this asana if you have low or high blood pressure, migraine, stress-related headaches, eye strain, rheumatoid arthritis, osteoarthritis of the knees, diarrhea, constipation, or if you are prone to alcohol abuse or insomnia. Do not practice the posture during menstruation.

PROPS (*See page* 164) A LOW, OPEN STOOL, A HALF-HALASANA STOOL, TWO BOLSTERS, AND TWO FOLDED BLANKETS. The stools support the back, gently massaging the heart and increasing coronary blood flow. This helps prevent arterial blockages and relieve anginal pain.

The posture lifts the torso and diaphragm, expands the lungs, and rests the brain. The bolsters, one placed on each stool, support the back and head, symmetrically curving the back in the posture. The blankets support the head and neck.

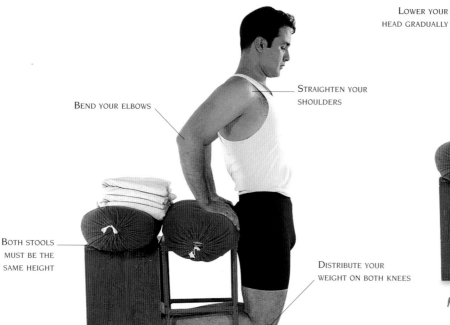

BEND YOUR ELBOWS

STRAIGHTEN YOUR SHOULDERS

BOTH STOOLS MUST BE THE SAME HEIGHT

DISTRIBUTE YOUR WEIGHT ON BOTH KNEES

LOWER YOUR HEAD GRADUALLY

LIFT YOUR STERNUM

1 Place the stool on the floor, with a bolster across its top. Place the second stool behind it. Position a bolster on this stool and put the blankets on it. Kneel in front of the stool with the open sides, and rest your palms on the bolster. Move your calves, one by one, between the legs of the stool. Your buttocks should touch the bolster on the stool.

2 Gradually arch your back, and lower your torso toward the bolster on the low, open stool. Broaden your chest as you move your elbows down on the first bolster. Then press your elbows down onto the bolster, and place your palms on your hips. Move your head back, toward the folded blankets on the second stool.

THE GURU'S ADVICE

"Once your head is placed on the folded blankets, you must ensure that you open the ribs, and move the shoulder blades into the body. Look at how I am pressing my student's shoulders back with my thumbs. Roll the armpits and chest forward and up. Lift your sternum. As your chest moves up, make sure that your head extends back on the blankets."

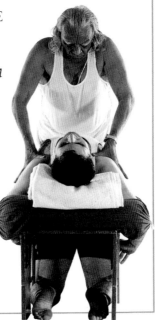

BENEFITS

◆

Enhances resistance to infections

◆

Stimulates the adrenal, pituitary, pineal, and thyroid glands

◆

Increases lung capacity, and helps maintain the elasticity of lung tissue

◆

Tones the liver, kidneys, and spleen

◆

Tones the spine, relieving lower backache and arthritic pain in the back

◆

Helps prevent varicose veins by toning the legs, hamstrings, and ankles

◆

Helps correct a prolapsed uterus by stretching the pelvic area

◆

Improves blood circulation to the ovaries and tones them

◆

Relieves menstrual pain and the symptoms of menopause

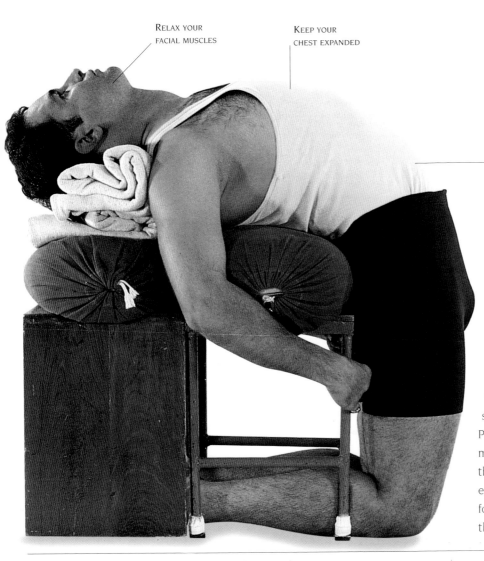

RELAX YOUR FACIAL MUSCLES

KEEP YOUR CHEST EXPANDED

STRETCH YOUR ABDOMEN

3 Lower your torso onto the bolster on the open stool until your head rests on the folded blankets on the second stool. Arch your neck, but do not strain your throat. Press your shins to the floor, and push the thighbones forward, away from the stool. Roll your shoulders back and move your shoulder blades toward your spine. Pull your spine, tailbone, and back muscles into your body. Stretch your thighs, hips, and buttocks. Close your eyes. Breathe evenly. Hold the posture for 1 minute. With practice, increase the duration to 3 minutes.

Supta Padangusthasana

- Reclining big toe posture -

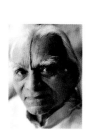

IN SANSKRIT, *supta* means "lying down," *pada* means "foot," and *angustha* means the big toe. These adapted postures work the whole foot, rather than just the toes. A yoga belt is placed around the sole of one foot. The resulting stretch to the legs increases flexibility in the pelvic area and improves blood circulation in the legs. It also makes the muscles of the legs stronger.

PROPS (*See page* 164)   A MAT, A WALL, AND A YOGA BELT. The wall steadies the outstretched foot, preventing it from tilting. It also ensures that the body is correctly aligned. The yoga belt, looped around the sole of the raised foot, makes the asana easier for those who are stiff in the hips and pelvic area.

CAUTIONS
◆

Do not practice this asana if you are recovering from a cardiac condition, or if you have blocked arteries, asthma, bronchitis, migraine, stress-related headaches, eye strain, or diarrhea. If you have high blood pressure, place a folded blanket under your head and neck.

DO NOT ALLOW YOUR HEAD TO TILT

PRESS THE BACK OF THE LEFT LEG DOWN ONTO THE MAT

STRAIGHTEN YOUR LEGS

2 Lower your back onto the mat supporting your torso on your palms until your head rests on the mat. Bend your right knee and bring it to your chest. Keep your left sole pressed against the wall. Loop the belt around the sole of your right foot. Hold one end of the belt in each hand. Make sure that you hold the yoga belt as close to your foot as possible. This opens your chest and keeps your breathing regular and even. Keep your extended leg pressed down on the mat.

1 Place a mat against a wall. Sit in Dandasana (*see page* 82) facing the wall. Keep a yoga belt beside you. The soles of your feet should touch the wall comfortably, toes pointing up. Press both your palms onto the mat.

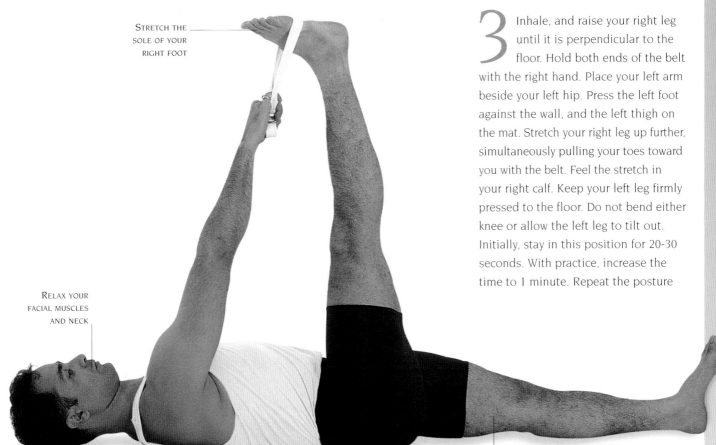

STRETCH THE
SOLE OF YOUR
RIGHT FOOT

RELAX YOUR
FACIAL MUSCLES
AND NECK

EXTEND THE
HAMSTRING MUSCLES
OF BOTH LEGS

3 Inhale, and raise your right leg until it is perpendicular to the floor. Hold both ends of the belt with the right hand. Place your left arm beside your left hip. Press the left foot against the wall, and the left thigh on the mat. Stretch your right leg up further, simultaneously pulling your toes toward you with the belt. Feel the stretch in your right calf. Keep your left leg firmly pressed to the floor. Do not bend either knee or allow the left leg to tilt out. Initially, stay in this position for 20-30 seconds. With practice, increase the time to 1 minute. Repeat the posture

BENEFITS

◆

Removes stiffness in the lower back, and relieves backache by helping align the pelvic area

◆

Prevents hernia

◆

Helps treat osteoarthritis of the hip and the knees by stretching the hamstrings and calf muscles, and strengthening the knees

◆

Strengthens the hip joint and tones the lower spine

◆

Relieves sciatic pain

◆

Helps relieve menstrual discomfort such as cramps, heavy bleeding, or pain during menstruation

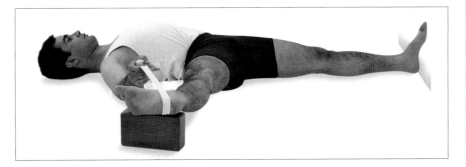

VARIATION 1 Foot on Block

PROPS (*See page* 164) A MAT, A WALL, A YOGA BELT, AND A WOODEN BLOCK. The block under the foot makes the posture easier for those who are stiff in the pelvic area.

SPECIFIC CAUTION You must keep your leg straight as you lower it onto the block. Allowing it to bend during this action might lead to injury.

GETTING INTO THE POSTURE Place the wooden block to your right. Follow Steps 1, 2, and 3 of the main asana. After you raise your right leg, exhale, then lower your leg to the right, keeping it absolutely straight. Place your right foot on the block. Pull on the belt and stretch your leg. Hold the posture for 20-30 seconds. Then repeat the posture on the other side.

Supta Baddhakonasana

- Reclining bound angle posture -

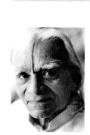

THE SANSKRIT WORD *supta* means "reclining," *baddha* means "fixed," while *kona* translates as "angle." This is a very restful asana that can be practiced even by those who have had bypass surgery. It gently massages the heart and helps open blocked arteries. The posture also improves blood circulation in the abdomen, massaging and toning the abdominal organs.

CAUTIONS
◆

Do not practice this asana if you have lower backache or poor bladder control. If you feel any strain while getting into the posture, use 2 bolsters instead of one. If you feel strain in the groin, place a folded towel or blanket on both blocks placed below the knees.

PROPS (*See page* 164) A BOLSTER, A BLANKET, A YOGA BELT, AND TWO WOODEN BLOCKS. The bolster supports the back and lifts the chest. The blanket supports the head, alleviating stress and heaviness in the head and neck. The belt helps maintain the angle of the legs easily and holds the feet together. The wooden blocks support the thighs, reducing strain in the groin.

GRIP THE SIDES OF THE YOGA BELT

RELAX YOUR SHOULDERS

POSITION YOUR KNEES ABOVE EACH BLOCK

PRESS YOUR SOLES TOGETHER

1 Sit in Dandasana (*see page* 82). Place a bolster behind you, its short end against your buttocks, and place a folded blanket on its far end. Place 2 wooden blocks on their broad sides on either side of your hips. Bend your knees, and join the soles of your feet together. Draw your heels toward your groin. Buckle the belt and loop it over your shoulders.

2 Bring the belt down below your waist. Pass it under both feet to stretch it over your ankles and the insides of the thighs. Move your feet closer to your groin. The belt should not feel too tight or too slack so adjust the buckle accordingly. Make sure that the end of the bolster touches your buttocks. Position a block under each thigh.

THE GURU'S ADVICE

"To bring your knees down to the floor, you must first widen the inside of your thighs and stretch the ligaments of the inner knees. Push the inner sides of your legs toward your knees and widen the groin. Then your knees will descend easily. The belt's position is also important. Here, I am adjusting the student's belt to flatten the thighs as much as possible."

BENEFITS

Regulates blood pressure

Prevents hernia as the hips and groin become more supple

Relieves varicose veins and sciatica

Reduces the pain caused by hemorrhoids

Relieves indigestion and flatulence

Tones the kidneys

Improves blood circulation in the ovarian region, and is particularly beneficial during puberty and menopause

Alleviates menstrual pain and leukorrhea

Corrects a prolapsed uterus

3 Place your elbows on the floor, and lower your head and back onto the bolster. Make sure that the bolster comfortably supports the length of your back and your head. Your spine should be on the center of the bolster. Stretch your arms out to the sides with the palms facing the ceiling. Relax, and extend your groin out to the sides. Feel the expansion of the pelvis and the release of tension in your ankles and knees. Initially, stay in the posture for 1 minute. With practice, increase the duration to 5-10 minutes.

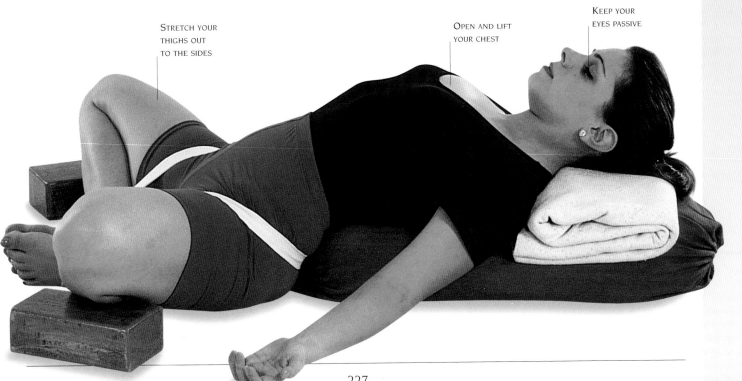

STRETCH YOUR THIGHS OUT TO THE SIDES

OPEN AND LIFT YOUR CHEST

KEEP YOUR EYES PASSIVE

Supta Virasana

- Reclining hero posture -

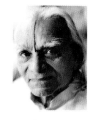

THIS ASANA IS LESS strenuous than the classic posture (*see page* 146). Practice the asana at the beginning of your yoga session since it calms a restless and agitated mind and induces the right mood for your practice. The posture reduces fatigue and stimulates the entire body. The chest expansion in the asana is particularly beneficial for the heart.

CAUTIONS
◆

Do not practice this asana if you have lower backache. Only practice the posture under expert supervision if you have angina or partially blocked arteries, or are recovering from bypass surgery.

PROPS (*See page* 164) A BOLSTER AND A ROLLED BLANKET. The bolster helps people with stiff backs to practice easily. It helps prevent the knees from lifting off the floor. It also helps maintain the lift of the chest and the stretch of the torso. The folded blanket under the head prevents eye strain and ensures that the head and neck do not tilt to one side.

PULL YOUR ABDOMEN UP TOWARD YOUR CHEST

KEEP YOUR KNEES PRESSED DOWN ONTO THE FLOOR

STRAIGHTEN YOUR SHOULDERS

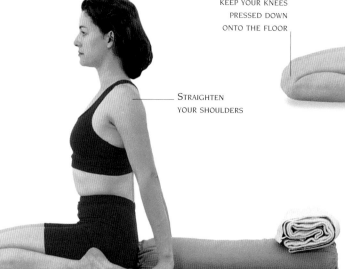

2 Press your palms onto the floor, bend both elbows, and lean back toward the bolster. Place your elbows and forearms on the floor one at a time. Gradually lower your back onto the bolster. To avoid strain in the pelvic area or the thighs, ensure that your knees remain firmly on the floor.

1 Kneel in Virasana (*see page* 84) and place a bolster behind you, the short end touching your buttocks. Place a rolled blanket on the far end. Make sure that the inner sides of your feet touch your hips. Keep your back straight. Place your fingers on the floor beside your toes.

FEEL THE STRETCH IN YOUR KNEES

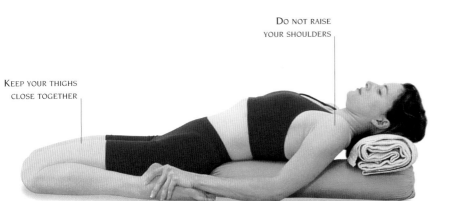

KEEP YOUR THIGHS
CLOSE TOGETHER

DO NOT RAISE
YOUR SHOULDERS

BENEFITS

◆

Helps prevent arterial blockages by gently massaging and strengthening the heart and increasing coronary blood flow

◆

Increases the elasticity of lung tissue

◆

Enhances resistance to infections

◆

Relieves indigestion, acidity, and flatulence

◆

Corrects a prolapsed uterus, and tones the pelvic organs

◆

Reduces inflammation in the knees, and relieves gout and rheumatic pain

◆

Relieves pain in the legs and feet and rests them, alleviating the effects of long hours of standing

◆

Helps correct flat feet

3 Once you lower your back onto the bolster, rest the back of your head on the rolled blanket. Keep your chest fully expanded. Press your shoulder blades down onto the bolster to lift your chest. Extend your toes and ankles toward the bolster. Push your feet closer to your hips with your hands. Extend the pelvis, and press your thighs close together.

4 Move your arms out to the sides, palms facing up. Extend your neck, but keep your throat relaxed. Drop your eyelids down gently. Experience the relaxation of the thighs and the abdomen, and the lift of the chest. Feel the continuous stretch from the cervical spine to the tailbone. Initially, stay in the posture for 1 minute. With practice, increase the duration to 5-10 minutes.

OPEN YOUR
CHEST, AND
LIFT YOUR RIBS

RELAX YOUR
FACIAL MUSCLES

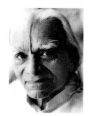

Ujjayi Pranayama

- Expanding conquest of life-force energy -

THIS IS THE BASIC FORM OF pranayama (*see page* 32). U*d* means "expand" in Sanskrit, *jaya* means "conquest," *prana* means "life-force," and *ayama* is the "distribution" of that force or energy. Pranayama is not just cycles of inhalation and exhalation, nor is it merely deep breathing. The practice of pranayama goes beyond these to link our physiological and spiritual dimensions. There are four stages to this pranayama. Attempt each stage sequentially, one at a time.

CAUTIONS

◆

This is not recommended for beginners. Intermediate students must practice with props. Never swallow saliva during or between inhalation and exhalation. Swallow after a complete exhalation. Do not practice if you have severe backache or constipation. Also do not practice if you are feeling tired, since exertion can be harmful for the lungs and the heart. Do not practice strenuous yoga asanas after pranayama. Before pranayama, practice a few reclining asanas to expand the abdominal cavity and the diaphragm.

PROPS (*see page* 164) TWO FOAM BLOCKS, TWO WOODEN BLOCKS, A ROLLED BLANKET, A CREPE BANDAGE, AND A MAT. The blanket and the two wooden blocks raise the head above the level of the chest, freeing and expanding the diaphragm. They also support the middle back and ribs and help stretch the intercostal muscles. The foam blocks lift the chest and keep the abdominal muscles soft. The rolled blanket helps relax the head and brain, stopping the flow of thought. The crepe bandage helps focus the mind and turn thoughts inward.

PREPARATION Hold one end of the bandage just above your ear and wrap it around your forehead 3 times, winding it over your eyes and ears. Make sure you tuck in the end of the bandage at your temple, as Geeta Iyengar (*see right*), demonstrates on the student. If you tuck it in at the back of the head, you will not be able to rest your head evenly on the blanket. Ensure that the bandage is neither too tight nor too loose. It should cover your forehead and eyes, but should not press down on your nose.

1 Spread a mat on the floor. Place 2 foam blocks about 1ft (30cm) from the mat's edge, the top one protruding over the right end of the lower one (*see inset*). Place the wooden blocks on their long sides, one parallel to the foam blocks, and the other at right angles to the first. Place a rolled blanket on the second wooden block.

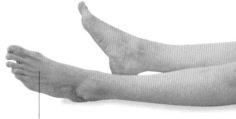

ALLOW YOUR
FEET TO TILT OUT

2 Sit in Dandasana (*see page* 82) and put on the bandage. Place your elbows and forearms on the mat and lower your back onto the foam blocks. There should be a slight gap between your buttocks and the blocks, as Geeta Iyengar demonstrates to the student (*see below*). Place your shoulders on the first wooden block, and push your lower shoulder blades into your chest, away from your spine and not toward your ears. This helps broaden your thoracic cavity, allowing you to inhale deeply. Rest the back of your head comfortably on the rolled blanket, but do not allow it to tilt back. Relax your jaws, and rest your tongue on your lower jaw, since this helps prevent the accumulation of saliva.

THE GURU'S ADVICE

" *Follow the instructions carefully. Remember that faulty practice can strain the lungs and diaphragm. Set aside 40-60 minutes at a fixed time of day for the pranayama. Never practice just after a meal or immediately after an energetic session of asanas.*"

3 Relax your throat. Stretch your legs out slowly, one at a time. Consciously relax every part of your body including your skin. Imagine you are pushing the skin of your scalp toward your brow. This calms the frontal brain while keeping it alert.

This is the key to complete physical, psychological, and neuro-physiological relaxation. Focus on an imaginary point inside your chest to exclude all external disturbances. Close your eyelids completely, but gently. Do not close your eyelids tightly. If your pupils move up, your mind will fill with thoughts and tension. Look inward and feel your senses withdraw.

RELAX YOUR
NECK MUSCLES

MAKE SURE THE
BANDAGE IS NOT
TOO TIGHT

MOVE YOUR SHOULDERS
AWAY FROM YOUR NECK

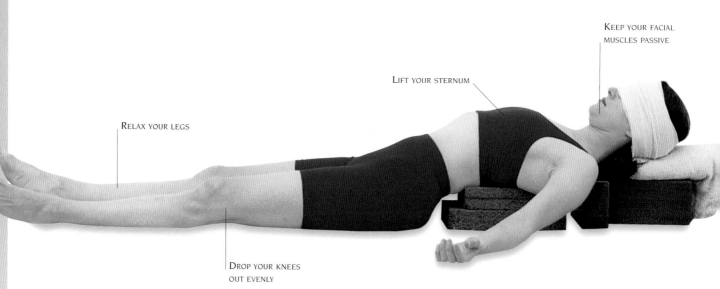

KEEP YOUR FACIAL
MUSCLES PASSIVE

LIFT YOUR STERNUM

RELAX YOUR LEGS

DROP YOUR KNEES
OUT EVENLY

STAGES Attempt the four stages in sequence. Each cycle of breath begins with an inhalation and ends with an exhalation, both of equal duration. Do not worry about the duration or retention of your breath; with practice, it will become steady, resonant, and rhythmic. Beginners should not attempt more than the advised cycles of the pranayama. Always stop before reaching the limit of your endurance. Practice each stage for 5-8 minutes.

1 This is a preparatory stage and consists of normal inhalation and exhalation. Breathe naturally, but consciously. When you inhale, expand your chest fully, but do not tense your diaphragm. Be conscious of your breathing, but do not breathe deeply. Practice 10 cycles.

2 This stage involves normal inhalation and deep exhalation. Inhale, then exhale slowly, deeply, and steadily, releasing all the air in your lungs. Keep your sternum lifted. Synchronize the movements of your diaphragm and abdomen, keeping the flow of breath smooth and uniform. Practice 15 cycles.

3 This stage involves deep inhalation and normal exhalation. Exhale without strain, then inhale slowly and deeply. Feel your breath move up from the pelvis to the pit of the throat, and then spread to each side of your torso. Practice 15-20 cycles.

4 The final stage consists of deep inhalation and deep exhalation. Exhale, emptying your lungs without strain. Then, inhale slowly, deeply, and smoothly. Exhale silently, until the lungs feel completely empty. Practice 15-20 cycles. End the pranayama with an exhalation.

BENEFITS
◆
Relieves depression and boosts confidence
◆
Alleviates cardiac disorders
◆
Normalizes blood pressure
◆
Relieves asthma
◆
Invigorates the nervous system

COMING OUT OF THE POSTURE
◆
Roll gently off the foam blocks onto your right side.
Sit up slowly and move the blocks away. Now lie down in Savasana (*see page* 150) with a blanket under your head and neck. Remain in the posture for 5 minutes, breathing normally. Then turn onto your right side again. Place your left hand on the right hand. Pause, then supporting yourself on your left hand, sit up slowly and sit cross-legged.
Remove the bandage and open your eyes gently.
Rest for a few moments.

Viloma 2 Pranayama

- Interrupted breathing cycle -

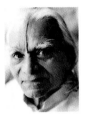

THIS PRANAYAMA IS PRACTICED in three stages and each stage can require 3-4 weeks to perfect. Each stage is more subtle than the preceding one and requires a greater level of awareness. *Viloma* means "against the natural course" in Sanskrit, and in this pranayama you have to hold your breath for two seconds during each breathing cycle.

PROPS (*see page* 164) TWO FOAM BLOCKS, TWO WOODEN BLOCKS, A CREPE BANDAGE, AND A MAT. The foam blocks support the back, lift the chest, and keep the abdominal muscles relaxed. The two wooden blocks lift the head above the chest, expanding the diaphragm, middle back, and ribs, helping stretch stiff intercostal muscles. The bandage helps to turn the mind inward.

CAUTIONS
◆

Do not practice if you have severe backache, constipation, or diarrhea. If you feel out of breath or fatigued, finish the cycle you are on, take a few normal breaths, and then resume your practice. Swallow your saliva only after a complete exhalation. Practice a few cycles of Stage 1, followed by Stage 2, before attempting all 3 stages sequentially. Never start your practice with Stage 3. Always stop before you reach your limit. Beginners should not practice more than 6 cycles.

BENEFITS
◆

Brings lightness to the body and serenity to the mind
◆
Regulates blood pressure
◆
Reduces eye strain and headaches
◆
Relieves symptoms of colds, coughs, and tonsillitis
◆
Helps treat menorrhagia and metrorrhagia
◆
Reduces mood-swings and PMS-related headaches
◆
Helps treat the symptoms of menopause

GETTING INTO THE POSTURE Place the foam and wooden blocks as in Ujjayi Pranayama (*see page* 230). Follow the steps for Savasana (*see page* 234). Then practice a few cycles of Ujjayi Pranayama. This will open your chest and stimulate your intercostal muscles.

1 Keep your sternum lifted and your diaphragm firm. Inhale and exhale without strain, slowly and deeply. Your exhalation should last for 2-3 seconds. Then, pause for 2 seconds before inhaling. This constitutes a single cycle. Repeat this 3-5 times.

2 Your breathing should now fade away effortlessly at each pause and resume equally easily. Follow the instructions for Stage 1, your exhalations longer than your pauses. Practice 15-20 cycles over 10 minutes. Rest in Savasana.

3 Do a few cycles of Steps 1 and 2. Focus on the silence of the pauses. Experience a feeling of serenity.

COMING OUT OF THE POSTURE
Practice a cycle of Ujjayi Pranayama (*see page* 230). Then follow the coming out of the posture sequence for Savasana (*see page* 235).

KEEP YOUR ABDOMEN SOFT AND RELAXED

Savasana

- Corpse posture -

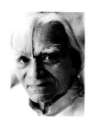

IN THIS VERSION OF the classic asana (*see page* 150), I subtle adjustments in the final posture are made easier with the help of props. The stillness in the posture is not meditation, but reflects a mastery of the inner self and a surrender to a higher, sublime consciousness. The steady, smooth breathing in the posture allows energy to flow into the body, invigorating it and reducing the stress of everyday life.

CAUTIONS
◆
This asana is usually practiced at the end of a yoga session. Do not practice it more than once in a single session. Beginners should practice Savasana without props for 5 weeks before attempting this version and should hold the posture for 5 minutes. For the first 10 weeks of practice with props, wrap the bandage around your forehead, but not your eyes. If at any time you experience feelings of isolation, anxiety, fear, or depression when your eyes are covered, practice without the bandage.

PROPS (*see page* 164) A FOLDED BLANKET, A BOLSTER, A CREPE BANDAGE, AND A MAT. The bolster supports the back and raises the diaphragm and chest. The folded blanket lifts the head and neck, soothing and clearing the mind. If you have a cold, cough, or asthma, keeping your head and chest raised in this posture, helps you breathe comfortably. The bandage shields the eyes from light. It also soothes the eyes, ears, and brain by softening and relaxing the facial skin, muscles, and ligaments.

EXTEND YOUR SPINE

STRETCH OUT YOUR LEGS

REST YOUR HEAD EVENLY ON THE BLANKET

1 Spread the mat on the floor. Place a bolster on the mat with its long sides parallel to the long sides of the mat. Sit in Dandasana (*see page* 82) with the short end of the bolster against your buttocks, and place the folded blanket on the far end. If you have osteoarthritis of the knees or if your legs are feeling tired, place a bolster under your knees (*see inset*).

2 Wrap the bandage around your forehead, following the instructions for Ujjayi Pranayama (*see page* 230). Now place your elbows and forearms on the mat. Lower your back, vertebra by vertebra, onto the bolster until your head rests comfortably on the folded blanket. Position your buttocks evenly on the center of the mat. Spread out your arms to the sides, palms facing up, and rest them on the floor.

BENEFITS

◆

Removes physical and mental fatigue

◆

Relaxes and soothes the sympathetic nervous system

◆

Helps treat high blood pressure, and relieves migraine and stress-related headaches

◆

Alleviates the symptoms of respiratory diseases and eases breathing

◆

Speeds recuperation after an illness

◆

Helps refresh dreamless sleep, especially for those with sleep disorders

COMING OUT OF THE POSTURE

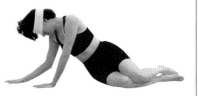

I When you come out of the posture do not tense your neck and throat. Bring your arms to your sides and bring your legs together. Gently roll off the bolster onto your right side, and place your right palm under your head. Keep your knees slightly bent. Pause for a few moments. Allow your body and mind to determine when you should sit up.

II When you feel ready push yourself into a sitting position with your left hand. Sit cross-legged and unwrap the bandage gently. Do not take it off when you are lying down since this can strain the facial and cranial nerves. Open your eyes slowly. If you open them too abruptly, your vision may blur. Straighten your legs and sit in Dandasana.

3 Straighten your legs and stretch them evenly away from each other without disturbing the extension of your waist. Exhale, focusing on your breathing, then lift and stretch your diaphragm, keeping it free of tension. Keep your arms at a comfortable distance from your body. If they are placed too near or too far away, your shoulders will lift off the bolster.

Stretch your shoulders away from your neck. The center of your back should be on the center of the bolster. Keep your abdomen soft and relaxed. Expand your chest and relax your throat, until you feel a soothing sensation in the neck. Ensure that your head does not tilt back. Relax your facial muscles and your jaw. Do not clench your teeth.

4 Keep your breathing smooth and free of tension, but do not breathe deeply. Let your eyeballs relax into their sockets, and allow external surroundings to recede. Feel the energy flow from your brain to your body as the physical, physiological, mental, intellectual, and spiritual planes come together. Stay in the posture for 5-10 minutes.

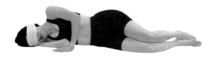

KEEP YOUR THIGH
MUSCLES RELAXED

LET YOUR FEET
DROP OUT TO THE
SIDES NATURALLY

CHAPTER 5

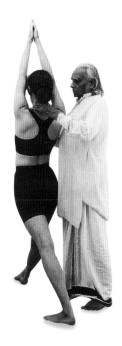

"Yoga is the golden key which unlocks the door to peace, tranquillity, and joy."

Yoga for Ailments

Yoga can heal parts of our bodies that have been injured, traumatized, or simply ignored and neglected. Medical treatment can accelerate the healing process but, all too often, cannot tackle the source of the problem. The ancient yogis realized that the cure for diseases lay within ourselves. They formulated a therapy which worked on our very natures, and enabled the systems of the body to function as effectively and efficiently as possible, both preventing and curing disease. Yoga asanas involve movements that stimulate injured parts of the body by increasing the blood supply to them. The practice of asanas also increases our ability to bear pain.

Yoga Therapy

Yoga's system of healing is based on the premise that the body should be allowed to function as naturally as possible. Practicing the recommended asanas will first rejuvenate your body, and then tackle the causes of the ailment.

The four pillars of yoga therapy are the physician, the medication, the attendant, and the patient. In the yogic worldview, the sage Patanjali is the physician, asanas are the medication, the yoga instructor is the attendant, and the student is the patient. Asanas are recommended to "patients" according to their ailment and their physical and emotional condition. This has to be done with care. If a doctor's diagnosis is wrong or the dosage is inappropriate, the treatment can actually harm the patient. Similarly, asanas that are not suited to an individual's requirements can adversely affect his or her health. Follow the recommended sequence of asanas carefully.

The human body is a very complex piece of machinery, a finely connected network of muscles, joints, nerves, veins, arteries, and capillaries. It is hard to keep all these elements coordinated and in good working order under the best circumstances. More often than not, ailments, whether minor or major, affect the body. The science of yoga, as well as that of Ayurveda, a traditional Indian system of healing based on herbal remedies, classify ailments that afflict the body and the mind under three basic categories. These are self-inflicted ailments, caused by neglect or abuse of the body, congenital ailments, present from birth, and ailments caused by the imbalance of any of the five elements of ether, air, fire, water, and earth, in our system. Yoga can treat all three, but the pace and effectiveness of the cure depends on the type of ailment, its progression, the patient's constitution, and his or her commitment to the treatment.

How the therapy works

The process of yoga therapy is based on selecting and sequencing asanas which stretch specified parts of the body, and block others. You must remember, however, that in the case of serious or congenital disabilities, yoga asanas may not effect a full recovery, but in many cases can alleviate some of the suffering associated with the condition. For instance, the asana sequence prescribed for AIDS (*see page 287*),

(*see page 287*)

YOGA THERAPY REJUVENATES THE BODY
Yogacharya Iyengar in a variation of Marichyasana

YOGA THERAPY

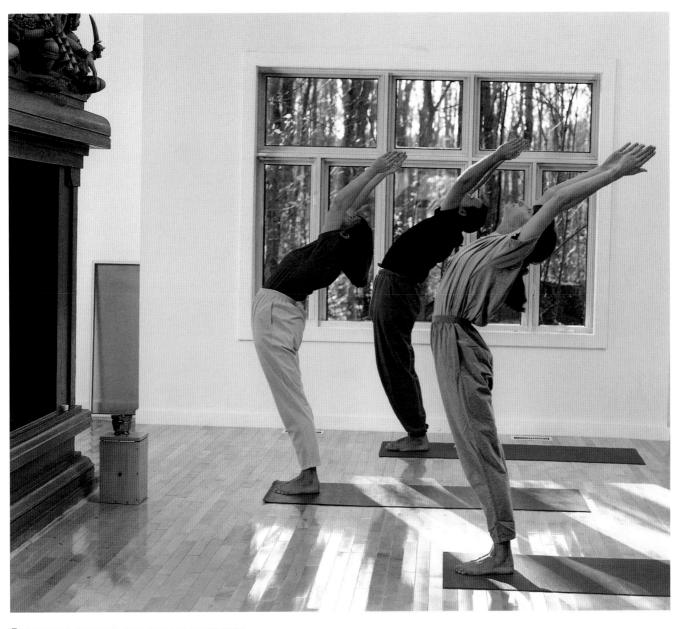

PRACTICING STEADILY AND WITH PERSISTENCE
Yoga therapy involves stretching certain parts of the body and relaxing others

may relieve some of the symptoms, and the relief can boost morale and self-confidence.

Another benefit of yoga therapy is that it has been known to raise the threshold of pain and endurance. However, this only happens if the recommended asanas are practiced with patience and dedication. Yoga calms the brain, soothes the nerves and reduces the apprehension of pain, which is, in many cases, as damaging as pain itself.

Medication accelerates the healing process, but is not a cure. Nature alone is the ultimate cure. The belief underlying yoga therapy is to enable the human system to function as efficiently, effectively, and naturally as it can. This natural process, however, operates at its own rhythm and pace, and the pace may be slow.

Yoga therapy begins with understanding the entire human body and the way it functions. The origins and development of the ailment in question are carefully studied, particularly the parts of the body most affected. The aim is not simply to cure the specific symptom, but to target the cause.

"Health is not a commodity to be bargained for. It has to be earned through sweat."

ASANAS AND HEALTH

Asanas make your body supple and bring alertness to your mind, while soothing your nerves and glands, relaxing your brain, and maintaining a physical, physiological, and emotional balance. Regular practice of asanas improves your will power and self-confidence. The practice of asanas lubricates joints and increases mobility, bringing about an awareness of each muscle, joint, and organ. Different combinations of asanas improve the range of movement for each muscle and joint, helping align the left and the right sides of the body.

HOW ASANAS HEAL YOU

Asanas are based on the simple principles of stretching, bending, rotating, and relaxing. These movements have diverse effects on the body's systems, and will either heal, stimulate, or seal off specific parts of the body. At the same time, the approach is holistic, and is aimed at purifying and strengthening each organ, bone, and cell of the body. Yoga is a combination of physiotherapy, psychotherapy, and spiritual therapy, a healing science which does not distinguish between the physical and physiological bodies. Asanas are bio-physio-psychological postures, through which we build many "dams" inside our body. Blood and energy are brought to these "dams," which then open gradually, and allow the organs to absorb fresh healing blood and energy. When a part of the body is affected by disease, it loses its sensitivity. During the practice of specifically therapeutic asanas, energy from these "dams" flows uninterruptedly to the affected area and allow the healing process to begin.

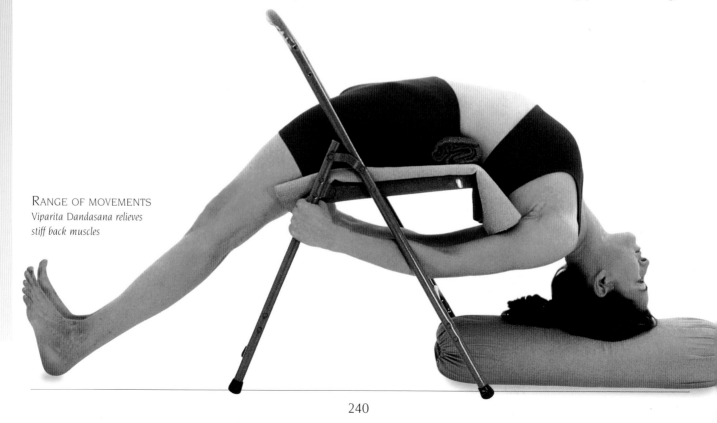

RANGE OF MOVEMENTS
Viparita Dandasana relieves stiff back muscles

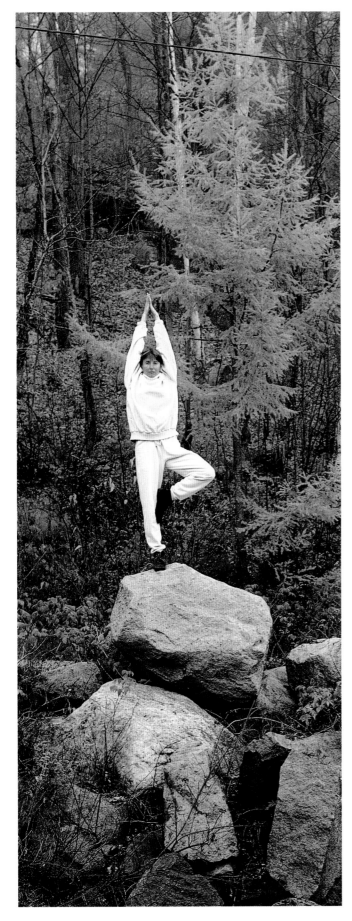

HOLISTIC THERAPY
Yoga addresses every organ, bone, muscle, and cell of the body

It is important to work gradually from the periphery to the affected area. First, the peripheral parts of the body should be toned, strengthened, and helped into good working order. Only then can the ailment be tackled. Sometimes, however, in the case of a new problem, the affected part should be worked on directly, before it degenerates further.

THE BRAIN AND THE BODY

A very important aspect of yoga therapy is that it teaches us to control the effect of the brain upon the body. The term "brain" is used here in the broadest sense, covering the mind and intellect, and including thought, experience, and imagination. Energy from the brain is diffused to various parts of the body in the form of vital, healing energy. Practicing yoga teaches the brain to be calm and passive, and to accept and subdue pain, not fight it. The energy that is otherwise dissipated in coping with stress and pain, is diverted to healing.

Ultimately, the aim of yoga therapy is to teach the brain and body to work in harmony. Specific asanas work on the various systems of the body, whether respiratory, circulatory, digestive, hormonal, immune, or reproductive. Therefore, the combination and sequencing of the asanas must be followed for the healing process to be effective. Follow the sequence prescribed for your particular ailment, and set up a schedule for practicing the recommended asanas (*see page* 386). Do not get discouraged if the healing of your ailment takes time. Remember, perseverance is the essence of yoga.

YOGA THERAPY

Heart & Circulation

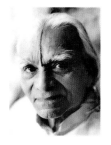

THE HEART IS THE ORGAN that pumps blood to all parts of the body. It is located in the thoracic cavity, nestled between the lungs. The circulatory system, composed of arteries, veins, and capillaries, carries blood to and from the heart to the entire body, supplying oxygen and nutrients, and carrying away waste products. The following sequences of asanas address some common disorders of this system.

Cold extremities

This is caused by a slowdown in circulation, when blood collects in the torso and fails to correctly reach the extremities. It gives rise to ailments of the chest and of the intestinal and abdominal organs. It is often the result of a sluggish thyroid, stress, or nervousness.

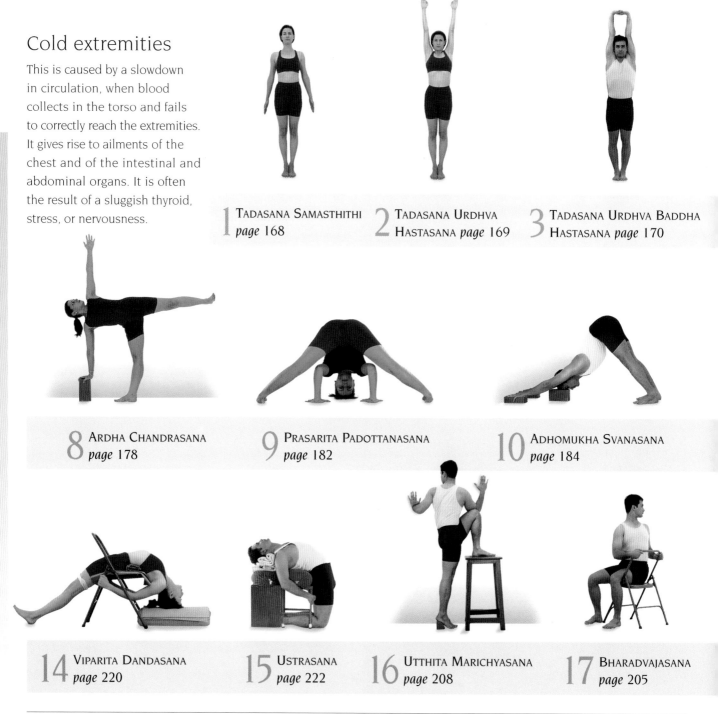

1 TADASANA SAMASTHITHI *page 168*

2 TADASANA URDHVA HASTASANA *page 169*

3 TADASANA URDHVA BADDHA HASTASANA *page 170*

8 ARDHA CHANDRASANA *page 178*

9 PRASARITA PADOTTANASANA *page 182*

10 ADHOMUKHA SVANASANA *page 184*

14 VIPARITA DANDASANA *page 220*

15 USTRASANA *page 222*

16 UTTHITA MARICHYASANA *page 208*

17 BHARADVAJASANA *page 205*

"Never perform asanas mechanically. If you do, your body stagnates."

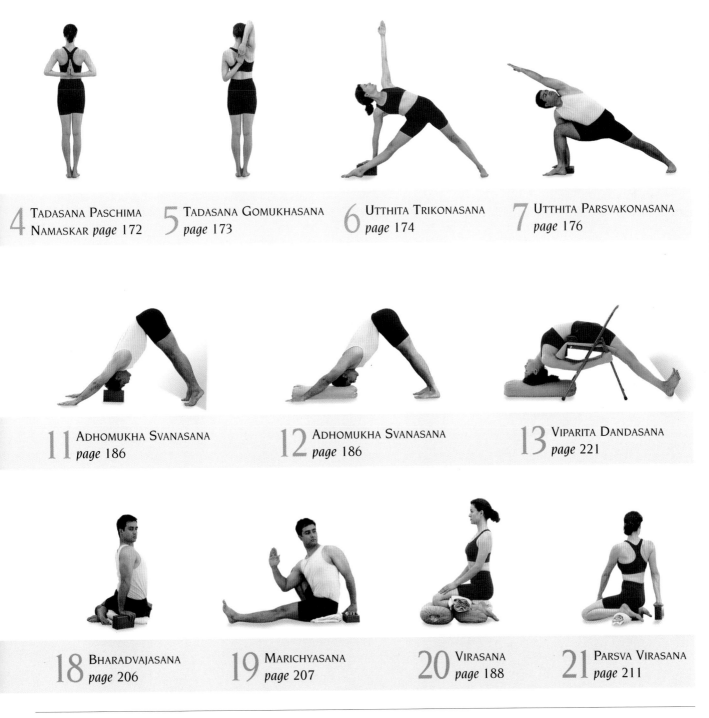

4 TADASANA PASCHIMA
NAMASKAR *page 172*

5 TADASANA GOMUKHASANA
page 173

6 UTTHITA TRIKONASANA
page 174

7 UTTHITA PARSVAKONASANA
page 176

11 ADHOMUKHA SVANASANA
page 186

12 ADHOMUKHA SVANASANA
page 186

13 VIPARITA DANDASANA
page 221

18 BHARADVAJASANA
page 206

19 MARICHYASANA
page 207

20 VIRASANA
page 188

21 PARSVA VIRASANA
page 211

HEART & CIRCULATION

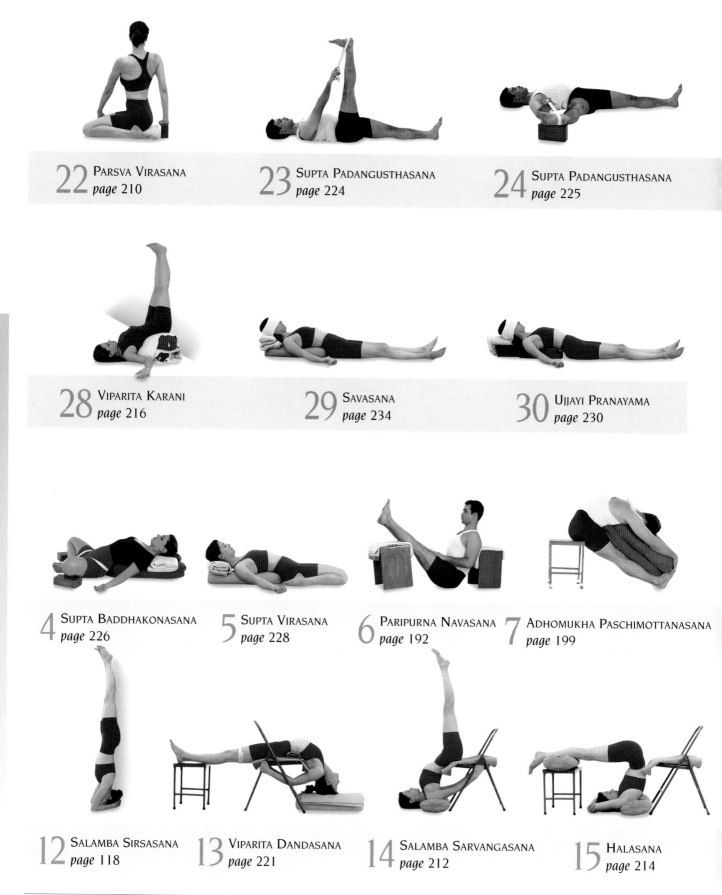

22 PARSVA VIRASANA
page 210

23 SUPTA PADANGUSTHASANA
page 224

24 SUPTA PADANGUSTHASANA
page 225

28 VIPARITA KARANI
page 216

29 SAVASANA
page 234

30 UJJAYI PRANAYAMA
page 230

4 SUPTA BADDHAKONASANA
page 226

5 SUPTA VIRASANA
page 228

6 PARIPURNA NAVASANA
page 192

7 ADHOMUKHA PASCHIMOTTANASANA
page 199

12 SALAMBA SIRSASANA
page 118

13 VIPARITA DANDASANA
page 221

14 SALAMBA SARVANGASANA
page 212

15 HALASANA
page 214

YOGA FOR AILMENTS

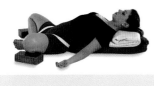

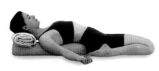

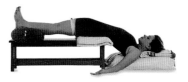

25 **SUPTA BADDHAKONASANA**
page 226

26 **SUPTA VIRASANA**
page 228

27 **SETUBANDHA SARVANGASANA**
page 219

Varicose veins

In this condition, veins just beneath the skin of the legs are elongated and dilated, leading to aching legs, fatigue, and muscle cramps. The condition often occurs during pregnancy and menstruation, and also affects those who have to stay on their feet for long periods.

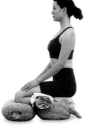

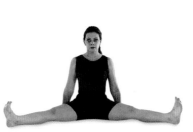

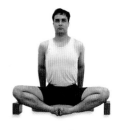

1 **VIRASANA**
page 188

2 **UPAVISTA KONASANA**
page 195

3 **BADDHAKONASANA**
page 190

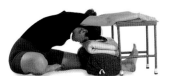

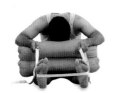

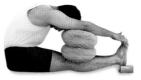

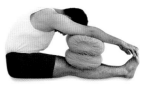

8 **JANU SIRSASANA**
page 200

9 **PASCHIMOTTANASANA**
page 198

10 **PASCHIMOTTANASANA**
page 197

11 **PASCHIMOTTANASANA**
page 196

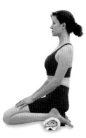

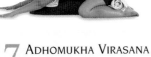

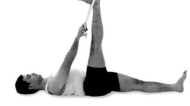

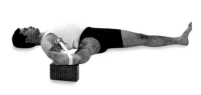

16 **VIRASANA**
page 188

17 **ADHOMUKHA VIRASANA**
page 202

18 **SUPTA PADANGUSTHASANA**
page 224

19 **SUPTA PADANGUSTHASANA**
page 225

HEART & CIRCULATION

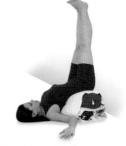

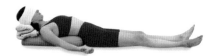

20 **SETUBANDHA SARVANGASANA**
page 219

21 **VIPARITA KARANI**
page 216

22 **SAVASANA**
page 234

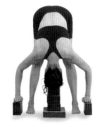

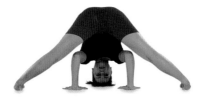

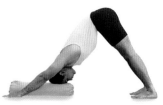

4 **UTTANASANA**
page 179

5 **PRASARITA PADOTTANASANA**
page 182

6 **ADHOMUKHA SVANASANA**
page 186

11 PASCHIMOTTANASANA
page 198

12 JANU SIRSASANA
page 200

13 PARIPURNA NAVASANA
page 192

14 PASCHIMOTTANASANA
page 198

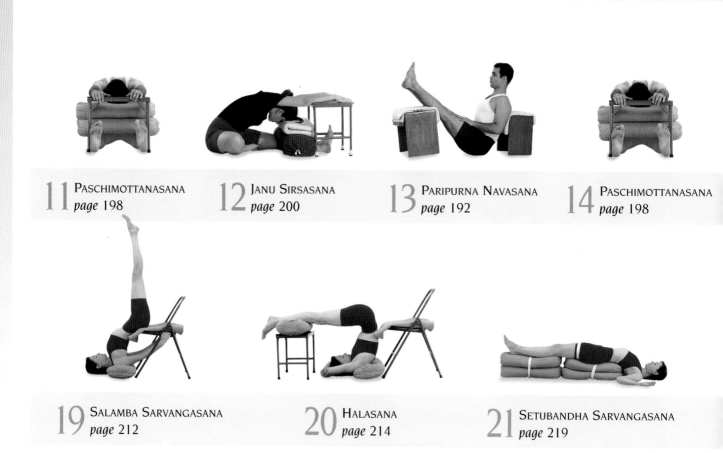

19 **SALAMBA SARVANGASANA**
page 212

20 **HALASANA**
page 214

21 **SETUBANDHA SARVANGASANA**
page 219

High blood pressure

This condition is defined as sustained, elevated blood pressure, and is also known as hypertension. It has many causes, which include psychological, physiological, and environmental factors.

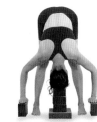

1 UTTANASANA
page 179

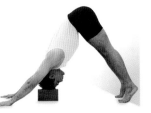

2 ADHOMUKHA SVANASANA
page 184

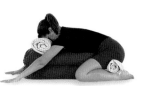

3 ADHOMUKHA SVANASANA
page 186

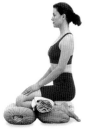

7 VIRASANA
page 188

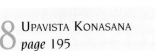

8 UPAVISTA KONASANA
page 195

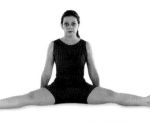

9 BADDHAKONASANA
page 190

10 ADHOMUKHA VIRASANA
page 203

15 SUPTA PADANGUSTHASANA
page 225

16 SUPTA BADDHAKONASANA
page 226

17 SUPTA VIRASANA
page 228

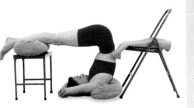

18 HALASANA
page 214

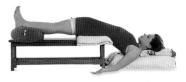

22 SETUBANDHA SARVANGASANA
page 219

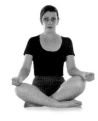

23 SWASTIKASANA
page 191

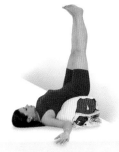

24 VIPARITA KARANI
page 216

HEART & CIRCULATION

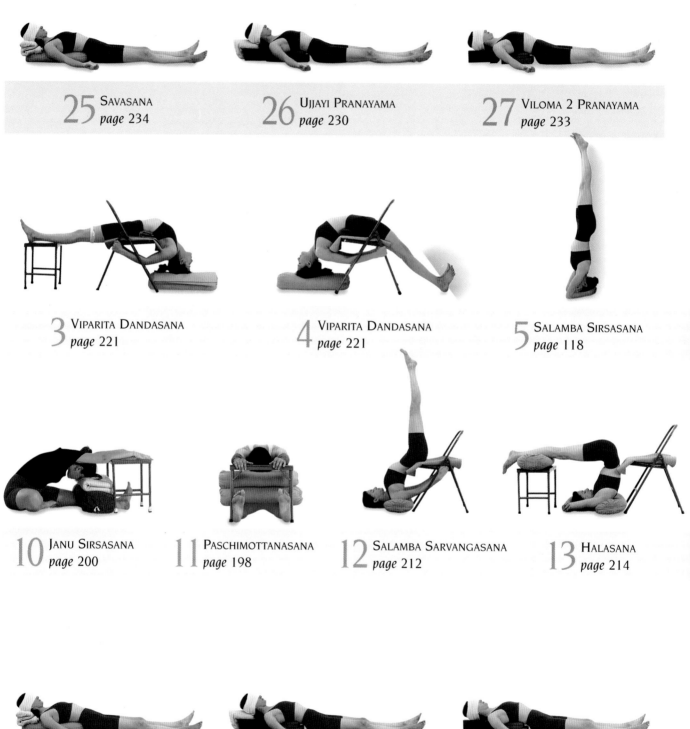

25 SAVASANA
page 234

26 UJJAYI PRANAYAMA
page 230

27 VILOMA 2 PRANAYAMA
page 233

3 VIPARITA DANDASANA
page 221

4 VIPARITA DANDASANA
page 221

5 SALAMBA SIRSASANA
page 118

10 JANU SIRSASANA
page 200

11 PASCHIMOTTANASANA
page 198

12 SALAMBA SARVANGASANA
page 212

13 HALASANA
page 214

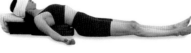

17 SAVASANA
page 234

18 UJJAYI PRANAYAMA
page 230

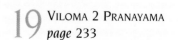

19 VILOMA 2 PRANAYAMA
page 233

Low blood pressure

This condition, also called hypotension, occurs when blood pressure is lower than what is normally required to transport blood to all parts of the body. This can reduce blood supply to the brain, resulting in fatigue, fainting spells, light-headedness, blurry vision, or nausea.

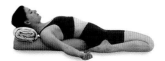

1 SUPTA BADDHAKONASANA
page 226

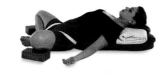

2 SUPTA VIRASANA
page 228

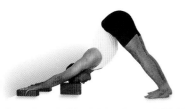

6 ADHOMUKHA SVANASANA
page 184

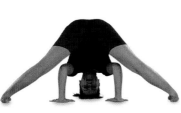

7 PRASARITA PADOTTANASANA
page 182

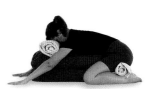

8 UTTANASANA
page 179

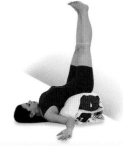

9 ADHOMUKHA VIRASANA
page 203

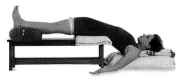

14 SETUBANDHA SARVANGASANA
page 219

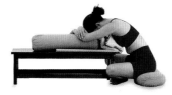

15 ADHOMUKHA SWASTIKASANA
page 204

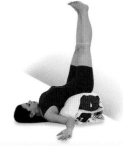

16 VIPARITA KARANI
page 216

Blocked arteries

This occurs when the coronary vessels are blocked, reducing blood flow to the cardiac muscles. This process eventually damages these muscles, and is a major cause of heart attacks. A common symptom is angina or chest pain (*see page 250*).

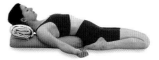

1 SUPTA BADDHAKONASANA
page 226

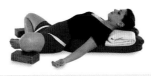

2 SUPTA VIRASANA
page 228

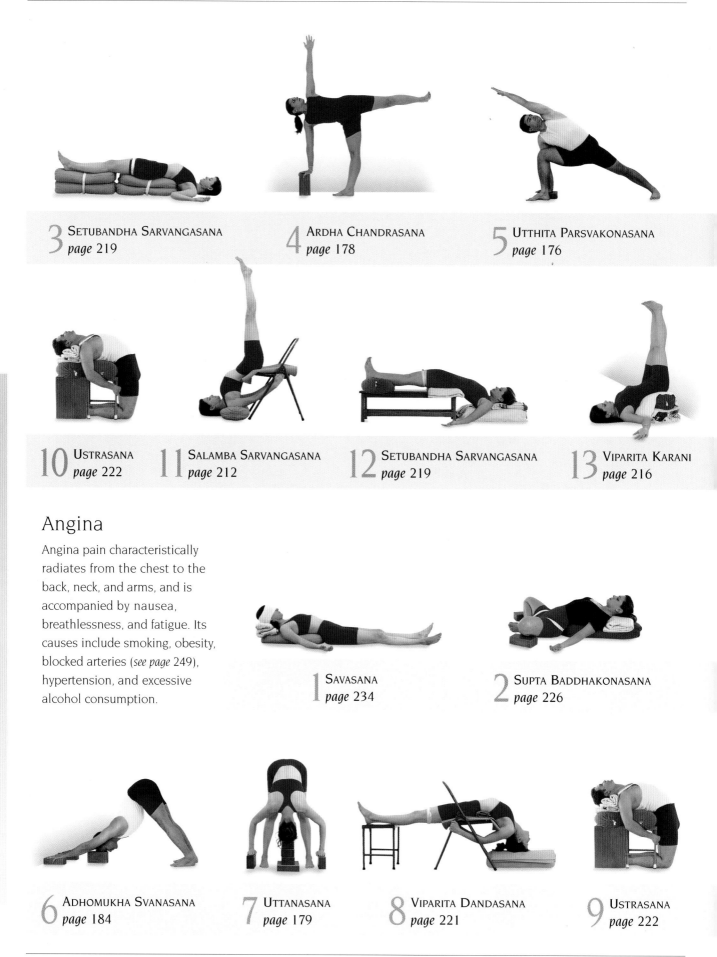

3 SETUBANDHA SARVANGASANA
page 219

4 ARDHA CHANDRASANA
page 178

5 UTTHITA PARSVAKONASANA
page 176

10 USTRASANA
page 222

11 SALAMBA SARVANGASANA
page 212

12 SETUBANDHA SARVANGASANA
page 219

13 VIPARITA KARANI
page 216

Angina

Angina pain characteristically radiates from the chest to the back, neck, and arms, and is accompanied by nausea, breathlessness, and fatigue. Its causes include smoking, obesity, blocked arteries (*see page* 249), hypertension, and excessive alcohol consumption.

1 SAVASANA
page 234

2 SUPTA BADDHAKONASANA
page 226

6 ADHOMUKHA SVANASANA
page 184

7 UTTANASANA
page 179

8 VIPARITA DANDASANA
page 221

9 USTRASANA
page 222

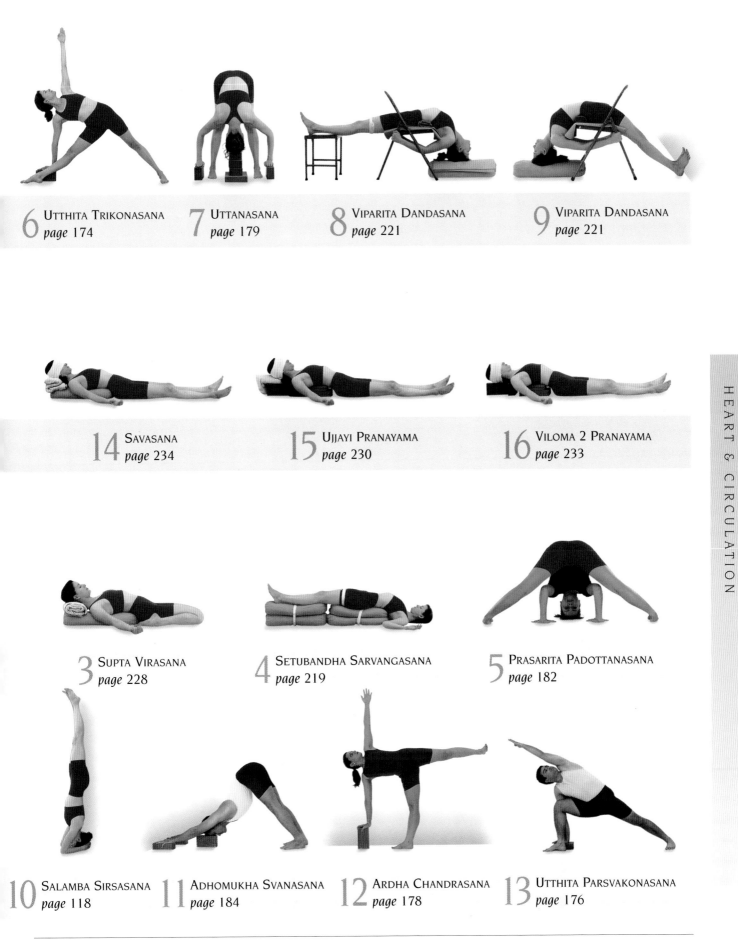

6 **UTTHITA TRIKONASANA**
page 174

7 **UTTANASANA**
page 179

8 **VIPARITA DANDASANA**
page 221

9 **VIPARITA DANDASANA**
page 221

14 **SAVASANA**
page 234

15 **UJJAYI PRANAYAMA**
page 230

16 **VILOMA 2 PRANAYAMA**
page 233

3 **SUPTA VIRASANA**
page 228

4 **SETUBANDHA SARVANGASANA**
page 219

5 **PRASARITA PADOTTANASANA**
page 182

10 **SALAMBA SIRSASANA**
page 118

11 **ADHOMUKHA SVANASANA**
page 184

12 **ARDHA CHANDRASANA**
page 178

13 **UTTHITA PARSVAKONASANA**
page 176

HEART & CIRCULATION

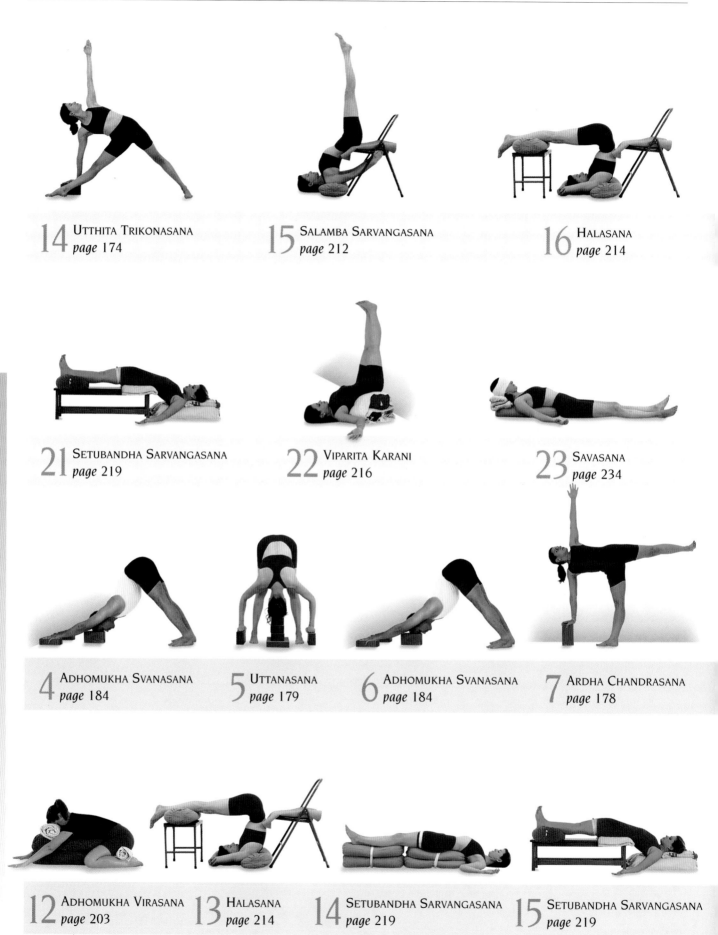

14 **UTTHITA TRIKONASANA**
page 174

15 **SALAMBA SARVANGASANA**
page 212

16 **HALASANA**
page 214

21 **SETUBANDHA SARVANGASANA**
page 219

22 **VIPARITA KARANI**
page 216

23 **SAVASANA**
page 234

4 **ADHOMUKHA SVANASANA**
page 184

5 **UTTANASANA**
page 179

6 **ADHOMUKHA SVANASANA**
page 184

7 **ARDHA CHANDRASANA**
page 178

12 **ADHOMUKHA VIRASANA**
page 203

13 **HALASANA**
page 214

14 **SETUBANDHA SARVANGASANA**
page 219

15 **SETUBANDHA SARVANGASANA**
page 219

YOGA FOR AILMENTS

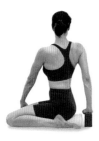

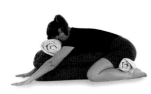

17 PARSVA VIRASANA
page 210

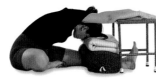

18 ADHOMUKHA VIRASANA
page 203

19 JANU SIRSASANA
page 200

20 PASCHIMOTTANASANA
page 198

Heart attack

Inadequate blood supply to the heart muscles results in myocardial infarction, or a heart attack. It is often due to the gradual blocking of the coronary arteries (*see page* 250).

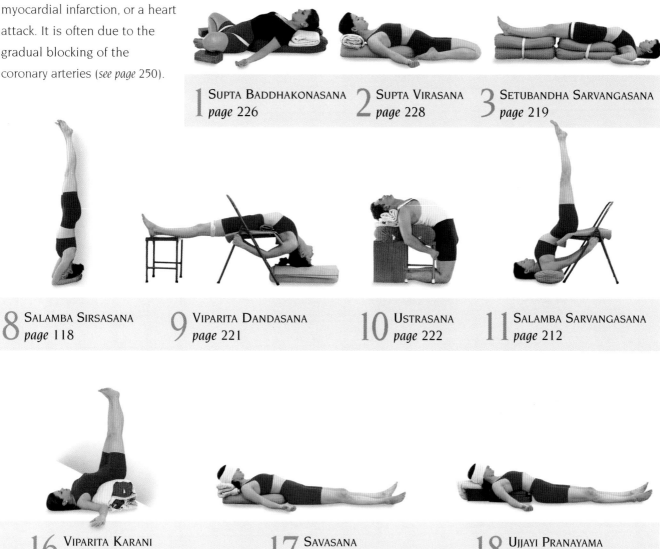

1 SUPTA BADDHAKONASANA
page 226

2 SUPTA VIRASANA
page 228

3 SETUBANDHA SARVANGASANA
page 219

8 SALAMBA SIRSASANA
page 118

9 VIPARITA DANDASANA
page 221

10 USTRASANA
page 222

11 SALAMBA SARVANGASANA
page 212

16 VIPARITA KARANI
page 216

17 SAVASANA
page 234

18 UJJAYI PRANAYAMA
page 230

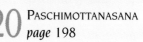

HEART & CIRCULATION

Respiratory System

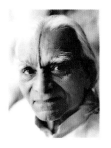

RESPIRATION STARTS FROM the upper respiratory tract in the nose and the pharynx (the throat). Then inhaled air passes through to the trachea (the wind-pipe), and the two major bronchi. These airways bring air into the lungs. Carbon dioxide from the body's cells is exhaled through the lungs. Yoga asanas are particularly beneficial for all respiratory disorders if the following recommended sequences are practiced regularly.

Colds

These are minor viral infections of the mucous membranes that line the upper respiratory tract, including the nose and throat. The most common symptoms are nasal obstruction and discharge, sinusitis, sore throat, sneezing, coughing, and headaches.

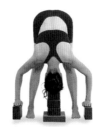

1 **UTTANASANA**
page 179

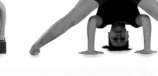

2 **PRASARITA PADOTTANASANA**
page 182

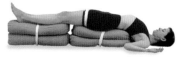

3 **ADHOMUKHA SVANASANA**
page 184

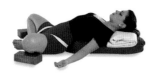

8 **SUPTA BADDHAKONASANA**
page 226

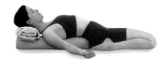

9 **SUPTA VIRASANA**
page 228

10 **SETUBANDHA SARVANGASANA**
page 219

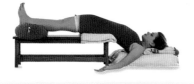

14 **SETUBANDHA SARVANGASANA**
page 219

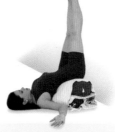

15 **VIPARITA KARANI**
page 216

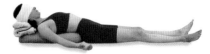

16 **SAVASANA**
page 234

"Like leaves move in the wind, your mind moves with your breath."

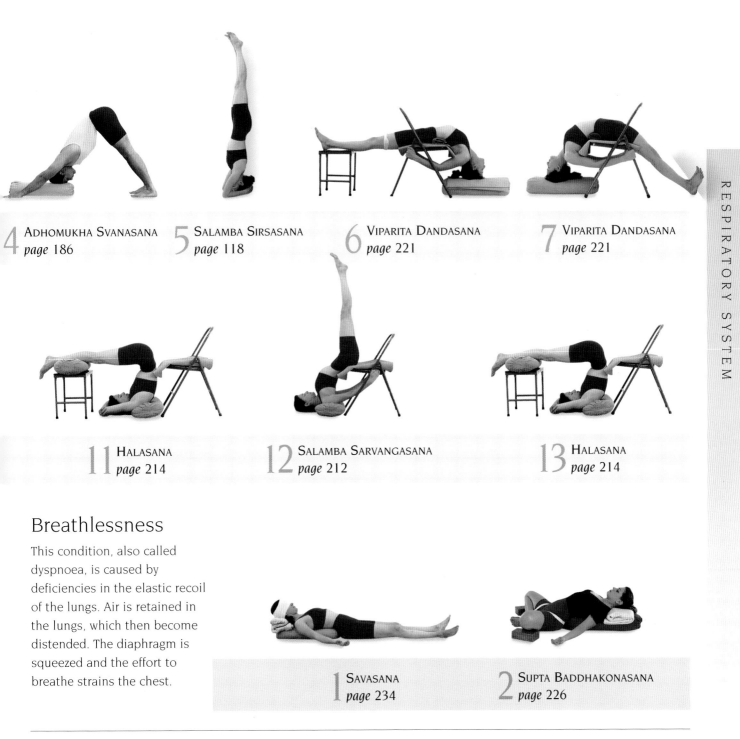

4 ADHOMUKHA SVANASANA
page 186

5 SALAMBA SIRSASANA
page 118

6 VIPARITA DANDASANA
page 221

7 VIPARITA DANDASANA
page 221

11 HALASANA
page 214

12 SALAMBA SARVANGASANA
page 212

13 HALASANA
page 214

Breathlessness

This condition, also called dyspnoea, is caused by deficiencies in the elastic recoil of the lungs. Air is retained in the lungs, which then become distended. The diaphragm is squeezed and the effort to breathe strains the chest.

1 SAVASANA
page 234

2 SUPTA BADDHAKONASANA
page 226

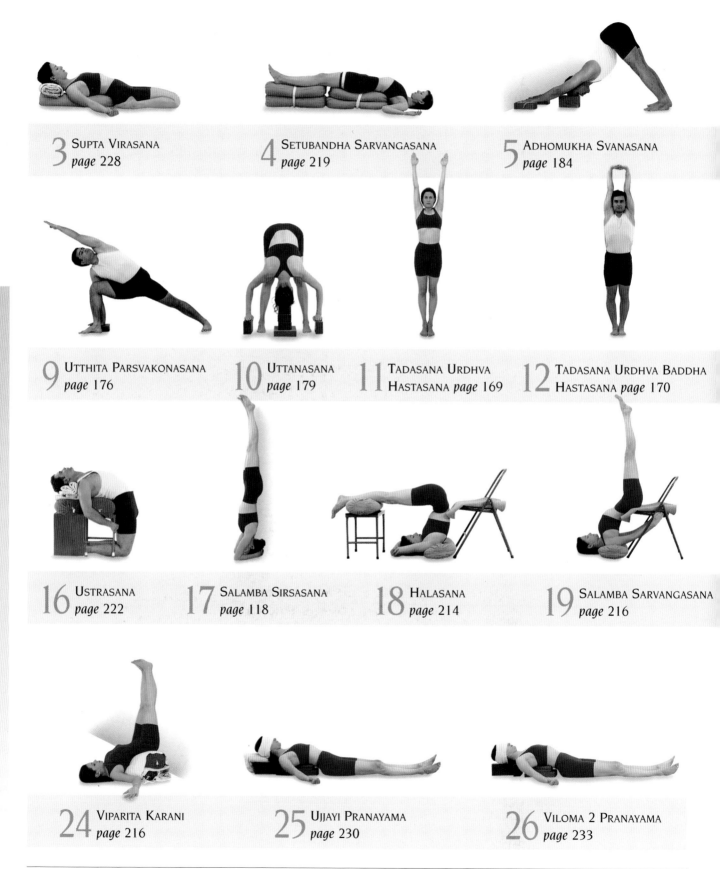

3 SUPTA VIRASANA
page 228

4 SETUBANDHA SARVANGASANA
page 219

5 ADHOMUKHA SVANASANA
page 184

9 UTTHITA PARSVAKONASANA
page 176

10 UTTANASANA
page 179

11 TADASANA URDHVA
HASTASANA *page* 169

12 TADASANA URDHVA BADDHA
HASTASANA *page* 170

16 USTRASANA
page 222

17 SALAMBA SIRSASANA
page 118

18 HALASANA
page 214

19 SALAMBA SARVANGASANA
page 216

24 VIPARITA KARANI
page 216

25 UJJAYI PRANAYAMA
page 230

26 VILOMA 2 PRANAYAMA
page 233

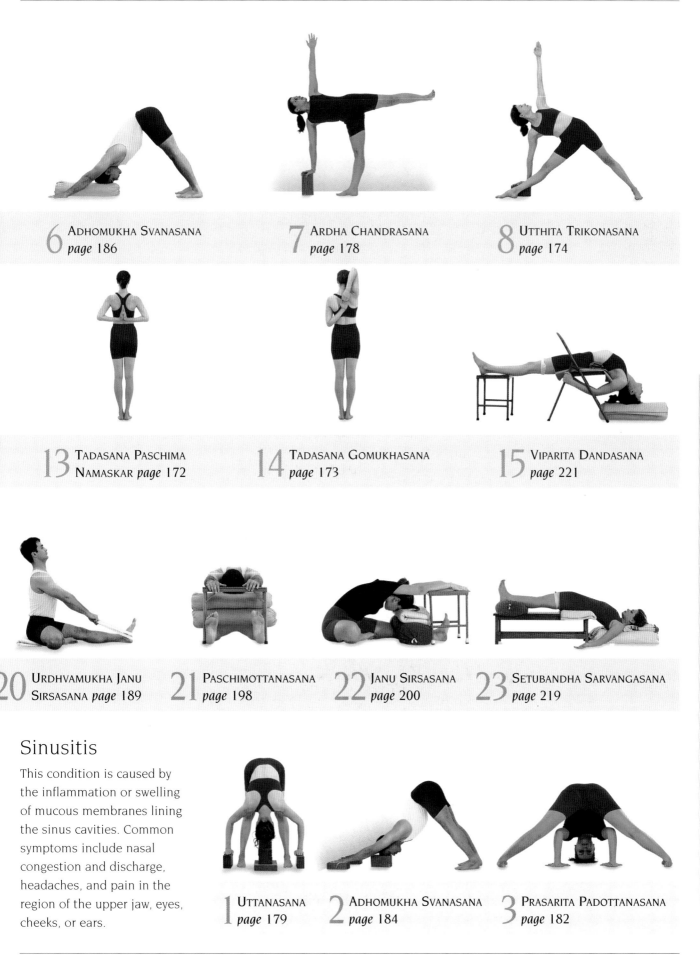

6 ADHOMUKHA SVANASANA *page* 186

7 ARDHA CHANDRASANA *page* 178

8 UTTHITA TRIKONASANA *page* 174

13 TADASANA PASCHIMA NAMASKAR *page* 172

14 TADASANA GOMUKHASANA *page* 173

15 VIPARITA DANDASANA *page* 221

20 URDHVAMUKHA JANU SIRSASANA *page* 189

21 PASCHIMOTTANASANA *page* 198

22 JANU SIRSASANA *page* 200

23 SETUBANDHA SARVANGASANA *page* 219

Sinusitis

This condition is caused by the inflammation or swelling of mucous membranes lining the sinus cavities. Common symptoms include nasal congestion and discharge, headaches, and pain in the region of the upper jaw, eyes, cheeks, or ears.

1 UTTANASANA *page* 179

2 ADHOMUKHA SVANASANA *page* 184

3 PRASARITA PADOTTANASANA *page* 182

RESPIRATORY SYSTEM

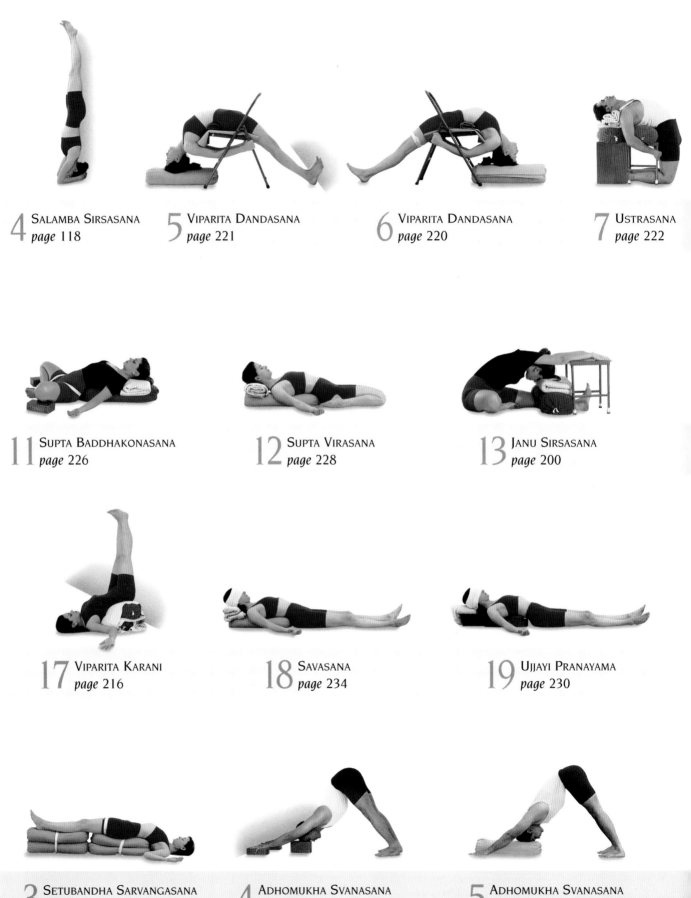

4 SALAMBA SIRSASANA
page 118

5 VIPARITA DANDASANA
page 221

6 VIPARITA DANDASANA
page 220

7 USTRASANA
page 222

11 SUPTA BADDHAKONASANA
page 226

12 SUPTA VIRASANA
page 228

13 JANU SIRSASANA
page 200

17 VIPARITA KARANI
page 216

18 SAVASANA
page 234

19 UJJAYI PRANAYAMA
page 230

3 SETUBANDHA SARVANGASANA
page 219

4 ADHOMUKHA SVANASANA
page 184

5 ADHOMUKHA SVANASANA
page 186

YOGA FOR AILMENTS

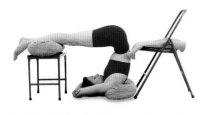

8 HALASANA
page 214

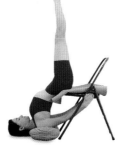

9 SALAMBA SARVANGASANA
page 212

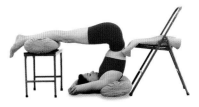

10 HALASANA
page 214

14 PASCHIMOTTANASANA
page 198

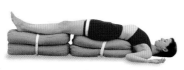

15 SETUBANDHA SARVANGASANA
page 219

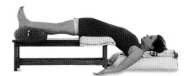

16 SETUBANDHA SARVANGASANA
page 219

RESPIRATORY SYSTEM

Bronchitis

This condition is caused by inflammation or excess mucus in the bronchi, the airways connecting the lungs to the trachea or wind-pipe. The common symptoms of this condition are shortness of breath, wheezing, and coughing.

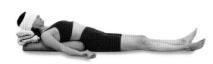

1 SAVASANA
page 234

2 SUPTA VIRASANA
page 228

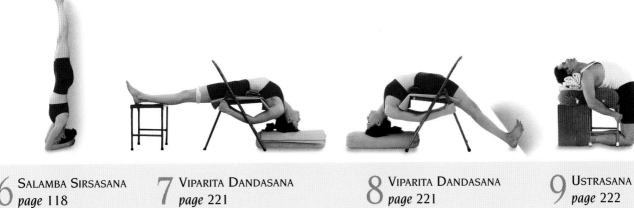

6 SALAMBA SIRSASANA
page 118

7 VIPARITA DANDASANA
page 221

8 VIPARITA DANDASANA
page 221

9 USTRASANA
page 222

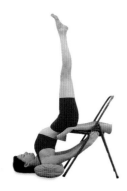
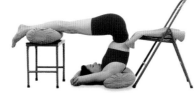
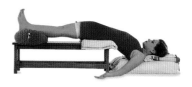

10 SALAMBA SARVANGASANA
page 212

11 HALASANA
page 214

12 SETUBANDHA SARVANGASANA
page 219

Asthma

In this condition, the airways of the lungs are constricted, causing tightness in the chest, bouts of coughing, wheezing, and breathing difficulties. The inflammation of the air passages can become chronic. Asthma is usually caused by allergies or stress.

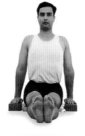
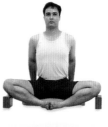
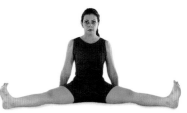

1 DANDASANA
page 187

2 BADDHAKONASANA
page 190

3 UPAVISTA KONASANA
page 195

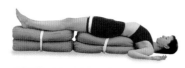
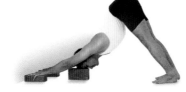
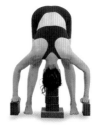

7 SETUBANDHA SARVANGASANA
page 219

8 ADHOMUKHA SVANASANA
page 184

9 UTTANASANA
page 179

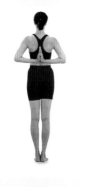
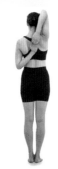
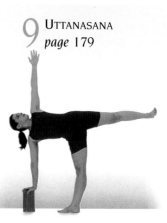

13 TADASANA PASCHIMA
NAMASKAR *page* 172

14 TADASANA GOMUKHASANA
page 173

15 ARDHA CHANDRASANA
page 178

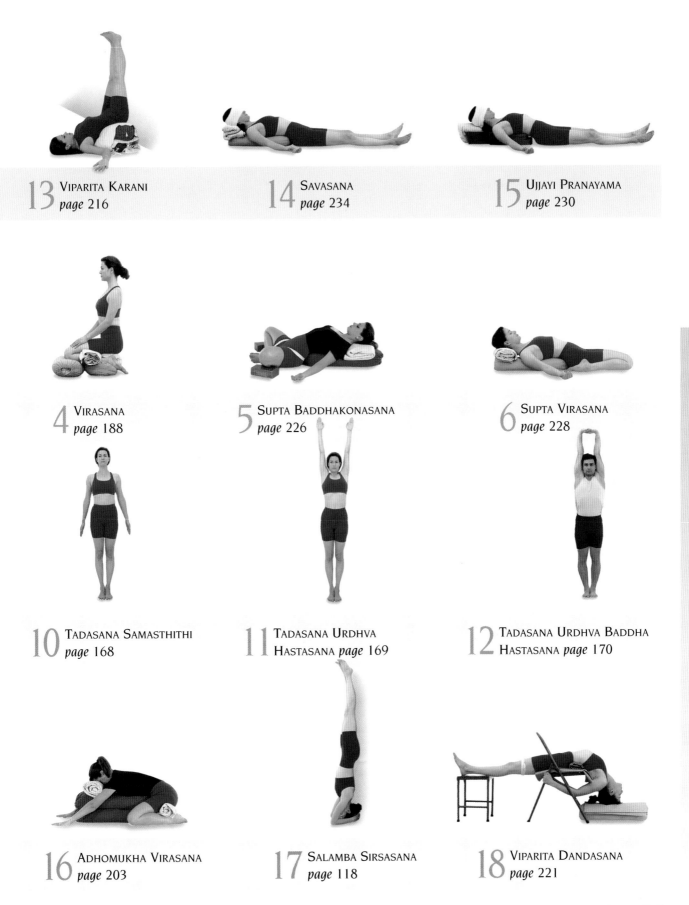

13 VIPARITA KARANI
page 216

14 SAVASANA
page 234

15 UJJAYI PRANAYAMA
page 230

4 VIRASANA
page 188

5 SUPTA BADDHAKONASANA
page 226

6 SUPTA VIRASANA
page 228

10 TADASANA SAMASTHITHI
page 168

11 TADASANA URDHVA
HASTASANA *page 169*

12 TADASANA URDHVA BADDHA
HASTASANA *page 170*

16 ADHOMUKHA VIRASANA
page 203

17 SALAMBA SIRSASANA
page 118

18 VIPARITA DANDASANA
page 221

RESPIRATORY SYSTEM

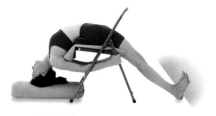

19 **VIPARITA DANDASANA**
page 221

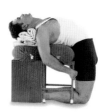

20 **USTRASANA**
page 222

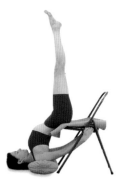

21 **SALAMBA SARVANGASANA**
page 212

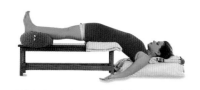

22 **SETUBANDHA SARVANGASANA**
page 219

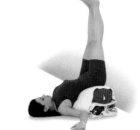

23 **VIPARITA KARANI**
page 216

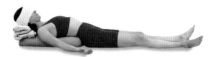

24 **SAVASANA**
page 234

"Fear and fatigue block the mind. Confront both, and courage and confidence will flow into you."

Digestive System

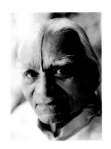

ALL THE FOOD WE EAT has to travel an average distance of almost 11yards through the body. It passes through the mouth, gullet, small intestine, and large intestine. Food interacts with the saliva and with the secretions of the pancreas, gall bladder, and liver, and is broken down by digestive enzymes and acids. During this process, nourishment is absorbed by the body. Regular practice of these recommended asanas effectively alleviates digestive disorders.

Indigestion

This condition is associated with upper abdominal pain, discomfort, or distension, which can be acute or chronic. Other indications are nausea, vomiting, belching, acidity, flatulence, and a constant feeling of being full.

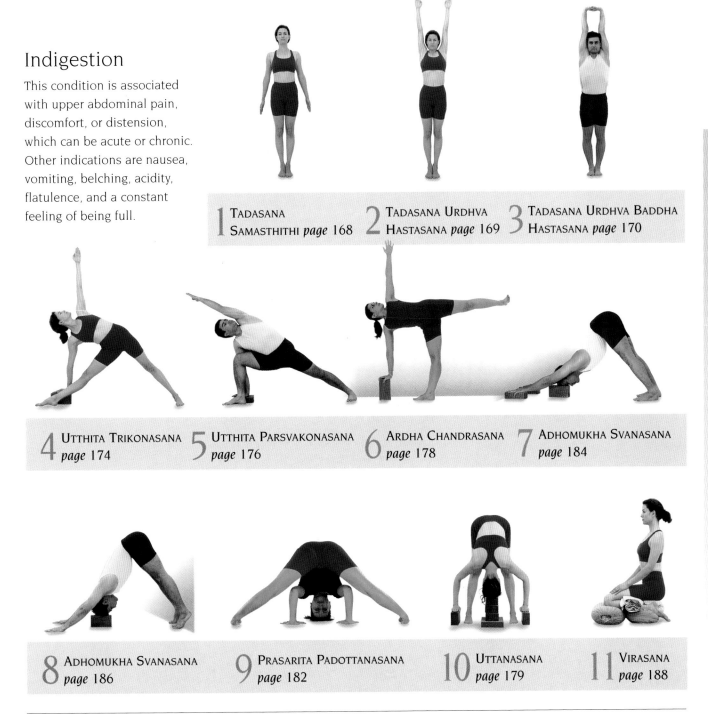

1 TADASANA SAMASTHITHI *page 168*

2 TADASANA URDHVA HASTASANA *page 169*

3 TADASANA URDHVA BADDHA HASTASANA *page 170*

4 UTTHITA TRIKONASANA *page 174*

5 UTTHITA PARSVAKONASANA *page 176*

6 ARDHA CHANDRASANA *page 178*

7 ADHOMUKHA SVANASANA *page 184*

8 ADHOMUKHA SVANASANA *page 186*

9 PRASARITA PADOTTANASANA *page 182*

10 UTTANASANA *page 179*

11 VIRASANA *page 188*

DIGESTIVE SYSTEM

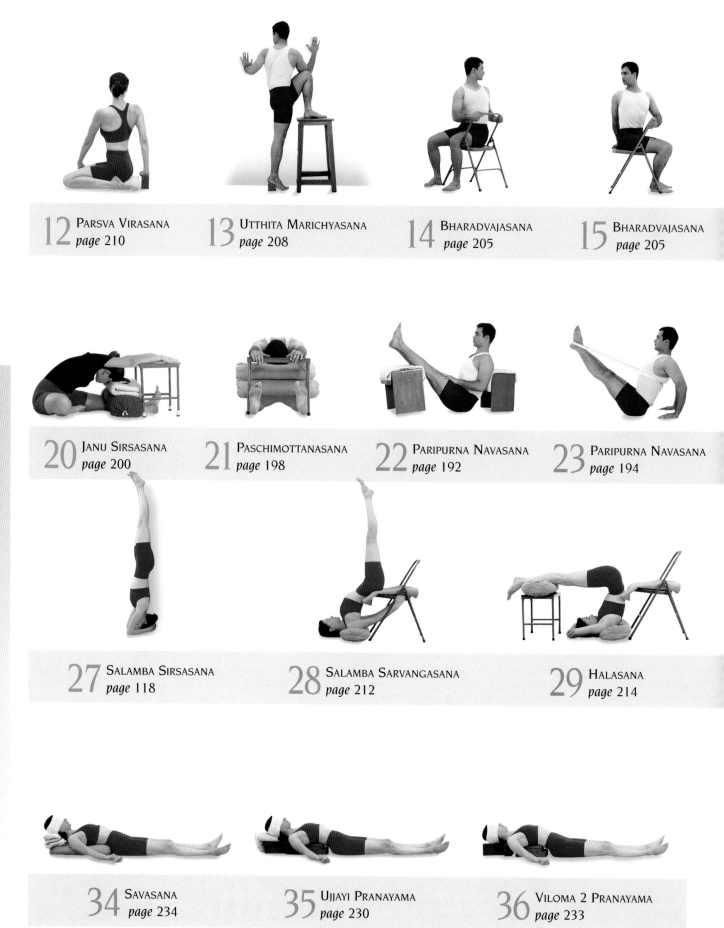

12 PARSVA VIRASANA
page 210

13 UTTHITA MARICHYASANA
page 208

14 BHARADVAJASANA
page 205

15 BHARADVAJASANA
page 205

20 JANU SIRSASANA
page 200

21 PASCHIMOTTANASANA
page 198

22 PARIPURNA NAVASANA
page 192

23 PARIPURNA NAVASANA
page 194

27 SALAMBA SIRSASANA
page 118

28 SALAMBA SARVANGASANA
page 212

29 HALASANA
page 214

34 SAVASANA
page 234

35 UJJAYI PRANAYAMA
page 230

36 VILOMA 2 PRANAYAMA
page 233

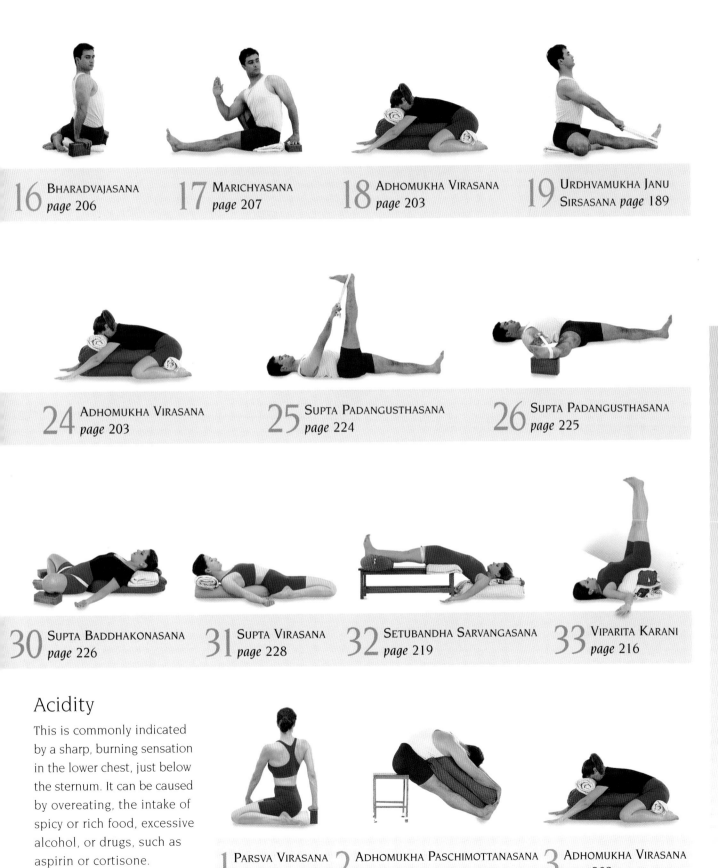

16 BHARADVAJASANA *page 206*

17 MARICHYASANA *page 207*

18 ADHOMUKHA VIRASANA *page 203*

19 URDHVAMUKHA JANU SIRSASANA *page 189*

24 ADHOMUKHA VIRASANA *page 203*

25 SUPTA PADANGUSTHASANA *page 224*

26 SUPTA PADANGUSTHASANA *page 225*

30 SUPTA BADDHAKONASANA *page 226*

31 SUPTA VIRASANA *page 228*

32 SETUBANDHA SARVANGASANA *page 219*

33 VIPARITA KARANI *page 216*

Acidity

This is commonly indicated by a sharp, burning sensation in the lower chest, just below the sternum. It can be caused by overeating, the intake of spicy or rich food, excessive alcohol, or drugs, such as aspirin or cortisone.

1 PARSVA VIRASANA *page 210*

2 ADHOMUKHA PASCHIMOTTANASANA *page 199*

3 ADHOMUKHA VIRASANA *page 203*

YOGA FOR AILMENTS

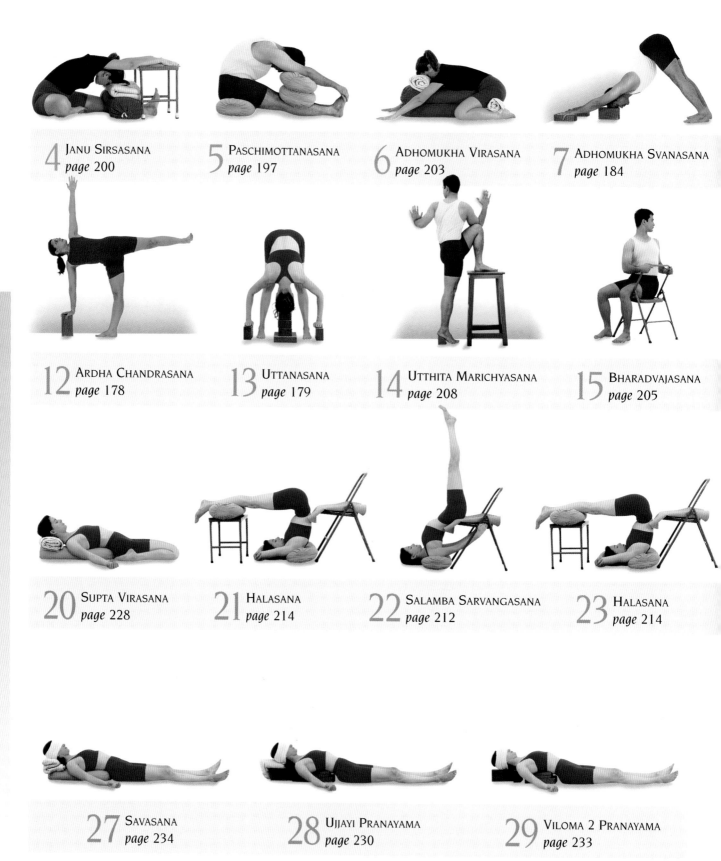

4 JANU SIRSASANA
page 200

5 PASCHIMOTTANASANA
page 197

6 ADHOMUKHA VIRASANA
page 203

7 ADHOMUKHA SVANASANA
page 184

12 ARDHA CHANDRASANA
page 178

13 UTTANASANA
page 179

14 UTTHITA MARICHYASANA
page 208

15 BHARADVAJASANA
page 205

20 SUPTA VIRASANA
page 228

21 HALASANA
page 214

22 SALAMBA SARVANGASANA
page 212

23 HALASANA
page 214

27 SAVASANA
page 234

28 UJJAYI PRANAYAMA
page 230

29 VILOMA 2 PRANAYAMA
page 233

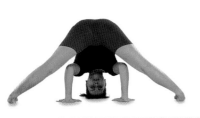

8 PRASARITA PADOTTANASANA
page 182

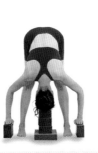

9 UTTANASANA
page 179

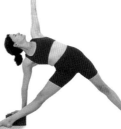

10 UTTHITA TRIKONASANA
page 174

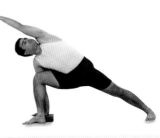

11 UTTHITA PARSVAKONASANA
page 176

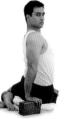

16 BHARADVAJASANA
page 206

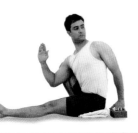

17 MARICHYASANA
page 207

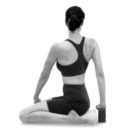

18 PARSVA VIRASANA
page 210

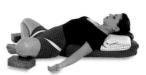

19 SUPTA BADDHAKONASANA
page 226

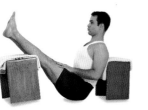

24 PARIPURNA NAVASANA
page 192

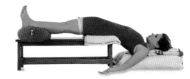

25 SETUBANDHA SARVANGASANA
page 219

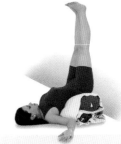
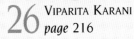

26 VIPARITA KARANI
page 216

Constipation

For some people, the elimination of waste from the body is difficult, infrequent, and sometimes painful. This is often accompanied by a feeling that the bowels have not been completely emptied.

1 UTTANASANA
page 179

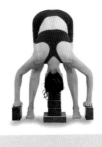

2 PRASARITA PADOTTANASANA
page 182

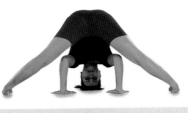

DIGESTIVE SYSTEM

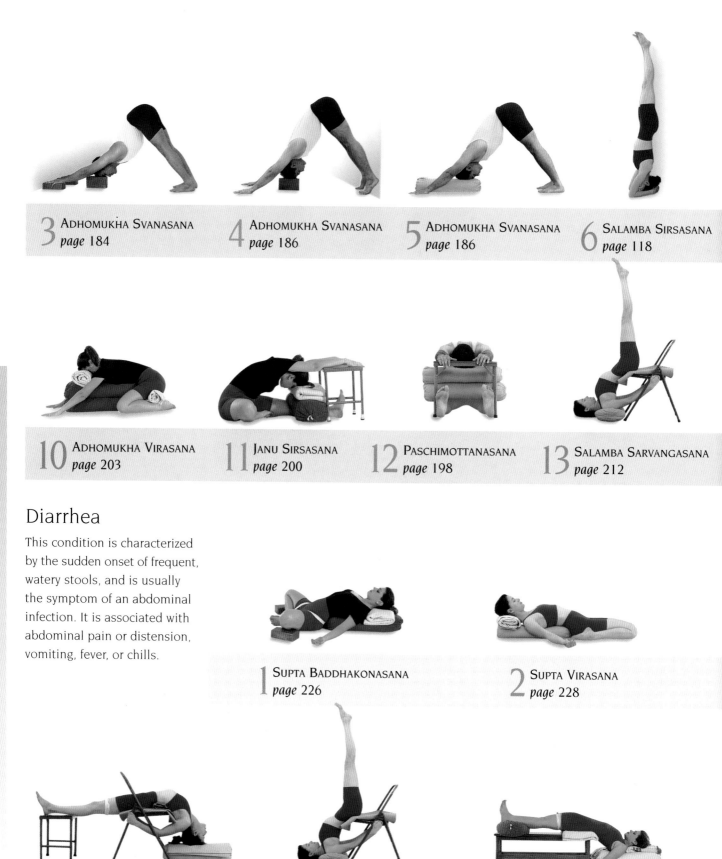

3 ADHOMUKHA SVANASANA
page 184

4 ADHOMUKHA SVANASANA
page 186

5 ADHOMUKHA SVANASANA
page 186

6 SALAMBA SIRSASANA
page 118

10 ADHOMUKHA VIRASANA
page 203

11 JANU SIRSASANA
page 200

12 PASCHIMOTTANASANA
page 198

13 SALAMBA SARVANGASANA
page 212

Diarrhea

This condition is characterized by the sudden onset of frequent, watery stools, and is usually the symptom of an abdominal infection. It is associated with abdominal pain or distension, vomiting, fever, or chills.

1 SUPTA BADDHAKONASANA
page 226

2 SUPTA VIRASANA
page 228

6 VIPARITA DANDASANA
page 221

7 SALAMBA SARVANGASANA
page 212

8 SETUBANDHA SARVANGASANA
page 219

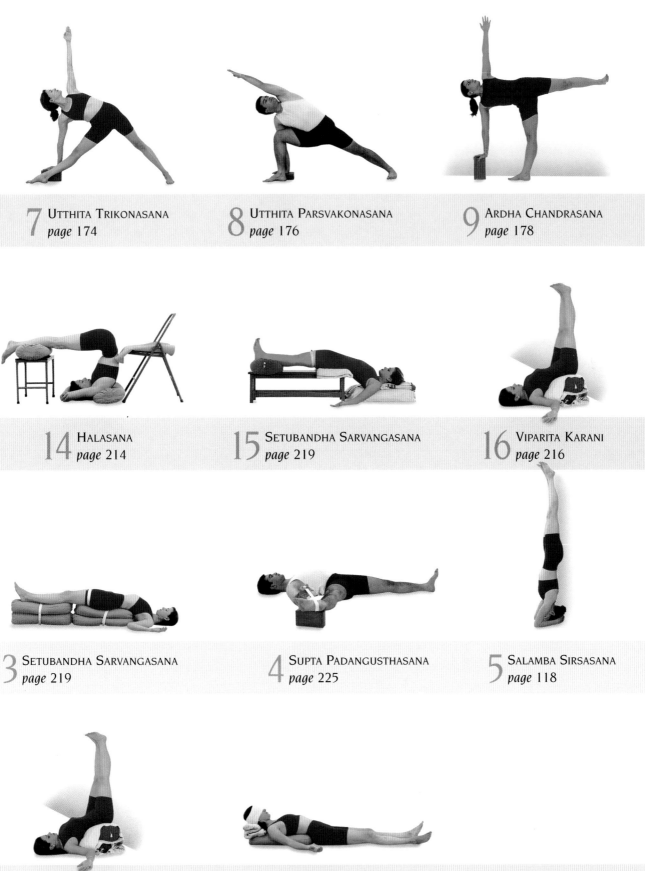

7 UTTHITA TRIKONASANA
page 174

8 UTTHITA PARSVAKONASANA
page 176

9 ARDHA CHANDRASANA
page 178

14 HALASANA
page 214

15 SETUBANDHA SARVANGASANA
page 219

16 VIPARITA KARANI
page 216

3 SETUBANDHA SARVANGASANA
page 219

4 SUPTA PADANGUSTHASANA
page 225

5 SALAMBA SIRSASANA
page 118

9 VIPARITA KARANI
page 216

10 SAVASANA
page 234

DIGESTIVE SYSTEM

Irritable bowel syndrome

Characterized by a combination of abdominal pain and altered bowel function, this syndrome is due to a disturbance in the muscle movements of the large intestine. Some predisposing factors are a low-fiber diet, the use of laxatives, or stress.

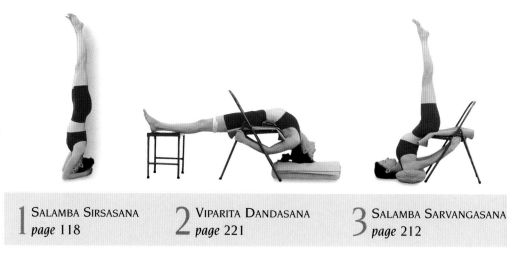

1 SALAMBA SIRSASANA
page 118

2 VIPARITA DANDASANA
page 221

3 SALAMBA SARVANGASANA
page 212

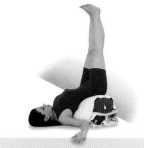

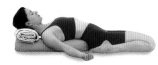

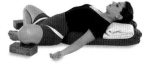

4 VIPARITA DANDASANA
page 221

5 BHARADVAJASANA
page 206

6 BHARADVAJASANA
page 205

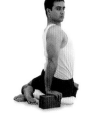

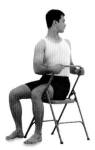

7 VIPARITA KARANI
page 216

8 SUPTA VIRASANA
page 228

9 SUPTA BADDHAKONASANA
page 226

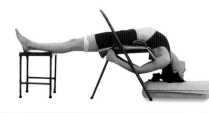

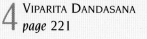

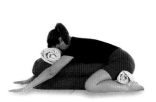

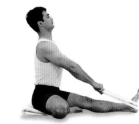

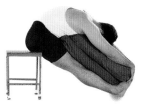

11 ADHOMUKHA VIRASANA
page 203

12 DANDASANA
page 187

13 URDHVAMUKHA JANU
SIRSASANA *page* 189

14 ADHOMUKHA PASCHIMOTTANASANA
page 199

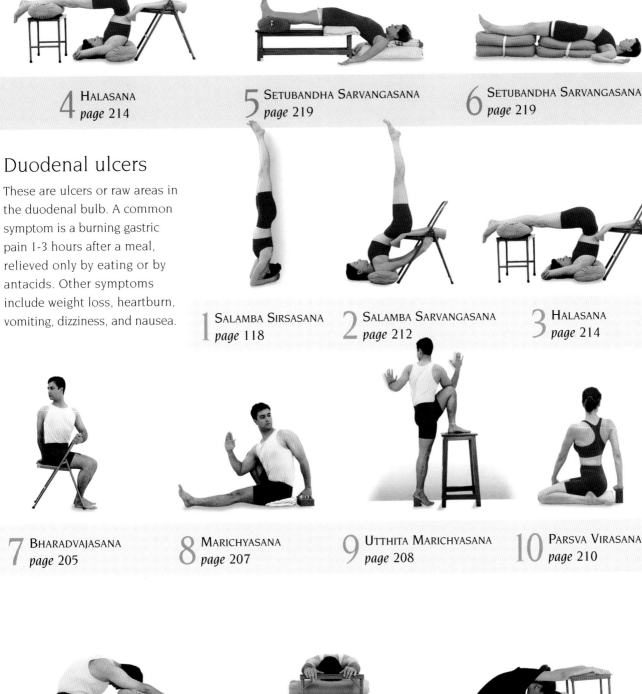

4 HALASANA
page 214

5 SETUBANDHA SARVANGASANA
page 219

6 SETUBANDHA SARVANGASANA
page 219

Duodenal ulcers

These are ulcers or raw areas in the duodenal bulb. A common symptom is a burning gastric pain 1-3 hours after a meal, relieved only by eating or by antacids. Other symptoms include weight loss, heartburn, vomiting, dizziness, and nausea.

1 SALAMBA SIRSASANA
page 118

2 SALAMBA SARVANGASANA
page 212

3 HALASANA
page 214

7 BHARADVAJASANA
page 205

8 MARICHYASANA
page 207

9 UTTHITA MARICHYASANA
page 208

10 PARSVA VIRASANA
page 210

15 PASCHIMOTTANASANA
page 197

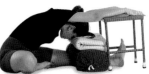

16 PASCHIMOTTANASANA
page 198

17 JANU SIRSASANA
page 200

DIGESTIVE SYSTEM

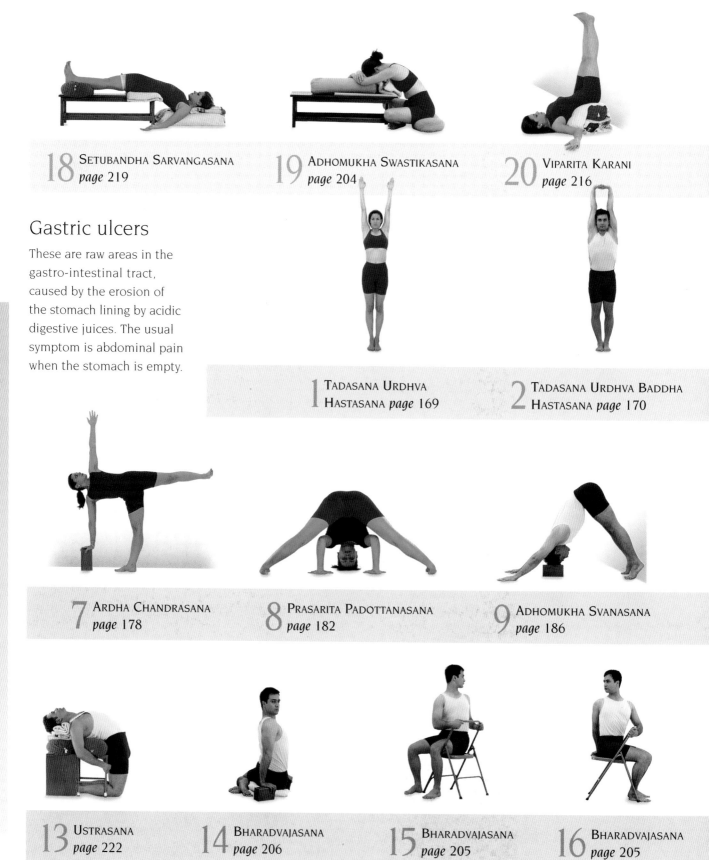

18 SETUBANDHA SARVANGASANA *page 219*

19 ADHOMUKHA SWASTIKASANA *page 204*

20 VIPARITA KARANI *page 216*

Gastric ulcers

These are raw areas in the gastro-intestinal tract, caused by the erosion of the stomach lining by acidic digestive juices. The usual symptom is abdominal pain when the stomach is empty.

1 TADASANA URDHVA HASTASANA *page 169*

2 TADASANA URDHVA BADDHA HASTASANA *page 170*

7 ARDHA CHANDRASANA *page 178*

8 PRASARITA PADOTTANASANA *page 182*

9 ADHOMUKHA SVANASANA *page 186*

13 USTRASANA *page 222*

14 BHARADVAJASANA *page 206*

15 BHARADVAJASANA *page 205*

16 BHARADVAJASANA *page 205*

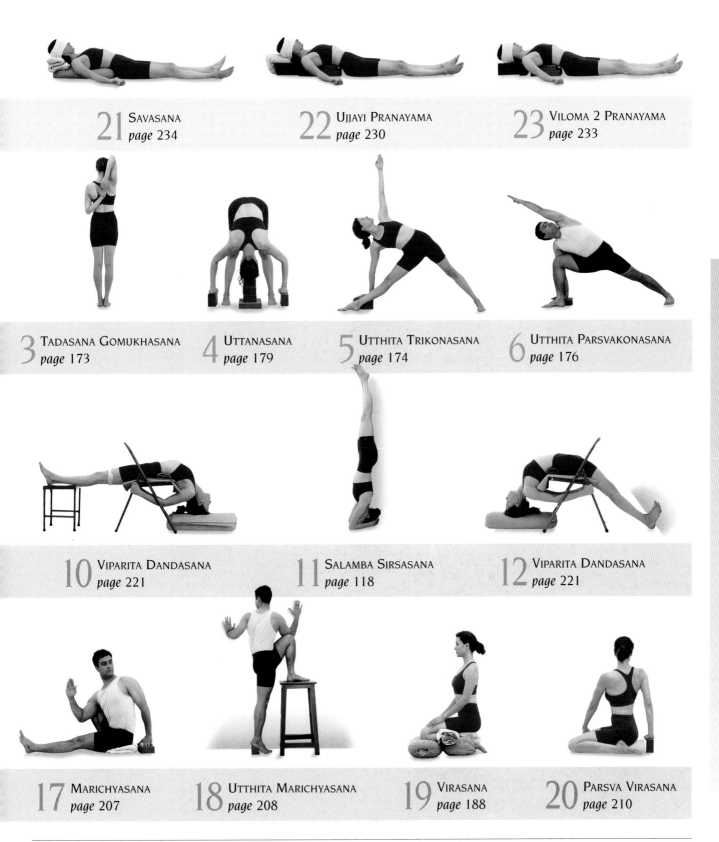

21 SAVASANA
page 234

22 UJJAYI PRANAYAMA
page 230

23 VILOMA 2 PRANAYAMA
page 233

3 TADASANA GOMUKHASANA
page 173

4 UTTANASANA
page 179

5 UTTHITA TRIKONASANA
page 174

6 UTTHITA PARSVAKONASANA
page 176

10 VIPARITA DANDASANA
page 221

11 SALAMBA SIRSASANA
page 118

12 VIPARITA DANDASANA
page 221

17 MARICHYASANA
page 207

18 UTTHITA MARICHYASANA
page 208

19 VIRASANA
page 188

20 PARSVA VIRASANA
page 210

DIGESTIVE SYSTEM

YOGA FOR AILMENTS

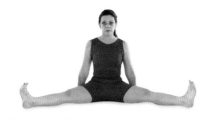

21 UPAVISTA KONASANA
page 195

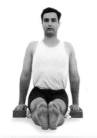

22 DANDASANA
page 187

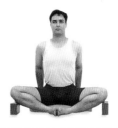

23 BADDHAKONASANA
page 190

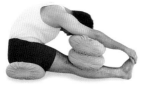

28 PASCHIMOTTANASANA
page 197

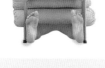

29 PASCHIMOTTANASANA
page 198

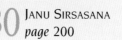

30 JANU SIRSASANA
page 200

31 PARIPURNA NAVASANA
page 192

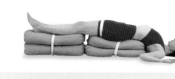

35 SETUBANDHA SARVANGASANA
page 219

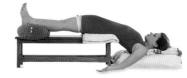

36 SETUBANDHA SARVANGASANA
page 219

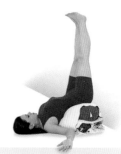

37 VIPARITA KARANI
page 216

Ulcerative colitis

This condition is caused by the inflammation of the colon and rectum. The common symptoms include diarrhea with blood in the stools, abdominal pain or cramps, and rectal bleeding. Attacks can be frequent or can occur after long intervals.

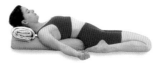

1 SUPTA VIRASANA
page 228

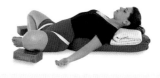

2 SUPTA BADDHAKONASANA
page 226

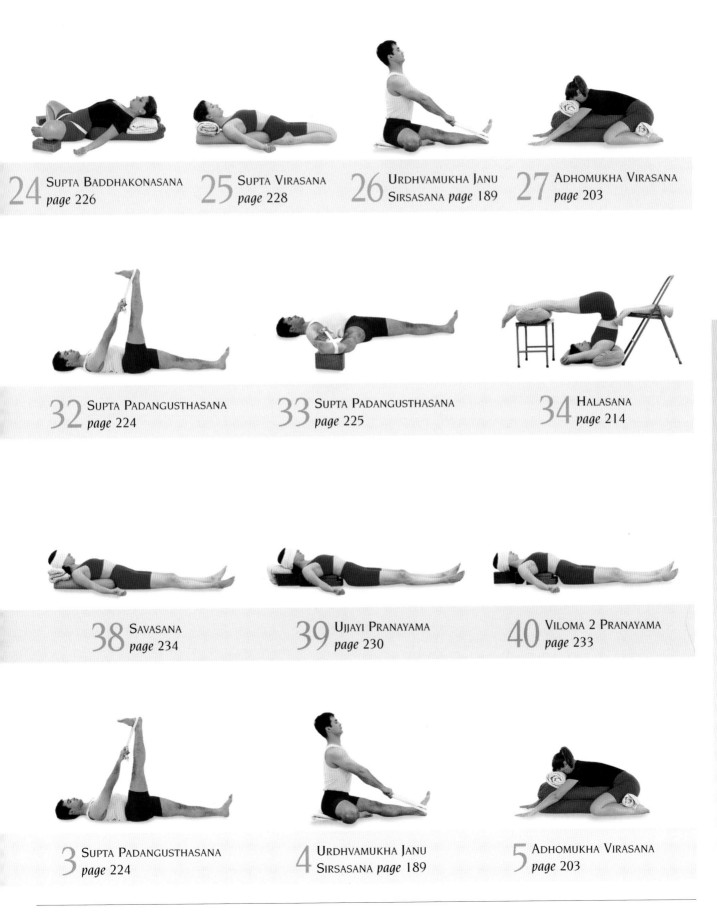

24 SUPTA BADDHAKONASANA
page 226

25 SUPTA VIRASANA
page 228

26 URDHVAMUKHA JANU
SIRSASANA *page 189*

27 ADHOMUKHA VIRASANA
page 203

32 SUPTA PADANGUSTHASANA
page 224

33 SUPTA PADANGUSTHASANA
page 225

34 HALASANA
page 214

38 SAVASANA
page 234

39 UJJAYI PRANAYAMA
page 230

40 VILOMA 2 PRANAYAMA
page 233

3 SUPTA PADANGUSTHASANA
page 224

4 URDHVAMUKHA JANU
SIRSASANA *page 189*

5 ADHOMUKHA VIRASANA
page 203

DIGESTIVE SYSTEM

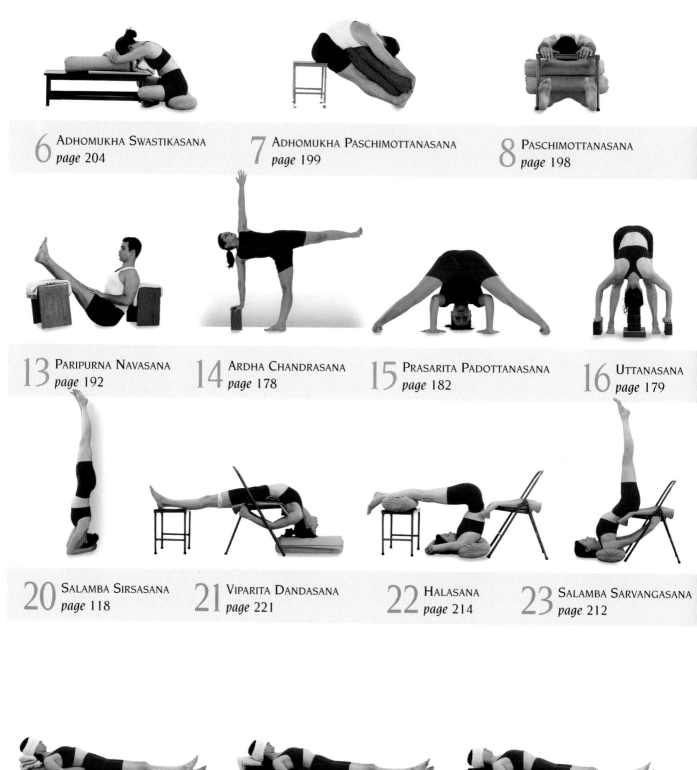

6 **ADHOMUKHA SWASTIKASANA**
page 204

7 **ADHOMUKHA PASCHIMOTTANASANA**
page 199

8 **PASCHIMOTTANASANA**
page 198

13 **PARIPURNA NAVASANA**
page 192

14 **ARDHA CHANDRASANA**
page 178

15 **PRASARITA PADOTTANASANA**
page 182

16 **UTTANASANA**
page 179

20 **SALAMBA SIRSASANA**
page 118

21 **VIPARITA DANDASANA**
page 221

22 **HALASANA**
page 214

23 **SALAMBA SARVANGASANA**
page 212

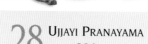

27 **SAVASANA**
page 234

28 **UJJAYI PRANAYAMA**
page 230

29 **VILOMA 2 PRANAYAMA**
page 233

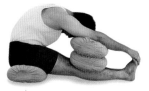
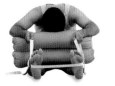
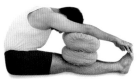
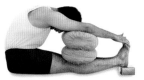

9 PASCHIMOTTANASANA
page 197

10 PASCHIMOTTANASANA
page 198

11 PASCHIMOTTANASANA
page 196

12 PASCHIMOTTANASANA
page 197

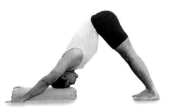
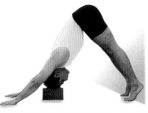
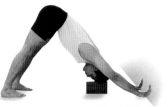

17 ADHOMUKHA SVANASANA
page 186

18 ADHOMUKHA SVANASANA
page 186

19 ADHOMUKHA SVANASANA
page 185

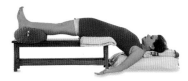
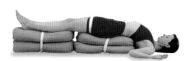
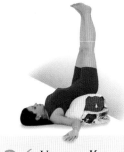

24 SETUBANDHA SARVANGASANA
page 219

25 SETUBANDHA SARVANGASANA
page 219

26 VIPARITA KARANI
page 216

"When stability becomes a habit, maturity and clarity follow."

Urinary System

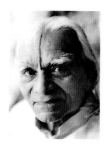

THIS SYSTEM COMPRISES THE kidneys, ureters, bladder, and the urethra. The kidneys manufacture urine, which consists of water and the waste products of metabolism, like protein. Urine is excreted from the body, enabling the kidneys to maintain a balance of the body's electrolytes and acid base. The ureters transport urine to the bladder, while the urethra is the canal for the passage of urine to the exterior. Yoga asanas help to treat many common urinary disorders.

Incontinence

This is the involuntary loss of urine from the bladder. The condition becomes more common with age. The causes include weakening of the pelvic floor muscles, strokes, bladder irritation, and loss of control in the central nervous system.

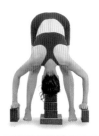

1 **UTTANASANA**
page 179

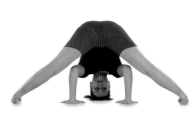

2 **PRASARITA PADOTTANASANA**
page 182

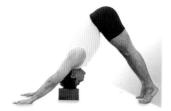

3 **ADHOMUKHA SVANASANA**
page 186

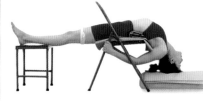

8 **VIPARITA DANDASANA**
page 221

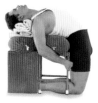

9 **USTRASANA**
page 222

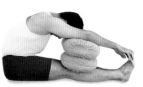

10 **PASCHIMOTTANASANA**
page 196

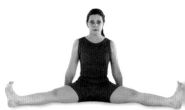

11 **UPAVISTA KONASANA**
page 195

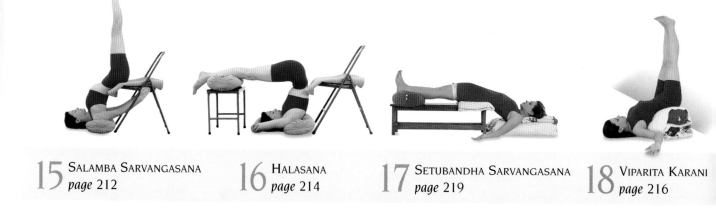

15 **SALAMBA SARVANGASANA**
page 212

16 **HALASANA**
page 214

17 **SETUBANDHA SARVANGASANA**
page 219

18 **VIPARITA KARANI**
page 216

"*Intensified action in yoga brings intensified intelligence.*"

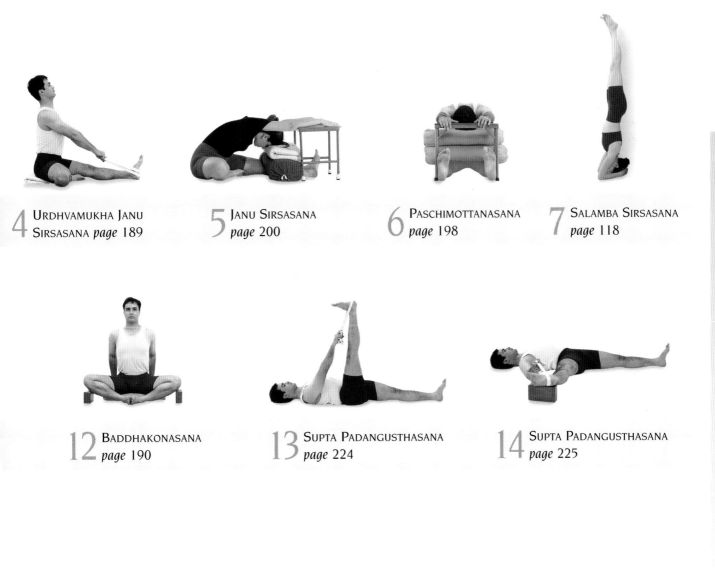

4 URDHVAMUKHA JANU
SIRSASANA *page* 189

5 JANU SIRSASANA
page 200

6 PASCHIMOTTANASANA
page 198

7 SALAMBA SIRSASANA
page 118

12 BADDHAKONASANA
page 190

13 SUPTA PADANGUSTHASANA
page 224

14 SUPTA PADANGUSTHASANA
page 225

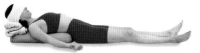

19 SAVASANA
page 234

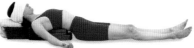

20 UJJAYI PRANAYAMA
page 230

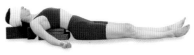

21 VILOMA 2 PRANAYAMA
page 233

Hormonal System

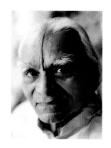

Hormones are natural chemical substances which control certain major functions of the body. Hormones are secreted by glands, which include the thyroid, parathyroid, pituitary, pineal, and adrenal glands, the testes and the ovaries, as well as the islets of Langerhans in the pancreas. Regular practice of the recommended asanas helps ensure an effective secretion of hormones into the bloodstream.

Obesity

This is a condition of excess body fat that is 20 percent greater than the individual's desired weight. Obesity is often caused by Cushing's syndrome, hypothalamic disorders, genetic factors, taking corticosteroid drugs, excess calorie intake, or lack of exercise.

1 TADASANA SAMASTHITHI *page* 168

2 TADASANA URDHVA HASTASANA *page* 169

3 TADASANA URDHVA BADDHA HASTASANA *page* 170

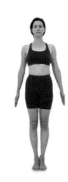

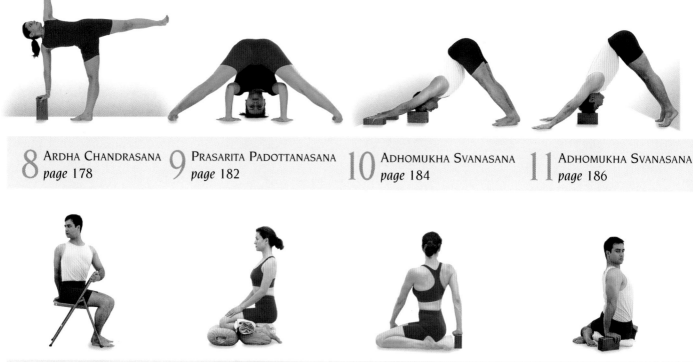

8 ARDHA CHANDRASANA *page* 178

9 PRASARITA PADOTTANASANA *page* 182

10 ADHOMUKHA SVANASANA *page* 184

11 ADHOMUKHA SVANASANA *page* 186

16 BHARADVAJASANA *page* 205

17 VIRASANA *page* 188

18 PARSVA VIRASANA *page* 210

19 BHARADVAJASANA *page* 206

"Yoga is a mirror to look at ourselves from within."

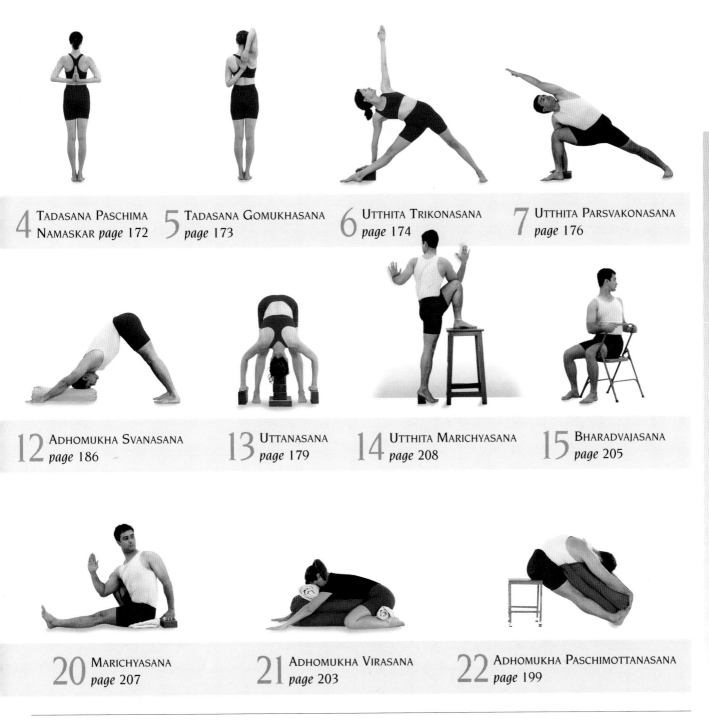

4 TADASANA PASCHIMA NAMASKAR *page* 172

5 TADASANA GOMUKHASANA *page* 173

6 UTTHITA TRIKONASANA *page* 174

7 UTTHITA PARSVAKONASANA *page* 176

12 ADHOMUKHA SVANASANA *page* 186

13 UTTANASANA *page* 179

14 UTTHITA MARICHYASANA *page* 208

15 BHARADVAJASANA *page* 205

20 MARICHYASANA *page* 207

21 ADHOMUKHA VIRASANA *page* 203

22 ADHOMUKHA PASCHIMOTTANASANA *page* 199

YOGA FOR AILMENTS

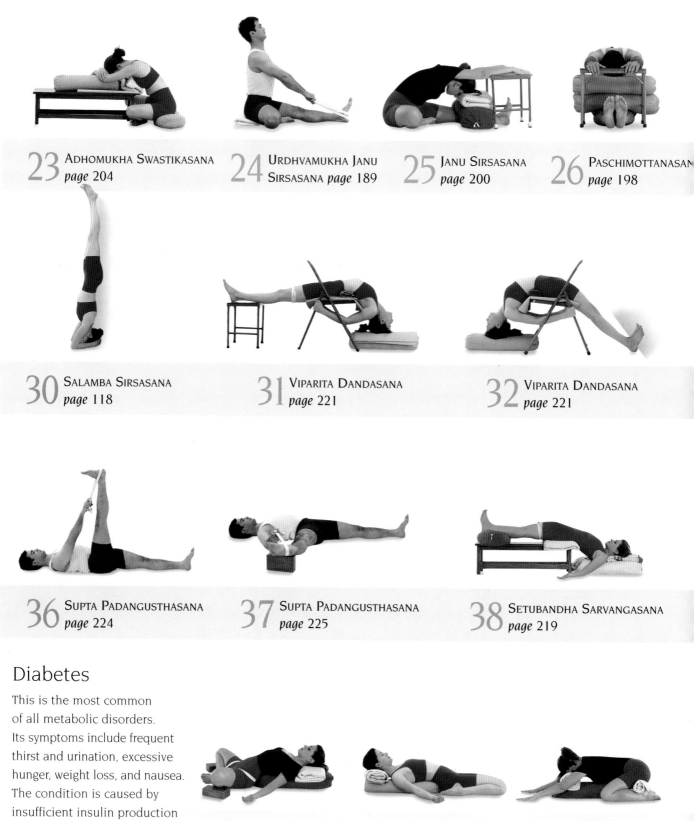

23 **ADHOMUKHA SWASTIKASANA** *page 204*

24 **URDHVAMUKHA JANU SIRSASANA** *page 189*

25 **JANU SIRSASANA** *page 200*

26 **PASCHIMOTTANASAN** *page 198*

30 **SALAMBA SIRSASANA** *page 118*

31 **VIPARITA DANDASANA** *page 221*

32 **VIPARITA DANDASANA** *page 221*

36 **SUPTA PADANGUSTHASANA** *page 224*

37 **SUPTA PADANGUSTHASANA** *page 225*

38 **SETUBANDHA SARVANGASANA** *page 219*

Diabetes

This is the most common of all metabolic disorders. Its symptoms include frequent thirst and urination, excessive hunger, weight loss, and nausea. The condition is caused by insufficient insulin production in the pancreas.

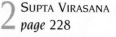

1 **SUPTA BADDHAKONASANA** *page 226*

2 **SUPTA VIRASANA** *page 228*

3 **ADHOMUKHA VIRASANA** *page 202*

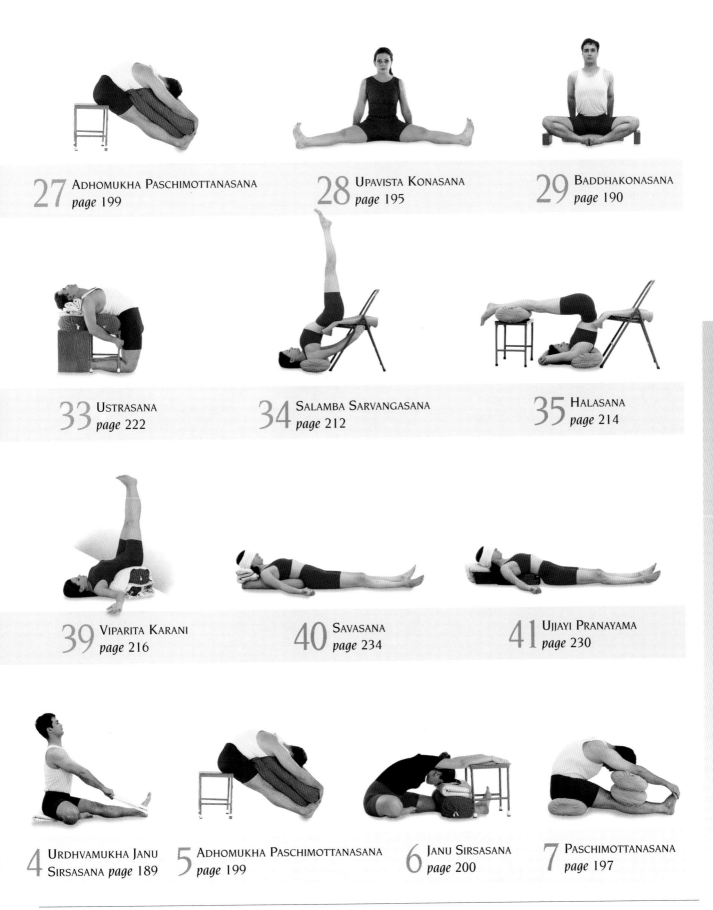

27 ADHOMUKHA PASCHIMOTTANASANA
page 199

28 UPAVISTA KONASANA
page 195

29 BADDHAKONASANA
page 190

33 USTRASANA
page 222

34 SALAMBA SARVANGASANA
page 212

35 HALASANA
page 214

39 VIPARITA KARANI
page 216

40 SAVASANA
page 234

41 UJJAYI PRANAYAMA
page 230

4 URDHVAMUKHA JANU
SIRSASANA page 189

5 ADHOMUKHA PASCHIMOTTANASANA
page 199

6 JANU SIRSASANA
page 200

7 PASCHIMOTTANASANA
page 197

HORMONAL SYSTEM

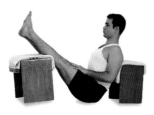

8 PARIPURNA NAVASANA
page 192

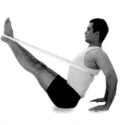

9 PARIPURNA NAVASANA
page 194

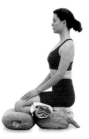

10 VIRASANA
page 188

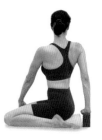

11 PARSVA VIRASANA
page 210

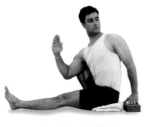

16 MARICHYASANA
page 207

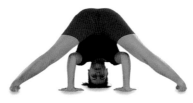

17 PRASARITA PADOTTANASANA
page 182

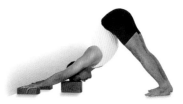

18 ADHOMUKHA SVANASANA
page 184

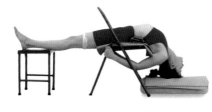

23 VIPARITA DANDASANA
page 221

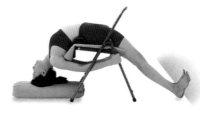

24 VIPARITA DANDASANA
page 221

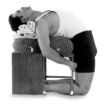

25 USTRASANA
page 222

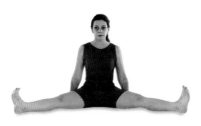

29 UPAVISTA KONASANA
page 195

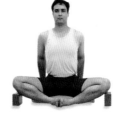

30 BADDHAKONASANA
page 190

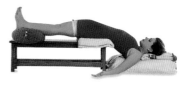

31 SETUBANDHA SARVANGASANA
page 219

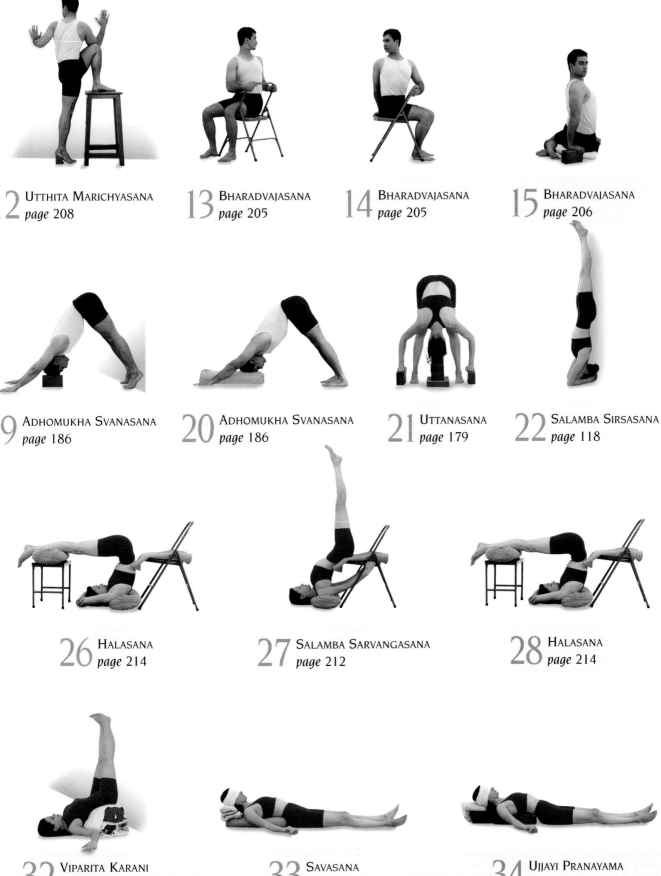

12 **UTTHITA MARICHYASANA**
page 208

13 **BHARADVAJASANA**
page 205

14 **BHARADVAJASANA**
page 205

15 **BHARADVAJASANA**
page 206

19 **ADHOMUKHA SVANASANA**
page 186

20 **ADHOMUKHA SVANASANA**
page 186

21 **UTTANASANA**
page 179

22 **SALAMBA SIRSASANA**
page 118

26 **HALASANA**
page 214

27 **SALAMBA SARVANGASANA**
page 212

28 **HALASANA**
page 214

32 **VIPARITA KARANI**
page 216

33 **SAVASANA**
page 234

34 **UJJAYI PRANAYAMA**
page 230

HORMONAL SYSTEM

Immune System

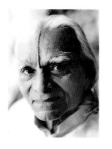

T HE IMMUNE SYSTEM IS THE defense mechanism of the body and protects us from disease. Its main agent is the blood, a fluid consisting of plasma and red and white blood cells. It is the white blood cells that inhibit the invasion of the bloodstream by micro-organisms. There are two types of immunity: natural and acquired. Yoga strengthens both, and regular practice of the recommended asanas can help counter the disorders that affect them.

Low immune system

In this condition, the body's immunity is impaired, resulting in a wide spectrum of illnesses. The symptoms include weight loss, increased susceptibility to infections, fatigue, fevers, and malignant disorders.

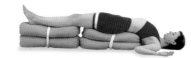

1 SETUBANDHA SARVANGASANA
 page 219

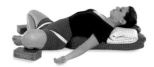

2 SUPTA BADDHAKONASANA
 page 226

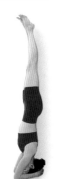

6 SALAMBA SIRSASANA
 page 118

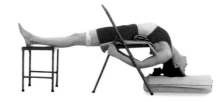

7 VIPARITA DANDASANA
 page 221

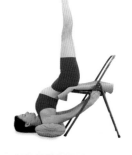

8 SALAMBA SARVANGASANA
 page 212

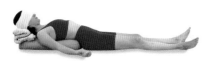

12 SAVASANA
 page 234

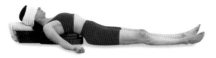

13 UJJAYI PRANAYAMA
 page 230

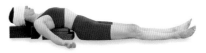

14 VILOMA 2 PRANAYAMA
 page 233

"Your whole body should be symmetrical. Yoga is symmetry."

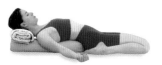

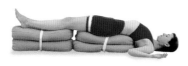

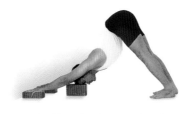

3 SUPTA VIRASANA
page 228

4 SETUBANDHA SARVANGASANA
page 219

5 ADHOMUKHA SVANASANA
page 184

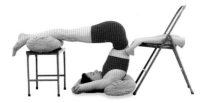

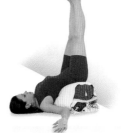

9 HALASANA
page 214

10 SETUBANDHA SARVANGASANA
page 219

11 VIPARITA KARANI
page 216

AIDS

Acquired Immune Deficiency Syndrome, or AIDS, is caused by the Human Immunodeficiency Virus (HIV) which attacks the immune system and leaves the human body vulnerable to many life-threatening diseases. The following sequence of asanas may help alleviate some of the symptoms of the condition.

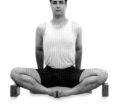

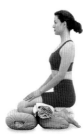

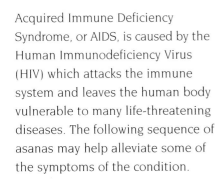

1 BADDHAKONASANA
page 190

2 VIRASANA
page 188

IMMUNE SYSTEM

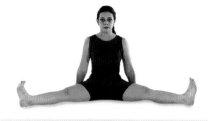

3 UPAVISTA KONASANA
page 195

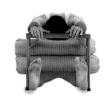

4 PASCHIMOTTANASANA
page 198

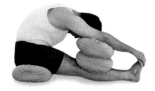

5 PASCHIMOTTANASANA
page 197

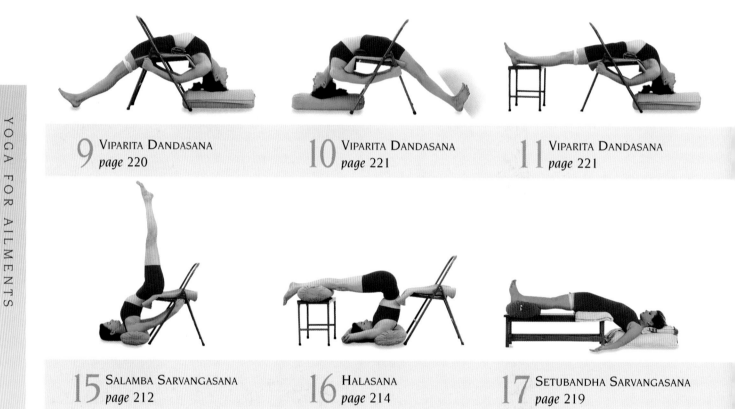

9 VIPARITA DANDASANA
page 220

10 VIPARITA DANDASANA
page 221

11 VIPARITA DANDASANA
page 221

15 SALAMBA SARVANGASANA
page 212

16 HALASANA
page 214

17 SETUBANDHA SARVANGASANA
page 219

"Yoga is for all of us. To limit

boundaries is the denial of

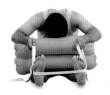
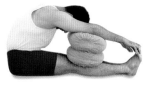
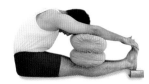

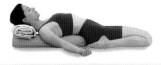
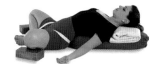
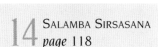

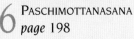
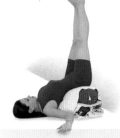
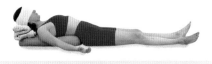

IMMUNE SYSTEM

yoga to national or cultural

universal consciousness."

Muscles, Bones, & Joints

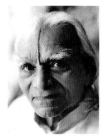

THE HUMAN BODY IS COMPOSED of bone and muscle. The bones that make up the skeletal frame of the body are attached to each other by joints which are held in place by strong ligaments and muscles. A muscle contracts or relaxes to move the bones connected to it. Better muscle function means a fitter, stronger body. Practicing yoga strengthens the bones, improves coordination of the muscles, and provides a non-invasive way of treating ailments that affect both.

Physical fatigue

Stressful physical exertion brings on this condition, characterized by exhaustion and a reluctance to exert oneself. If unrelieved by rest, and the removal of stress factors, the condition may lead to chronic fatigue syndrome.

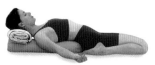
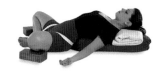

1 SUPTA BADDHAKONASANA *page 226*

2 SUPTA VIRASANA *page 228*

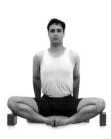
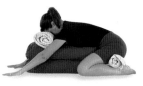

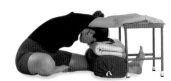

7 BADDHAKONASANA *page 190*

8 ADHOMUKHA VIRASANA *page 203*

9 PASCHIMOTTANASANA *page 198*

10 JANU SIRSASANA *page 200*

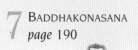
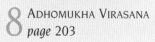
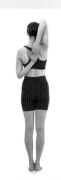
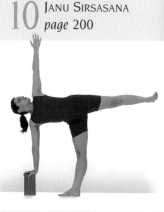

15 TADASANA URDHVA BADDHA HASTASANA *page 170*

16 TADASANA PASCHIMA NAMASKAR *page 172*

17 TADASANA GOMUKHASANA *page 173*

18 ARDHA CHANDRASANA *page 178*

"Freedom with true discipline is true freedom."

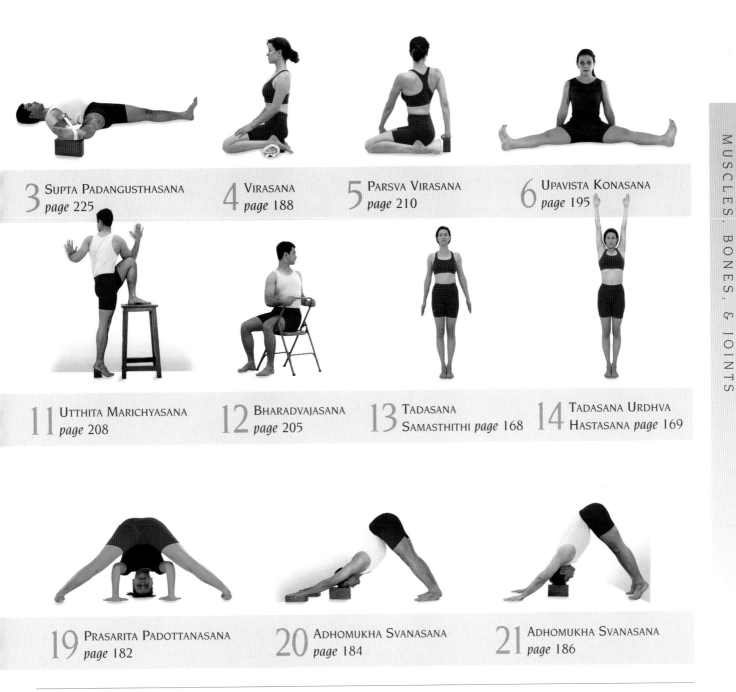

3 SUPTA PADANGUSTHASANA *page* 225

4 VIRASANA *page* 188

5 PARSVA VIRASANA *page* 210

6 UPAVISTA KONASANA *page* 195

11 UTTHITA MARICHYASANA *page* 208

12 BHARADVAJASANA *page* 205

13 TADASANA SAMASTHITHI *page* 168

14 TADASANA URDHVA HASTASANA *page* 169

19 PRASARITA PADOTTANASANA *page* 182

20 ADHOMUKHA SVANASANA *page* 184

21 ADHOMUKHA SVANASANA *page* 186

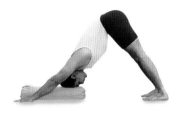

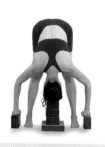

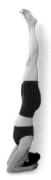

22 ADHOMUKHA SVANASANA *page 186*

23 UTTANASANA *page 179*

24 SALAMBA SIRSASANA *page 118*

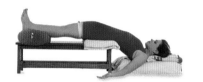

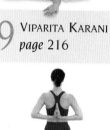

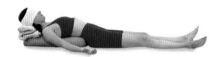

28 SETUBANDHA SARVANGASANA *page 219*

29 VIPARITA KARANI *page 216*

30 SAVASANA *page 234*

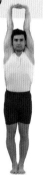

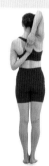

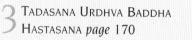

3 TADASANA URDHVA BADDHA HASTASANA *page 170*

4 TADASANA PASCHIMA NAMASKAR *page 172*

5 TADASANA GOMUKHASANA *page 173*

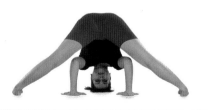

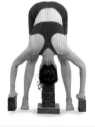

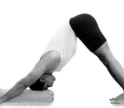

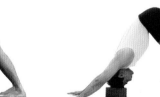

10 PRASARITA PADOTTANASANA *page 182*

11 UTTANASANA *page 179*

12 ADHOMUKHA SVANASANA *page 186*

13 ADHOMUKHA SVANASANA *page 186*

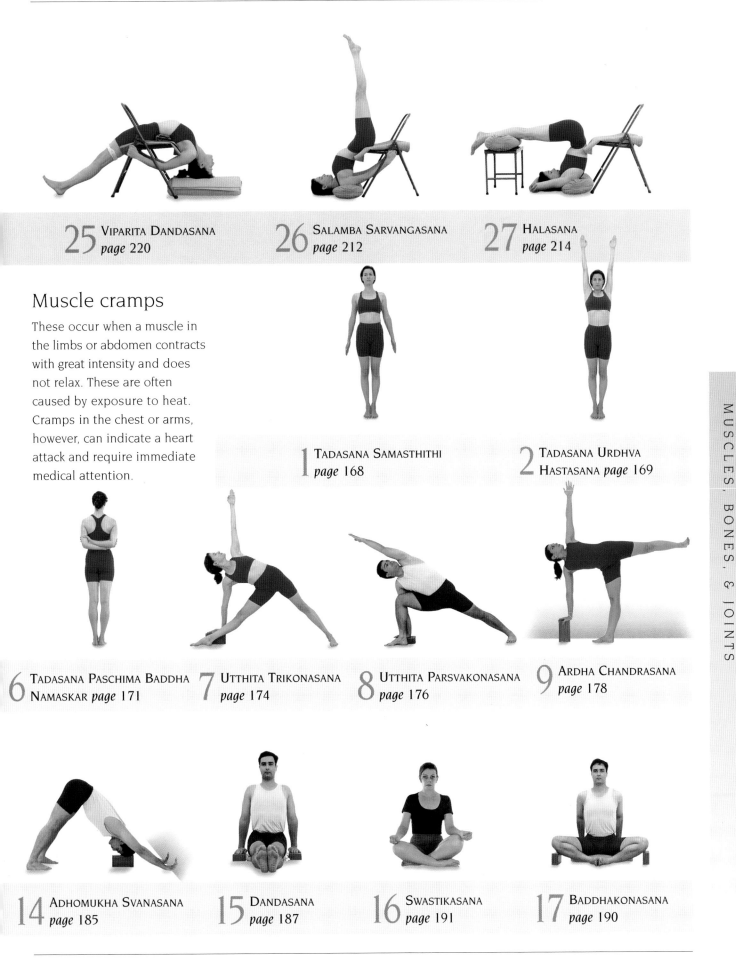

25 VIPARITA DANDASANA *page 220*

26 SALAMBA SARVANGASANA *page 212*

27 HALASANA *page 214*

Muscle cramps

These occur when a muscle in the limbs or abdomen contracts with great intensity and does not relax. These are often caused by exposure to heat. Cramps in the chest or arms, however, can indicate a heart attack and require immediate medical attention.

1 TADASANA SAMASTHITHI *page 168*

2 TADASANA URDHVA HASTASANA *page 169*

6 TADASANA PASCHIMA BADDHA NAMASKAR *page 171*

7 UTTHITA TRIKONASANA *page 174*

8 UTTHITA PARSVAKONASANA *page 176*

9 ARDHA CHANDRASANA *page 178*

14 ADHOMUKHA SVANASANA *page 185*

15 DANDASANA *page 187*

16 SWASTIKASANA *page 191*

17 BADDHAKONASANA *page 190*

MUSCLES, BONES, & JOINTS

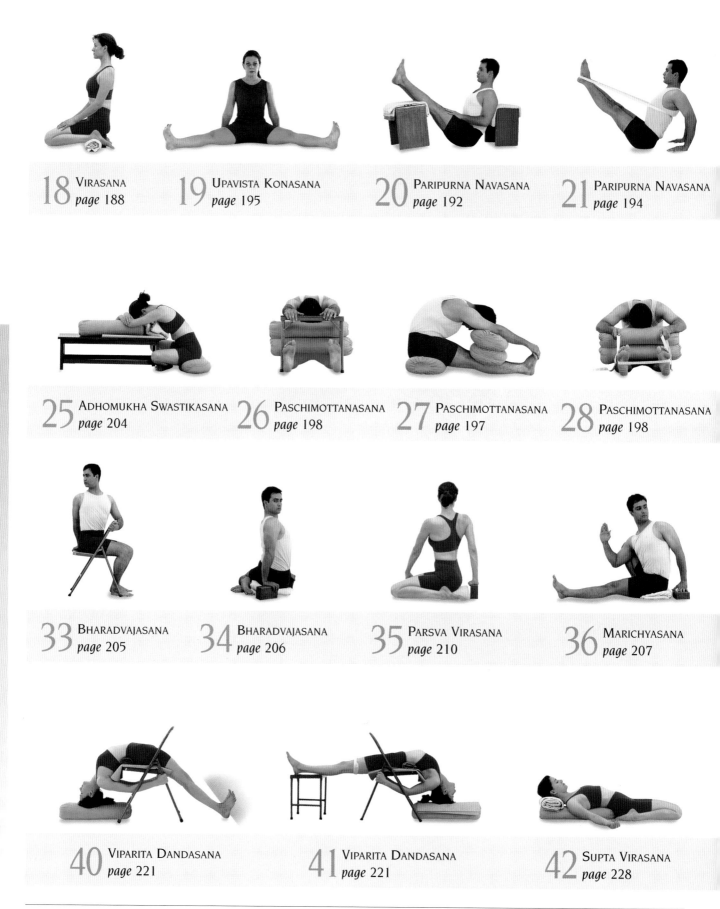

18 VIRASANA
page 188

19 UPAVISTA KONASANA
page 195

20 PARIPURNA NAVASANA
page 192

21 PARIPURNA NAVASANA
page 194

25 ADHOMUKHA SWASTIKASANA
page 204

26 PASCHIMOTTANASANA
page 198

27 PASCHIMOTTANASANA
page 197

28 PASCHIMOTTANASANA
page 198

33 BHARADVAJASANA
page 205

34 BHARADVAJASANA
page 206

35 PARSVA VIRASANA
page 210

36 MARICHYASANA
page 207

40 VIPARITA DANDASANA
page 221

41 VIPARITA DANDASANA
page 221

42 SUPTA VIRASANA
page 228

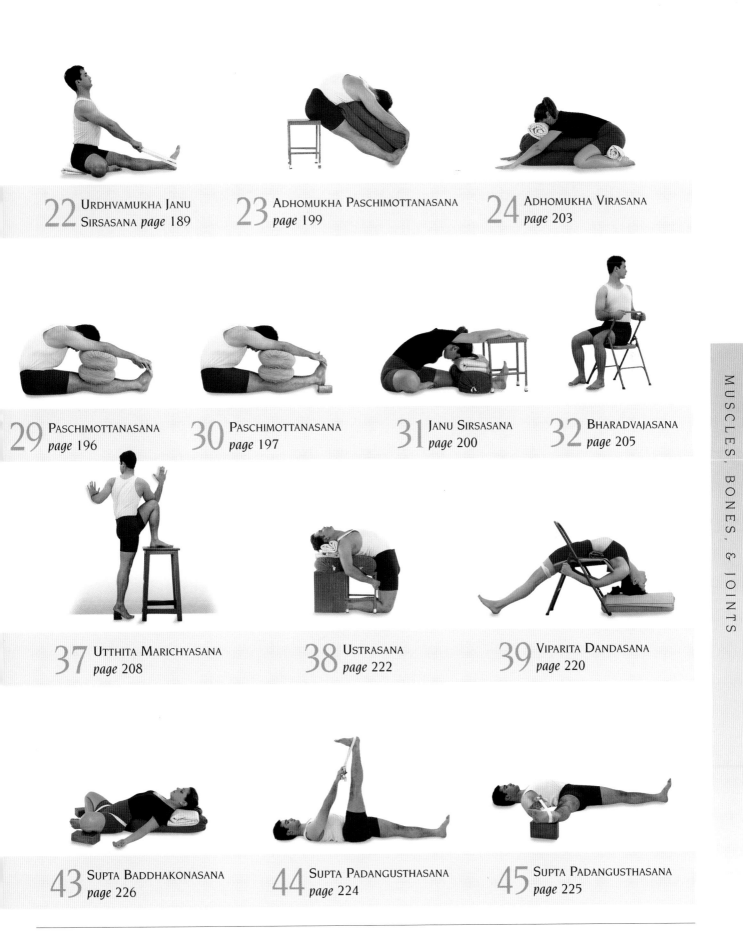

22 URDHVAMUKHA JANU
SIRSASANA *page* 189

23 ADHOMUKHA PASCHIMOTTANASANA
page 199

24 ADHOMUKHA VIRASANA
page 203

29 PASCHIMOTTANASANA
page 196

30 PASCHIMOTTANASANA
page 197

31 JANU SIRSASANA
page 200

32 BHARADVAJASANA
page 205

37 UTTHITA MARICHYASANA
page 208

38 USTRASANA
page 222

39 VIPARITA DANDASANA
page 220

43 SUPTA BADDHAKONASANA
page 226

44 SUPTA PADANGUSTHASANA
page 224

45 SUPTA PADANGUSTHASANA
page 225

MUSCLES, BONES, & JOINTS

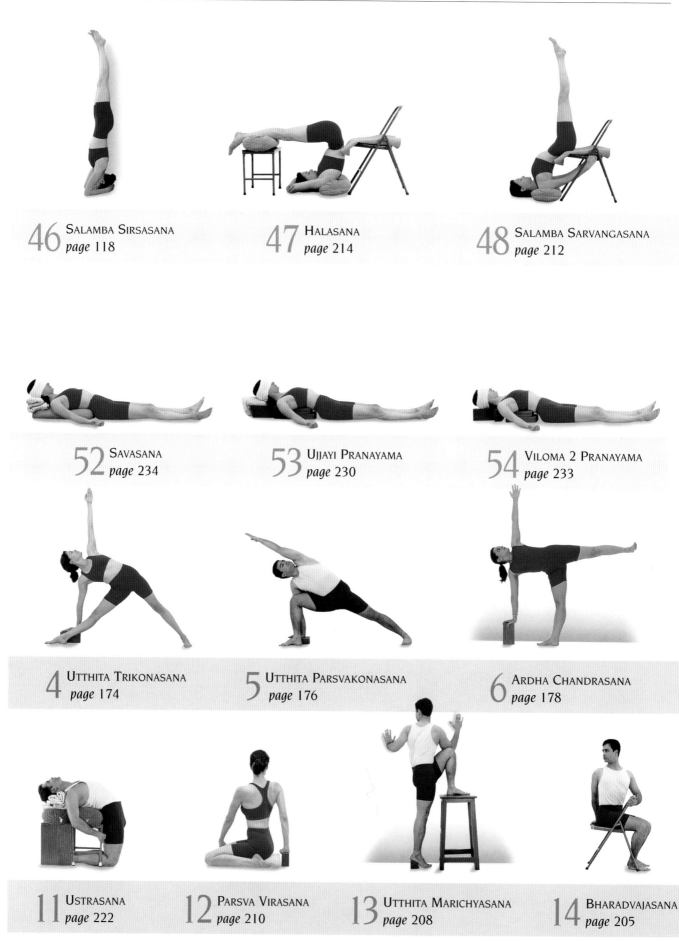

46 SALAMBA SIRSASANA
page 118

47 HALASANA
page 214

48 SALAMBA SARVANGASANA
page 212

52 SAVASANA
page 234

53 UJJAYI PRANAYAMA
page 230

54 VILOMA 2 PRANAYAMA
page 233

4 UTTHITA TRIKONASANA
page 174

5 UTTHITA PARSVAKONASANA
page 176

6 ARDHA CHANDRASANA
page 178

11 USTRASANA
page 222

12 PARSVA VIRASANA
page 210

13 UTTHITA MARICHYASANA
page 208

14 BHARADVAJASANA
page 205

YOGA FOR AILMENTS

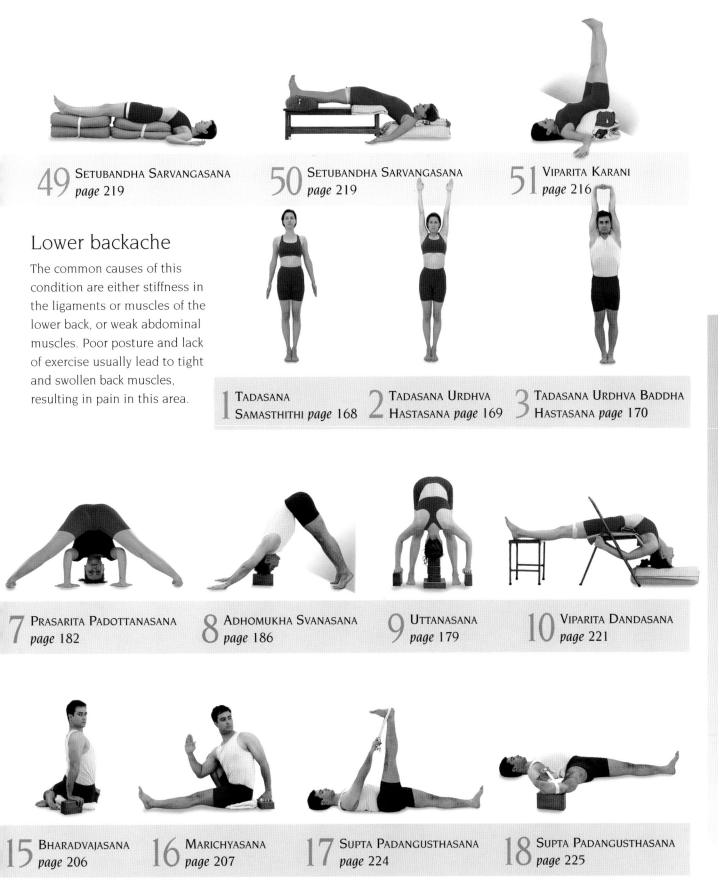

49 SETUBANDHA SARVANGASANA
page 219

50 SETUBANDHA SARVANGASANA
page 219

51 VIPARITA KARANI
page 216

Lower backache

The common causes of this condition are either stiffness in the ligaments or muscles of the lower back, or weak abdominal muscles. Poor posture and lack of exercise usually lead to tight and swollen back muscles, resulting in pain in this area.

1 TADASANA
SAMASTHITHI *page* 168

2 TADASANA URDHVA
HASTASANA *page* 169

3 TADASANA URDHVA BADDHA
HASTASANA *page* 170

7 PRASARITA PADOTTANASANA
page 182

8 ADHOMUKHA SVANASANA
page 186

9 UTTANASANA
page 179

10 VIPARITA DANDASANA
page 221

15 BHARADVAJASANA
page 206

16 MARICHYASANA
page 207

17 SUPTA PADANGUSTHASANA
page 224

18 SUPTA PADANGUSTHASANA
page 225

MUSCLES, BONES, & JOINTS

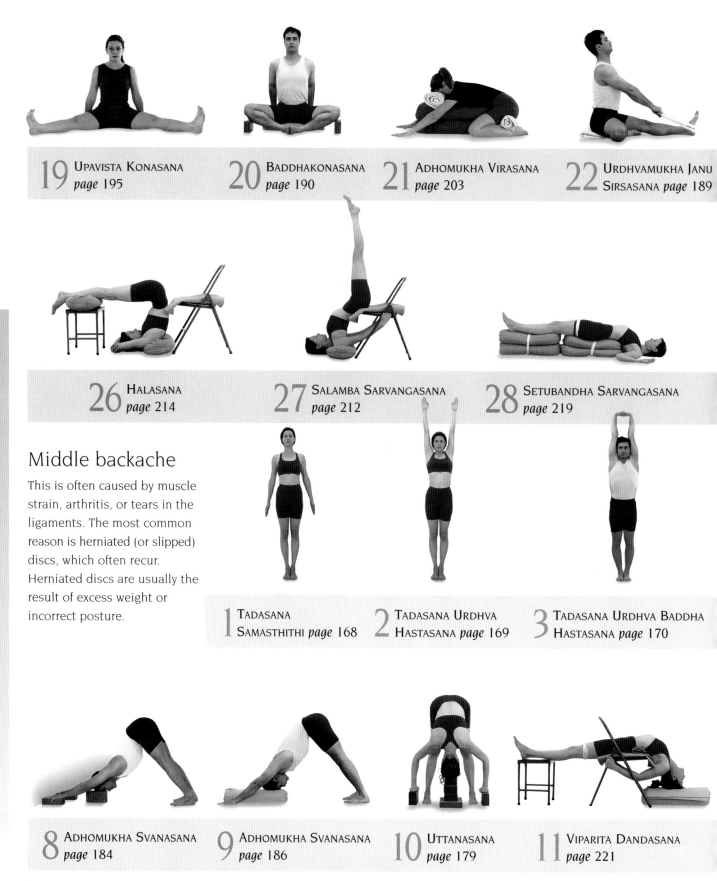

19 UPAVISTA KONASANA *page 195*

20 BADDHAKONASANA *page 190*

21 ADHOMUKHA VIRASANA *page 203*

22 URDHVAMUKHA JANU SIRSASANA *page 189*

26 HALASANA *page 214*

27 SALAMBA SARVANGASANA *page 212*

28 SETUBANDHA SARVANGASANA *page 219*

Middle backache

This is often caused by muscle strain, arthritis, or tears in the ligaments. The most common reason is herniated (or slipped) discs, which often recur. Herniated discs are usually the result of excess weight or incorrect posture.

1 TADASANA SAMASTHITHI *page 168*

2 TADASANA URDHVA HASTASANA *page 169*

3 TADASANA URDHVA BADDHA HASTASANA *page 170*

8 ADHOMUKHA SVANASANA *page 184*

9 ADHOMUKHA SVANASANA *page 186*

10 UTTANASANA *page 179*

11 VIPARITA DANDASANA *page 221*

YOGA FOR AILMENTS

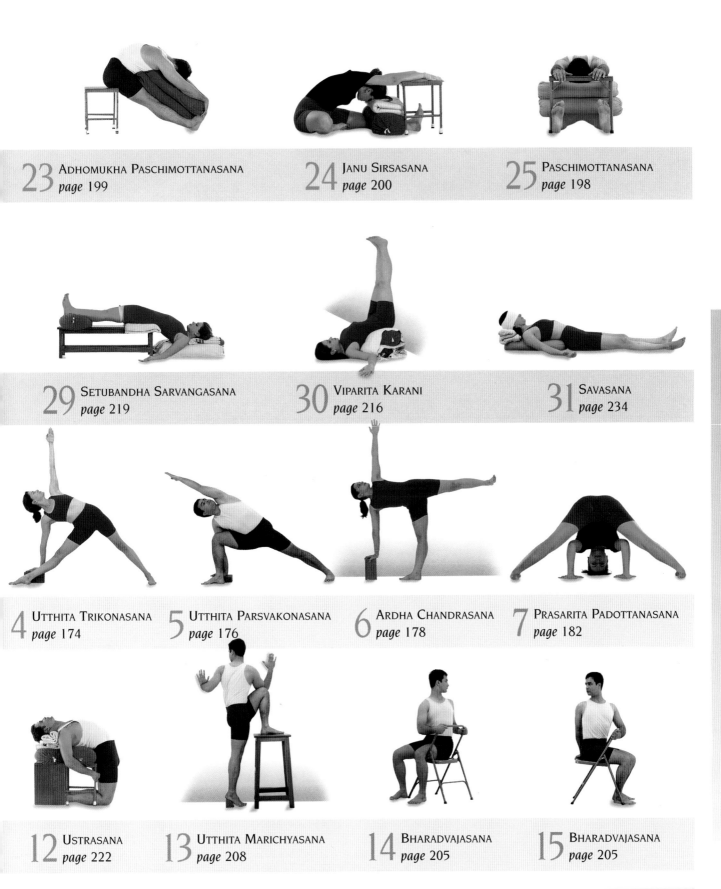

23 ADHOMUKHA PASCHIMOTTANASANA
page 199

24 JANU SIRSASANA
page 200

25 PASCHIMOTTANASANA
page 198

29 SETUBANDHA SARVANGASANA
page 219

30 VIPARITA KARANI
page 216

31 SAVASANA
page 234

4 UTTHITA TRIKONASANA
page 174

5 UTTHITA PARSVAKONASANA
page 176

6 ARDHA CHANDRASANA
page 178

7 PRASARITA PADOTTANASANA
page 182

12 USTRASANA
page 222

13 UTTHITA MARICHYASANA
page 208

14 BHARADVAJASANA
page 205

15 BHARADVAJASANA
page 205

MUSCLES, BONES, & JOINTS

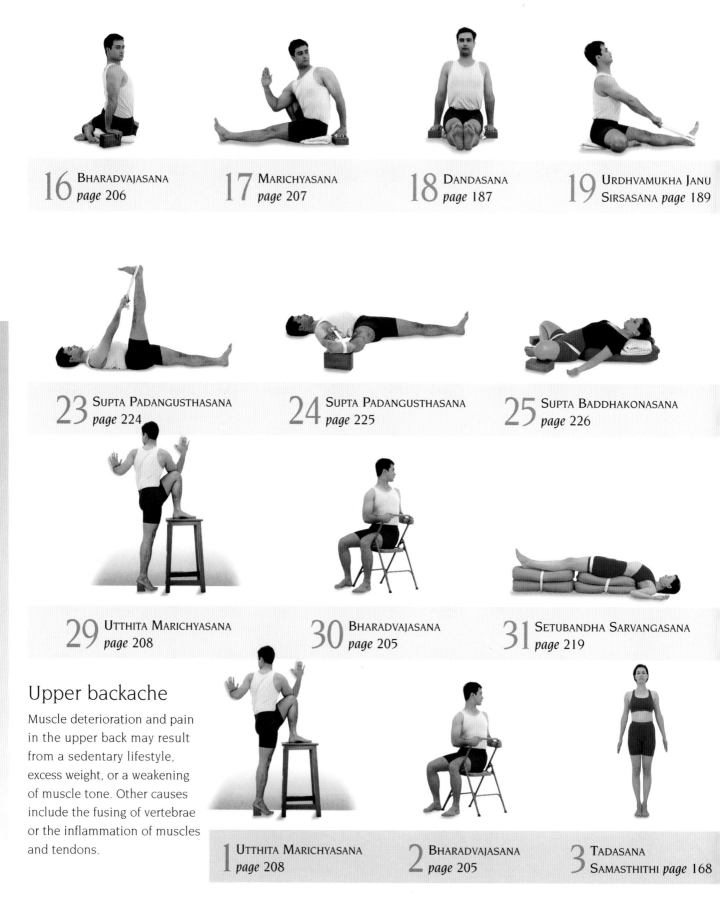

16 BHARADVAJASANA
page 206

17 MARICHYASANA
page 207

18 DANDASANA
page 187

19 URDHVAMUKHA JANU
SIRSASANA page 189

23 SUPTA PADANGUSTHASANA
page 224

24 SUPTA PADANGUSTHASANA
page 225

25 SUPTA BADDHAKONASANA
page 226

29 UTTHITA MARICHYASANA
page 208

30 BHARADVAJASANA
page 205

31 SETUBANDHA SARVANGASANA
page 219

Upper backache

Muscle deterioration and pain in the upper back may result from a sedentary lifestyle, excess weight, or a weakening of muscle tone. Other causes include the fusing of vertebrae or the inflammation of muscles and tendons.

1 UTTHITA MARICHYASANA
page 208

2 BHARADVAJASANA
page 205

3 TADASANA
SAMASTHITHI page 168

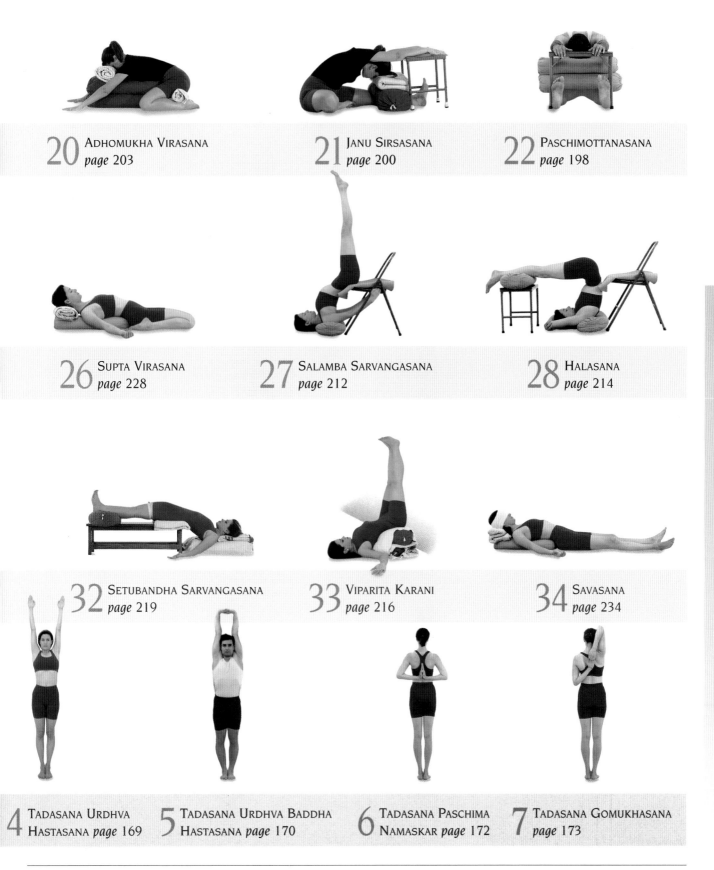

20 ADHOMUKHA VIRASANA
page 203

21 JANU SIRSASANA
page 200

22 PASCHIMOTTANASANA
page 198

26 SUPTA VIRASANA
page 228

27 SALAMBA SARVANGASANA
page 212

28 HALASANA
page 214

32 SETUBANDHA SARVANGASANA
page 219

33 VIPARITA KARANI
page 216

34 SAVASANA
page 234

4 TADASANA URDHVA
HASTASANA *page* 169

5 TADASANA URDHVA BADDHA
HASTASANA *page* 170

6 TADASANA PASCHIMA
NAMASKAR *page* 172

7 TADASANA GOMUKHASANA
page 173

MUSCLES, BONES, & JOINTS

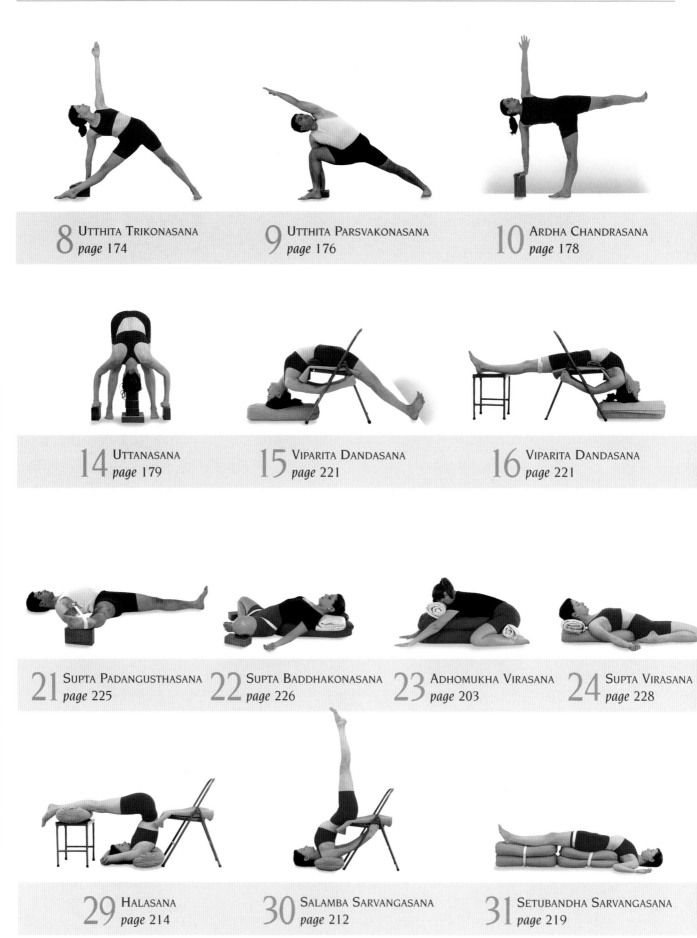

YOGA FOR AILMENTS

8 UTTHITA TRIKONASANA
page 174

9 UTTHITA PARSVAKONASANA
page 176

10 ARDHA CHANDRASANA
page 178

14 UTTANASANA
page 179

15 VIPARITA DANDASANA
page 221

16 VIPARITA DANDASANA
page 221

21 SUPTA PADANGUSTHASANA
page 225

22 SUPTA BADDHAKONASANA
page 226

23 ADHOMUKHA VIRASANA
page 203

24 SUPTA VIRASANA
page 228

29 HALASANA
page 214

30 SALAMBA SARVANGASANA
page 212

31 SETUBANDHA SARVANGASANA
page 219

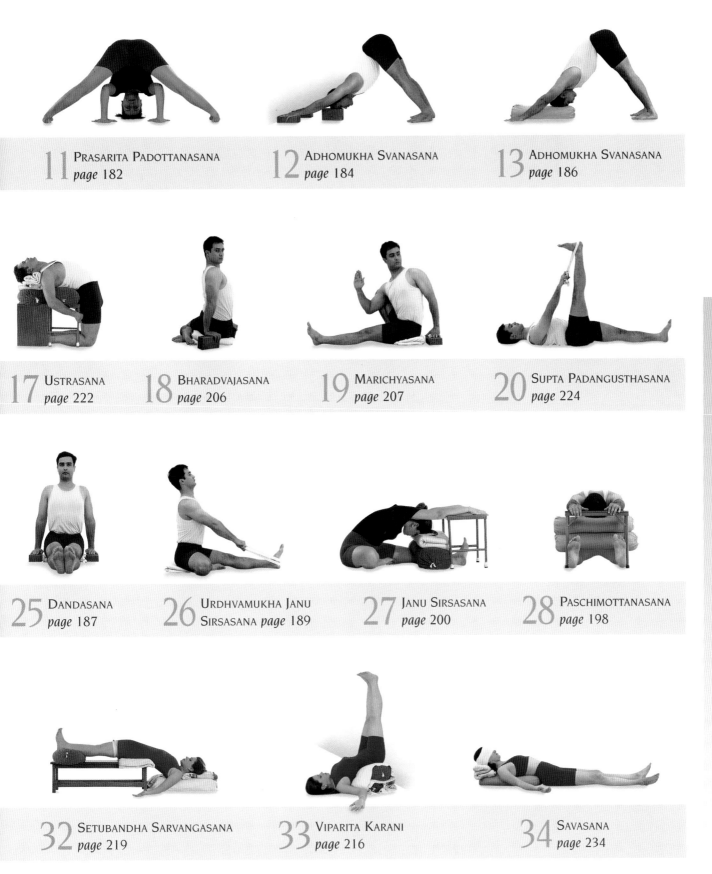

11 PRASARITA PADOTTANASANA
page 182

12 ADHOMUKHA SVANASANA
page 184

13 ADHOMUKHA SVANASANA
page 186

17 USTRASANA
page 222

18 BHARADVAJASANA
page 206

19 MARICHYASANA
page 207

20 SUPTA PADANGUSTHASANA
page 224

25 DANDASANA
page 187

26 URDHVAMUKHA JANU
SIRSASANA *page* 189

27 JANU SIRSASANA
page 200

28 PASCHIMOTTANASANA
page 198

32 SETUBANDHA SARVANGASANA
page 219

33 VIPARITA KARANI
page 216

34 SAVASANA
page 234

MUSCLES, BONES, & JOINTS

Cervical spondylosis

This is a degenerative disease of the spine caused by wear and tear on the joints between the cervical vertebrae. Also called cervical osteoarthritis, the symptoms include pain in the arms and neck, headaches, and dizziness.

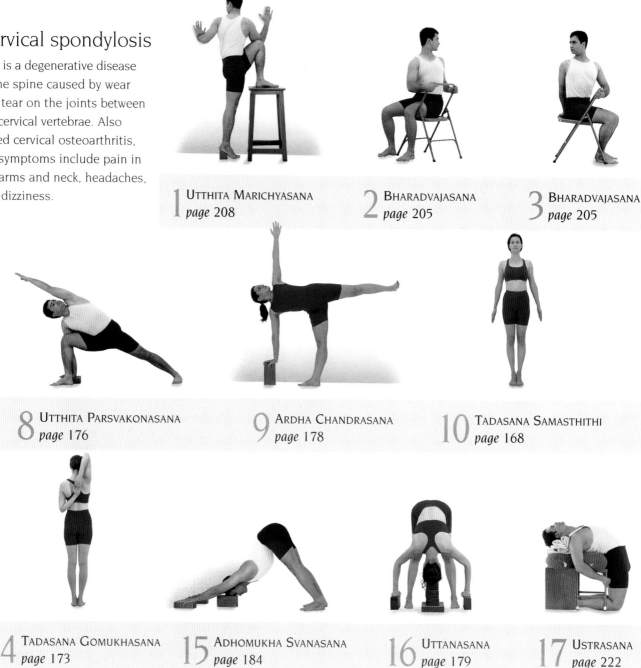

1 **UTTHITA MARICHYASANA**
page 208

2 **BHARADVAJASANA**
page 205

3 **BHARADVAJASANA**
page 205

8 **UTTHITA PARSVAKONASANA**
page 176

9 **ARDHA CHANDRASANA**
page 178

10 **TADASANA SAMASTHITHI**
page 168

14 **TADASANA GOMUKHASANA**
page 173

15 **ADHOMUKHA SVANASANA**
page 184

16 **UTTANASANA**
page 179

17 **USTRASANA**
page 222

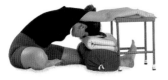

21 **JANU SIRSASANA**
PAGE 200

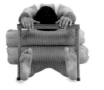

22 **PASCHIMOTTANASANA**
page 198

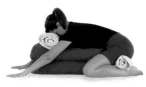

23 **ADHOMUKHA VIRASANA**
page 203

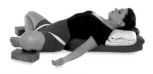

24 **SUPTA BADDHAKONASANA**
page 226

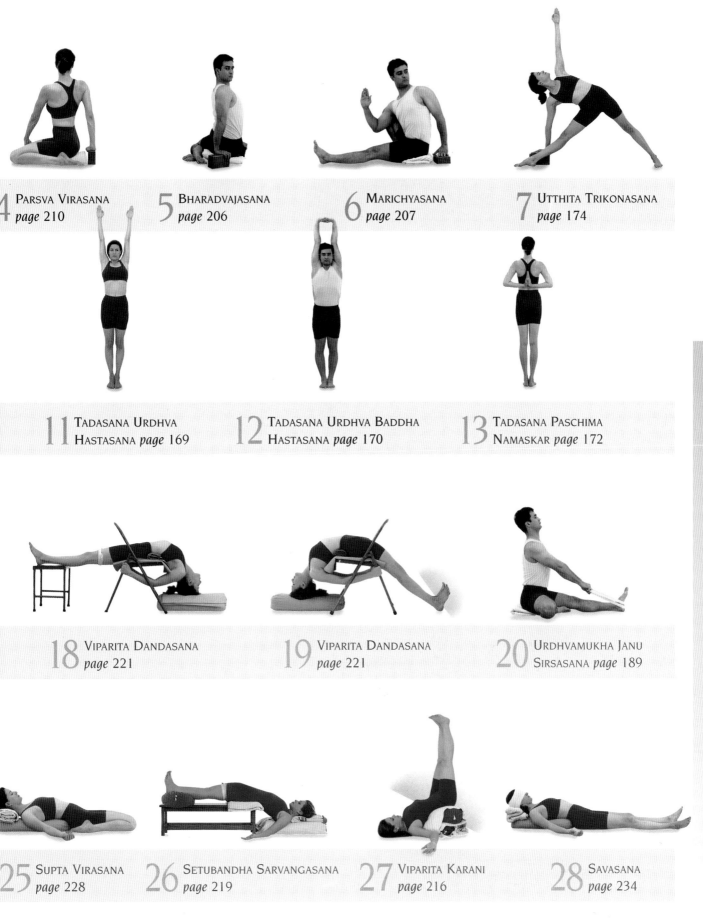

4 PARSVA VIRASANA
page 210

5 BHARADVAJASANA
page 206

6 MARICHYASANA
page 207

7 UTTHITA TRIKONASANA
page 174

11 TADASANA URDHVA
HASTASANA *page* 169

12 TADASANA URDHVA BADDHA
HASTASANA *page* 170

13 TADASANA PASCHIMA
NAMASKAR *page* 172

18 VIPARITA DANDASANA
page 221

19 VIPARITA DANDASANA
page 221

20 URDHVAMUKHA JANU
SIRSASANA *page* 189

25 SUPTA VIRASANA
page 228

26 SETUBANDHA SARVANGASANA
page 219

27 VIPARITA KARANI
page 216

28 SAVASANA
page 234

MUSCLES, BONES, & JOINTS

Osteoarthritis

SHOULDERS This condition is caused by the erosion of cartilage between joints causing the bones to press against each other. The narrowing of joint space due to calcification, along with the thickening of tendons in the shoulder joint, cause severe pain.

YOGA FOR AILMENTS

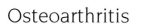

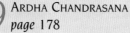

1 TADASANA SAMASTHITHI *page* 168

2 TADASANA URDHVA HASTASANA *page* 170

3 TADASANA URDHVA BADDHA HASTASANA *page* 170

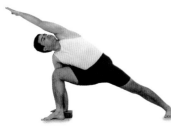

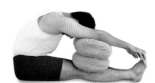

8 UTTHITA PARSVAKONASANA *page* 176

9 ARDHA CHANDRASANA *page* 178

10 ADHOMUKHA SVANASANA *page* 184

11 UTTHITA MARICHYASANA *page* 208

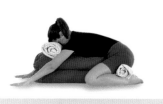

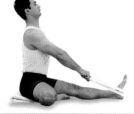

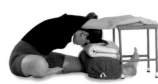

16 ADHOMUKHA VIRASANA *page* 203

17 URDHVAMUKHA JANU SIRSASANA *page* 189

18 JANU SIRSASANA *page* 200

19 PASCHIMOTTANASANA *page* 196

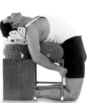

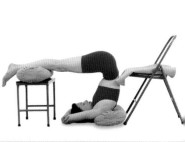

24 SALAMBA SIRSASANA *page* 118

25 USTRASANA *page* 222

26 SALAMBA SARVANGASANA *page* 212

27 HALASANA *page* 214

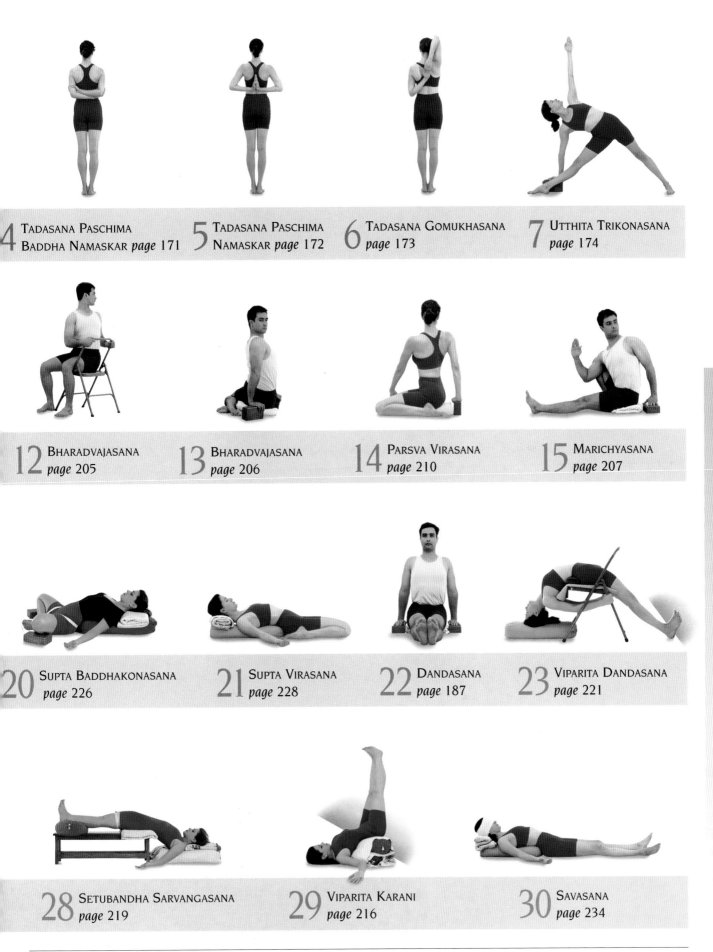

4 TADASANA PASCHIMA BADDHA NAMASKAR *page* 171

5 TADASANA PASCHIMA NAMASKAR *page* 172

6 TADASANA GOMUKHASANA *page* 173

7 UTTHITA TRIKONASANA *page* 174

12 BHARADVAJASANA *page* 205

13 BHARADVAJASANA *page* 206

14 PARSVA VIRASANA *page* 210

15 MARICHYASANA *page* 207

20 SUPTA BADDHAKONASANA *page* 226

21 SUPTA VIRASANA *page* 228

22 DANDASANA *page* 187

23 VIPARITA DANDASANA *page* 221

28 SETUBANDHA SARVANGASANA *page* 219

29 VIPARITA KARANI *page* 216

30 SAVASANA *page* 234

MUSCLES, BONES, & JOINTS

Osteoarthritis

ELBOWS In this condition, the cartilage between the joints of the elbows wears out, causing inflammation and pain. This can lead to the formation of bone spurs, or the condition of tennis elbow, the latter usually indicated by severe pain in the forearm and elbow.

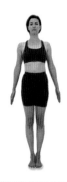
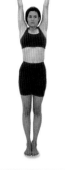

1 TADASANA SAMASTHITHI *page* 168

2 TADASANA URDHVA HASTASANA *page* 169

3 TADASANA URDHVA BADDHA HASTASANA *page* 170

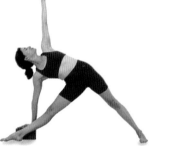
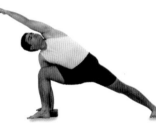
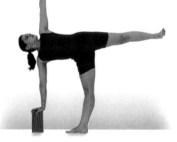

7 UTTHITA TRIKONASANA *page* 174

8 UTTHITA PARSVAKONASANA *page* 176

9 ARDHA CHANDRASANA *page* 178

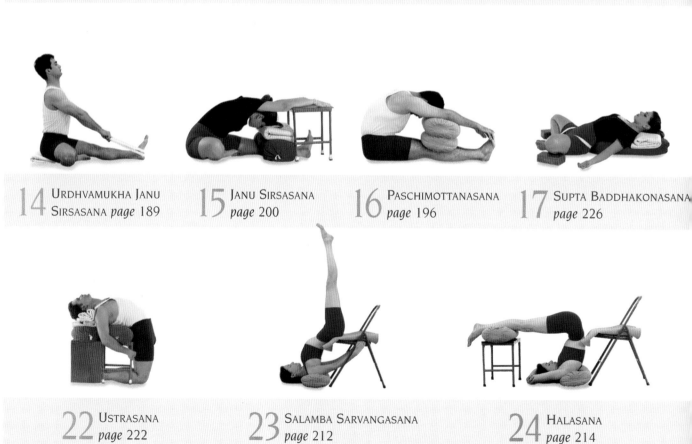

14 URDHVAMUKHA JANU SIRSASANA *page* 189

15 JANU SIRSASANA *page* 200

16 PASCHIMOTTANASANA *page* 196

17 SUPTA BADDHAKONASANA *page* 226

22 USTRASANA *page* 222

23 SALAMBA SARVANGASANA *page* 212

24 HALASANA *page* 214

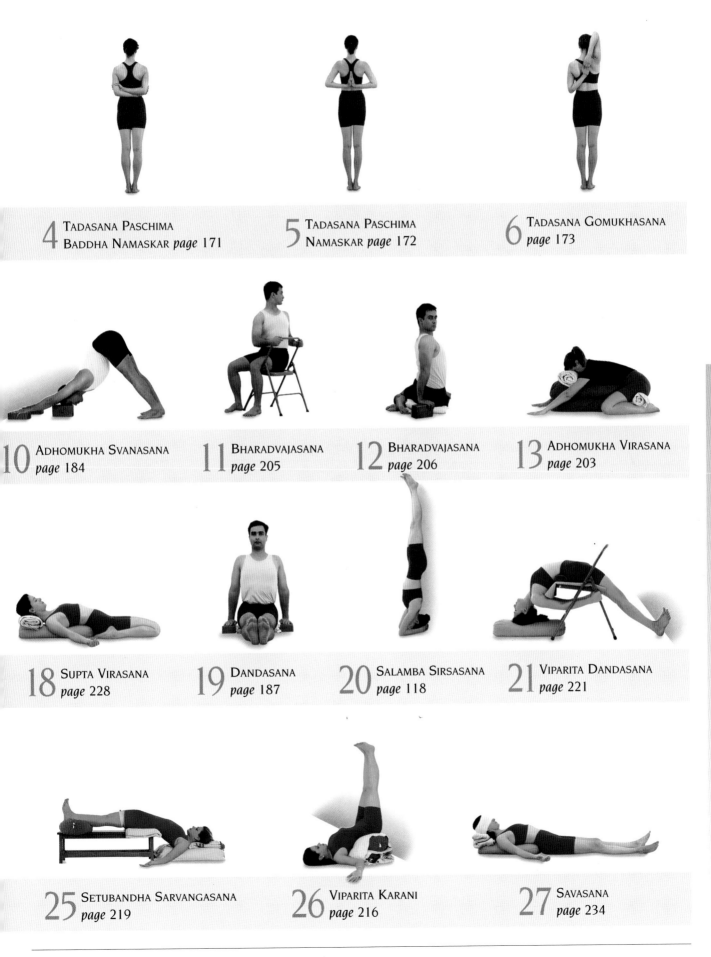

4 TADASANA PASCHIMA BADDHA NAMASKAR *page* 171

5 TADASANA PASCHIMA NAMASKAR *page* 172

6 TADASANA GOMUKHASANA *page* 173

10 ADHOMUKHA SVANASANA *page* 184

11 BHARADVAJASANA *page* 205

12 BHARADVAJASANA *page* 206

13 ADHOMUKHA VIRASANA *page* 203

18 SUPTA VIRASANA *page* 228

19 DANDASANA *page* 187

20 SALAMBA SIRSASANA *page* 118

21 VIPARITA DANDASANA *page* 221

25 SETUBANDHA SARVANGASANA *page* 219

26 VIPARITA KARANI *page* 216

27 SAVASANA *page* 234

MUSCLES, BONES, & JOINTS

Osteoarthritis

WRISTS AND FINGERS In the wrist, this condition is usually the result of an old injury and is characterized by restricted movement and pain in the joint. In the fingers, osteoarthritis is most common at the base of the thumb.

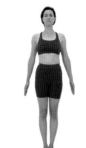
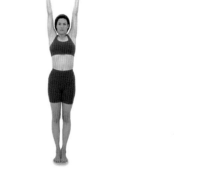
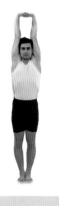

1 TADASANA SAMASTHITHI *page* 168

2 TADASANA URDHVA HASTASANA *page* 169

3 TADASANA URDHVA BADDHA HASTASANA *page* 170

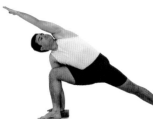
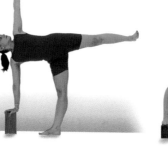
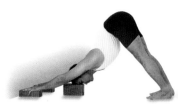

8 UTTHITA PARSVAKONASANA *page* 176

9 ARDHA CHANDRASANA *page* 178

10 UTTANASANA *page* 179

11 ADHOMUKHA SVANASANA *page* 184

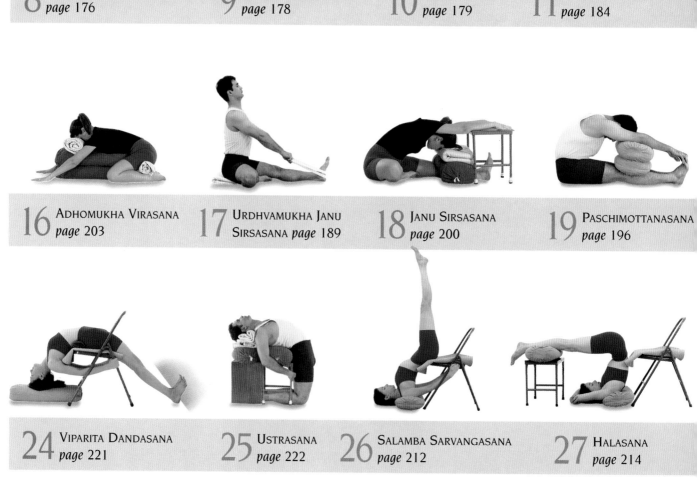

16 ADHOMUKHA VIRASANA *page* 203

17 URDHVAMUKHA JANU SIRSASANA *page* 189

18 JANU SIRSASANA *page* 200

19 PASCHIMOTTANASANA *page* 196

24 VIPARITA DANDASANA *page* 221

25 USTRASANA *page* 222

26 SALAMBA SARVANGASANA *page* 212

27 HALASANA *page* 214

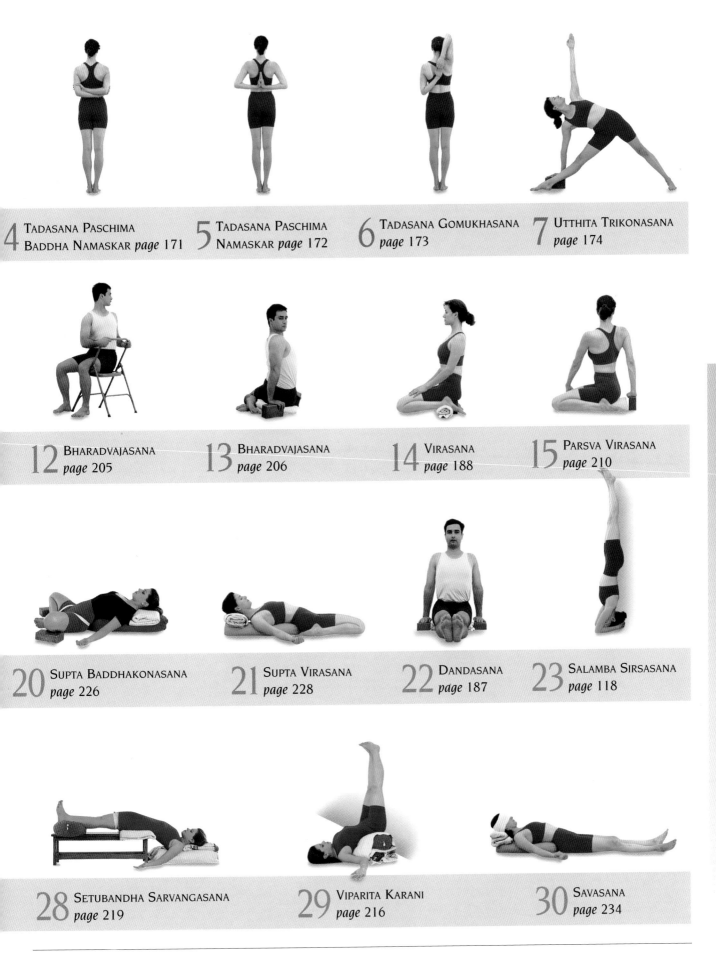

4 TADASANA PASCHIMA
BADDHA NAMASKAR *page 171*

5 TADASANA PASCHIMA
NAMASKAR *page 172*

6 TADASANA GOMUKHASANA
page 173

7 UTTHITA TRIKONASANA
page 174

12 BHARADVAJASANA
page 205

13 BHARADVAJASANA
page 206

14 VIRASANA
page 188

15 PARSVA VIRASANA
page 210

20 SUPTA BADDHAKONASANA
page 226

21 SUPTA VIRASANA
page 228

22 DANDASANA
page 187

23 SALAMBA SIRSASANA
page 118

28 SETUBANDHA SARVANGASANA
page 219

29 VIPARITA KARANI
page 216

30 SAVASANA
page 234

MUSCLES, BONES, & JOINTS

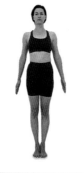
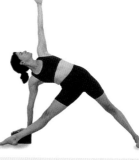
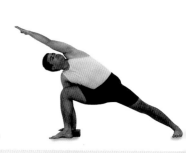

Osteoarthritis

HIPS This joint is particularly prone to this condition since it bears a lot of weight. Pain is experienced in surrounding areas such as the groin, outer hips, and knees. This can result in a vicious circle. Reduced movement due to pain, leads to more stiffness due to inactivity.

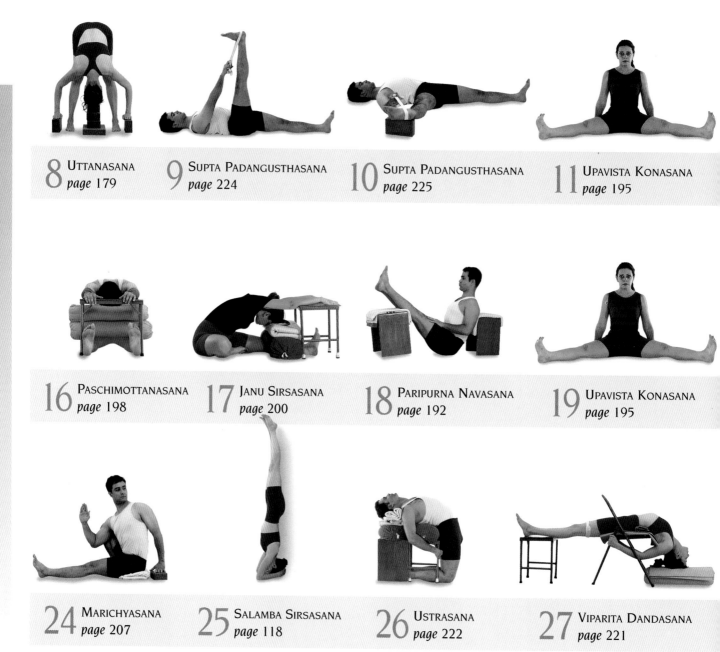

1 **TADASANA SAMASTHITHI** *page 168*

2 **UTTHITA TRIKONASANA** *page 174*

3 **UTTHITA PARSVAKONASANA** *page 176*

8 **UTTANASANA** *page 179*

9 **SUPTA PADANGUSTHASANA** *page 224*

10 **SUPTA PADANGUSTHASANA** *page 225*

11 **UPAVISTA KONASANA** *page 195*

16 **PASCHIMOTTANASANA** *page 198*

17 **JANU SIRSASANA** *page 200*

18 **PARIPURNA NAVASANA** *page 192*

19 **UPAVISTA KONASANA** *page 195*

24 **MARICHYASANA** *page 207*

25 **SALAMBA SIRSASANA** *page 118*

26 **USTRASANA** *page 222*

27 **VIPARITA DANDASANA** *page 221*

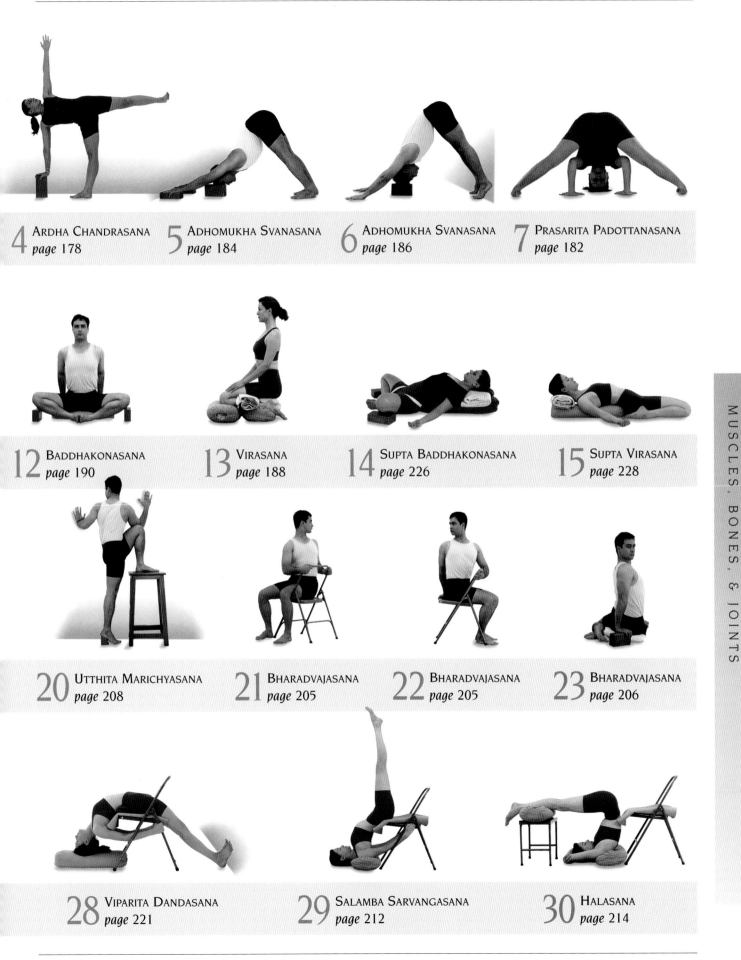

4 ARDHA CHANDRASANA
page 178

5 ADHOMUKHA SVANASANA
page 184

6 ADHOMUKHA SVANASANA
page 186

7 PRASARITA PADOTTANASANA
page 182

12 BADDHAKONASANA
page 190

13 VIRASANA
page 188

14 SUPTA BADDHAKONASANA
page 226

15 SUPTA VIRASANA
page 228

20 UTTHITA MARICHYASANA
page 208

21 BHARADVAJASANA
page 205

22 BHARADVAJASANA
page 205

23 BHARADVAJASANA
page 206

28 VIPARITA DANDASANA
page 221

29 SALAMBA SARVANGASANA
page 212

30 HALASANA
page 214

MUSCLES, BONES, & JOINTS

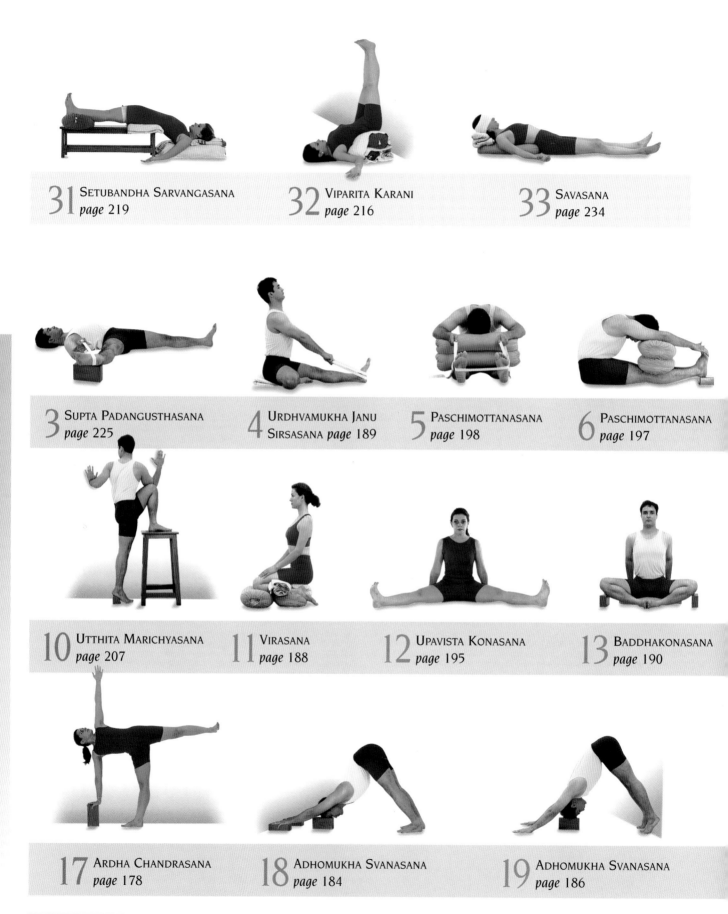

31 SETUBANDHA SARVANGASANA
page 219

32 VIPARITA KARANI
page 216

33 SAVASANA
page 234

3 SUPTA PADANGUSTHASANA
page 225

4 URDHVAMUKHA JANU
SIRSASANA *page* 189

5 PASCHIMOTTANASANA
page 198

6 PASCHIMOTTANASANA
page 197

10 UTTHITA MARICHYASANA
page 207

11 VIRASANA
page 188

12 UPAVISTA KONASANA
page 195

13 BADDHAKONASANA
page 190

17 ARDHA CHANDRASANA
page 178

18 ADHOMUKHA SVANASANA
page 184

19 ADHOMUKHA SVANASANA
page 186

Osteoarthritis

KNEES A decrease in the synovial fluid that lubricates the knee joint leads to this condition. The cartilage in the area becomes rough and tends to flake off. The knee looks swollen, and the joint loses flexibility and the ability to stretch and bend.

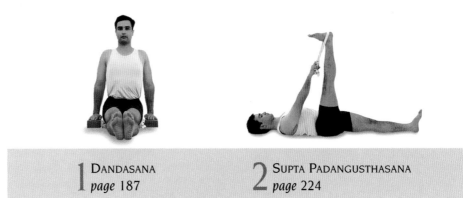

1 DANDASANA
page 187

2 SUPTA PADANGUSTHASANA
page 224

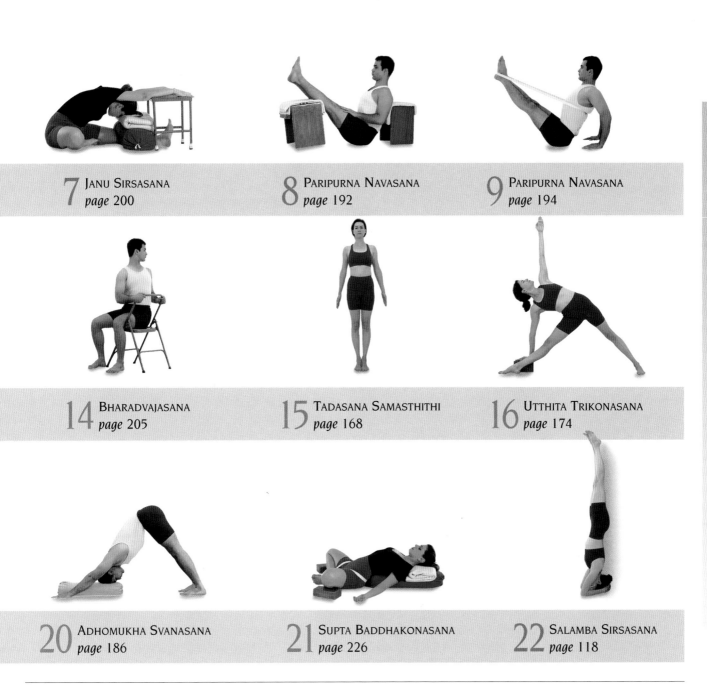

7 JANU SIRSASANA
page 200

8 PARIPURNA NAVASANA
page 192

9 PARIPURNA NAVASANA
page 194

14 BHARADVAJASANA
page 205

15 TADASANA SAMASTHITHI
page 168

16 UTTHITA TRIKONASANA
page 174

20 ADHOMUKHA SVANASANA
page 186

21 SUPTA BADDHAKONASANA
page 226

22 SALAMBA SIRSASANA
page 118

MUSCLES, BONES, & JOINTS

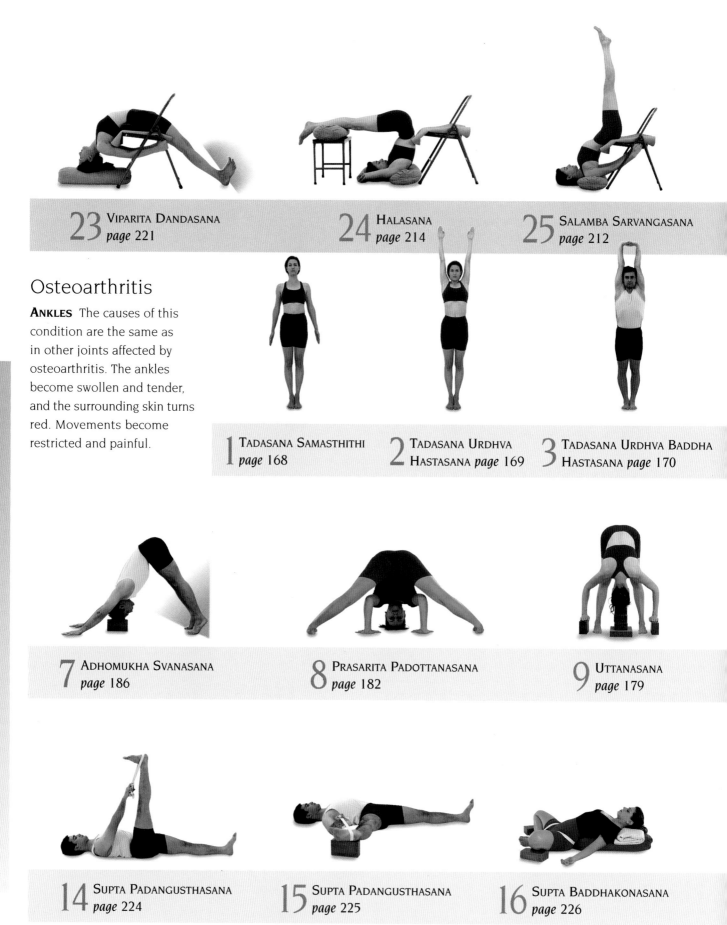

23 VIPARITA DANDASANA
page 221

24 HALASANA
page 214

25 SALAMBA SARVANGASANA
page 212

Osteoarthritis

ANKLES The causes of this condition are the same as in other joints affected by osteoarthritis. The ankles become swollen and tender, and the surrounding skin turns red. Movements become restricted and painful.

1 TADASANA SAMASTHITHI
page 168

2 TADASANA URDHVA HASTASANA *page 169*

3 TADASANA URDHVA BADDHA HASTASANA *page 170*

7 ADHOMUKHA SVANASANA
page 186

8 PRASARITA PADOTTANASANA
page 182

9 UTTANASANA
page 179

14 SUPTA PADANGUSTHASANA
page 224

15 SUPTA PADANGUSTHASANA
page 225

16 SUPTA BADDHAKONASANA
page 226

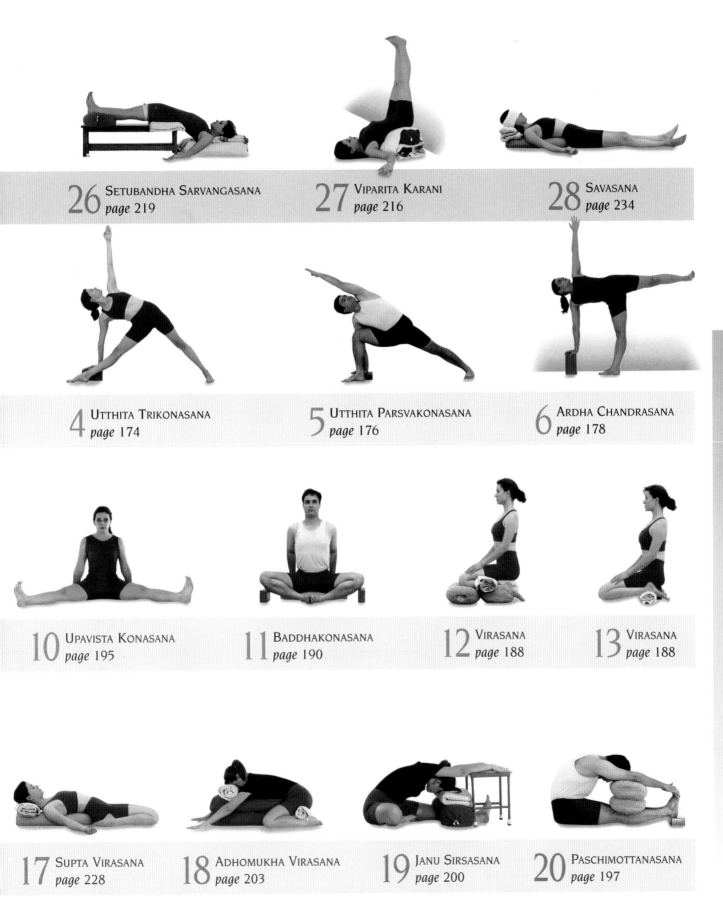

26 SETUBANDHA SARVANGASANA
page 219

27 VIPARITA KARANI
page 216

28 SAVASANA
page 234

4 UTTHITA TRIKONASANA
page 174

5 UTTHITA PARSVAKONASANA
page 176

6 ARDHA CHANDRASANA
page 178

10 UPAVISTA KONASANA
page 195

11 BADDHAKONASANA
page 190

12 VIRASANA
page 188

13 VIRASANA
page 188

17 SUPTA VIRASANA
page 228

18 ADHOMUKHA VIRASANA
page 203

19 JANU SIRSASANA
page 200

20 PASCHIMOTTANASANA
page 197

MUSCLES, BONES, & JOINTS

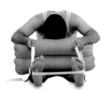

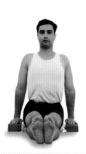

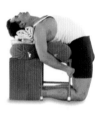

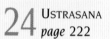

21 **PASCHIMOTTANASANA** *page 198*

22 **DANDASANA** *page 187*

23 **SALAMBA SIRSASANA** *page 118*

24 **USTRASANA** *page 222*

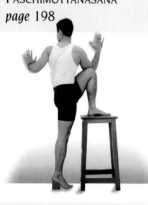

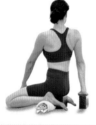

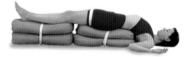

28 **UTTHITA MARICHYASANA** *page 208*

29 **PARSVA VIRASANA** *page 211*

30 **SETUBANDHA SARVANGASANA** *page 219*

Rheumatoid arthritis

This is a chronic, systemic, inflammatory condition, which leads to the eventual disability of the joints. The symptoms are stiffness in the mornings, fatigue, burning and swelling of the joints, and the appearance of rheumatoid nodules.

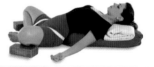

1 **SAVASANA** *page 234*

2 **SUPTA BADDHAKONASANA** *page 226*

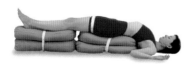

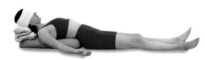

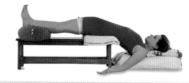

6 **SETUBANDHA SARVANGASANA** *page 219*

7 **SETUBANDHA SARVANGASANA** *page 219*

8 **UPAVISTA KONASANA** *page 195*

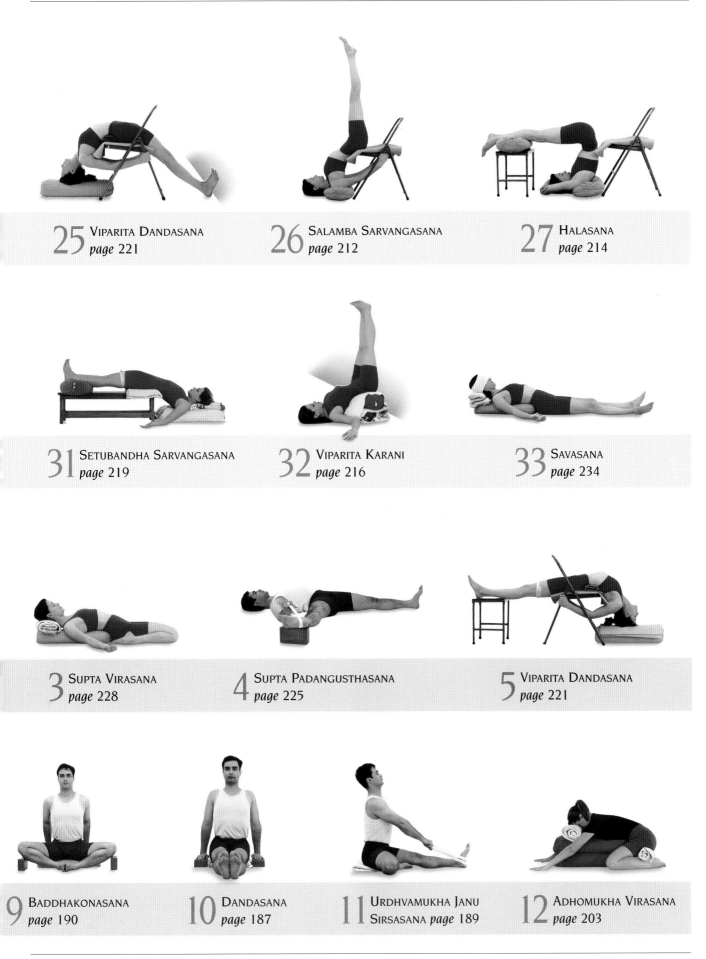

25 VIPARITA DANDASANA
page 221

26 SALAMBA SARVANGASANA
page 212

27 HALASANA
page 214

31 SETUBANDHA SARVANGASANA
page 219

32 VIPARITA KARANI
page 216

33 SAVASANA
page 234

3 SUPTA VIRASANA
page 228

4 SUPTA PADANGUSTHASANA
page 225

5 VIPARITA DANDASANA
page 221

9 BADDHAKONASANA
page 190

10 DANDASANA
page 187

11 URDHVAMUKHA JANU
SIRSASANA *page* 189

12 ADHOMUKHA VIRASANA
page 203

MUSCLES, BONES, & JOINTS

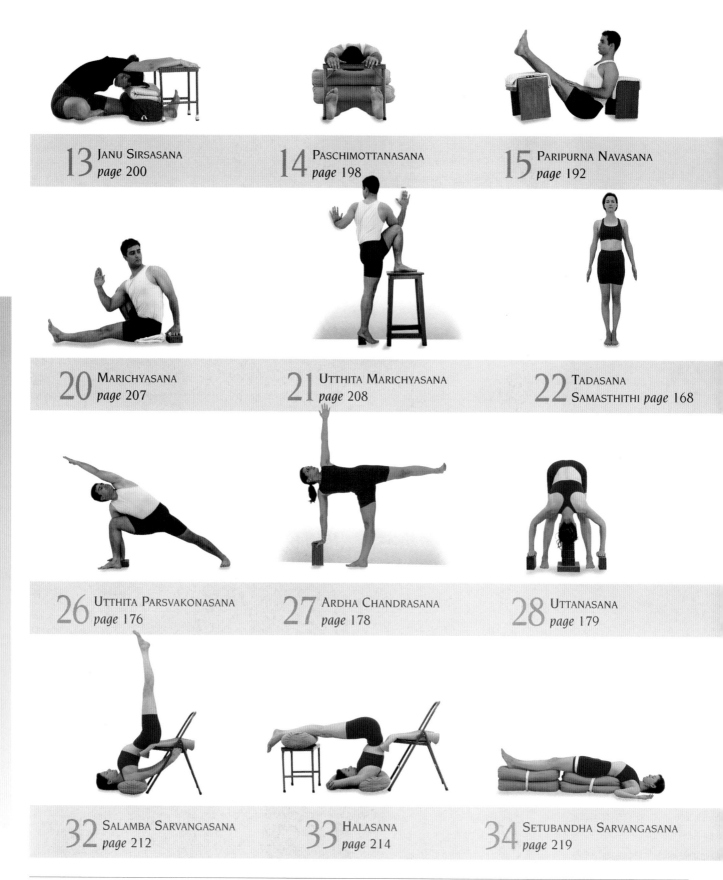

YOGA FOR AILMENTS

13 JANU SIRSASANA
page 200

14 PASCHIMOTTANASANA
page 198

15 PARIPURNA NAVASANA
page 192

20 MARICHYASANA
page 207

21 UTTHITA MARICHYASANA
page 208

22 TADASANA
SAMASTHITHI *page 168*

26 UTTHITA PARSVAKONASANA
page 176

27 ARDHA CHANDRASANA
page 178

28 UTTANASANA
page 179

32 SALAMBA SARVANGASANA
page 212

33 HALASANA
page 214

34 SETUBANDHA SARVANGASANA
page 219

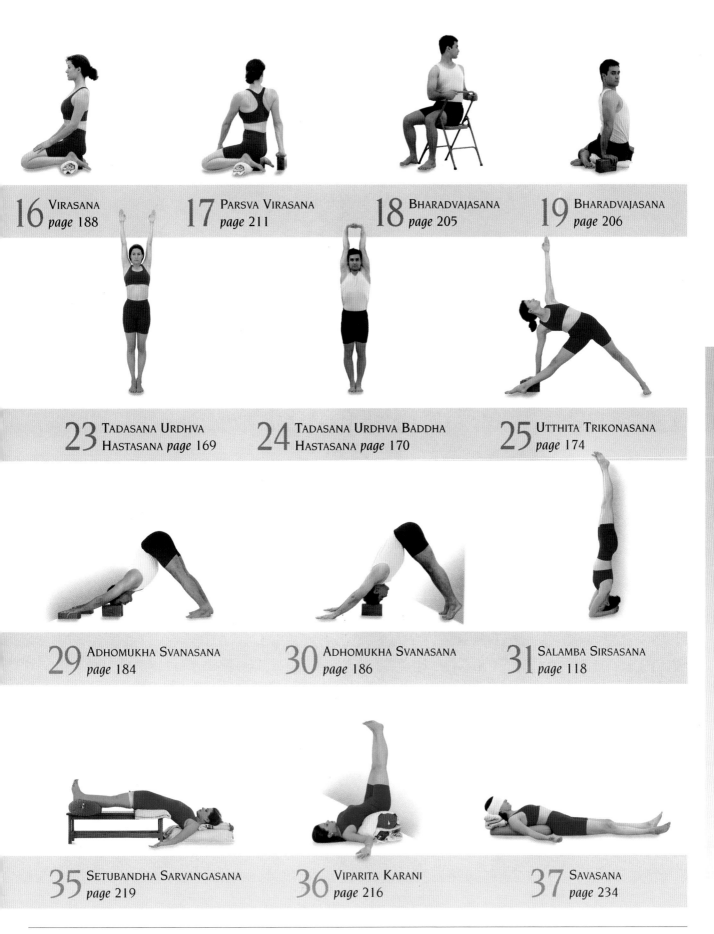

16 VIRASANA *page* 188

17 PARSVA VIRASANA *page* 211

18 BHARADVAJASANA *page* 205

19 BHARADVAJASANA *page* 206

23 TADASANA URDHVA HASTASANA *page* 169

24 TADASANA URDHVA BADDHA HASTASANA *page* 170

25 UTTHITA TRIKONASANA *page* 174

29 ADHOMUKHA SVANASANA *page* 184

30 ADHOMUKHA SVANASANA *page* 186

31 SALAMBA SIRSASANA *page* 118

35 SETUBANDHA SARVANGASANA *page* 219

36 VIPARITA KARANI *page* 216

37 SAVASANA *page* 234

MUSCLES, BONES, & JOINTS

Skin

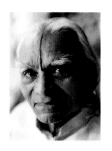

THE SKIN, THE LARGEST ORGAN OF THE BODY, is part of the sensory system. It is the principal organ of the sense of touch and it serves to protect the internal organs. The skin also regulates body temperature. It consists of a vascular layer called the dermis, and an external covering called the epidermis. The sweat glands, hair follicles, and sebaceous glands are embedded in the dermis. Disorders of the skin are common, and yoga asanas offer a healthy and effective form of treatment.

Acne

This is a skin disorder caused by inflammation of the sebaceous glands or hair follicles. Acne, appearing as boils, pimples, pustules, spots, or whiteheads, is sometimes triggered by anxiety. It usually affects adolescents, but may persist in later age.

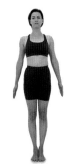
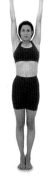
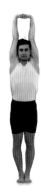

1 TADASANA SAMASTHITHI *page* 168

2 TADASANA URDHVA HASTASANA *page* 169

3 TADASANA URDHVA BADDHA HASTASANA *page* 170

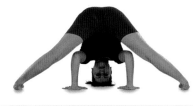
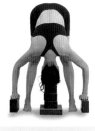
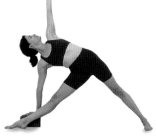

8 PRASARITA PADOTTANASANA *page* 182

9 UTTANASANA *page* 179

10 UTTHITA TRIKONASANA *page* 174

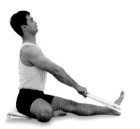
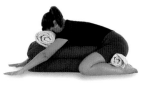
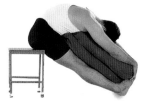

14 URDHVAMUKHA JANU SIRSASANA *page* 189

15 ADHOMUKHA VIRASANA *page* 203

16 ADHOMUKHA PASCHIMOTTANASANA *page* 199

"Keep your brain calm and quiet. Let your body be active."

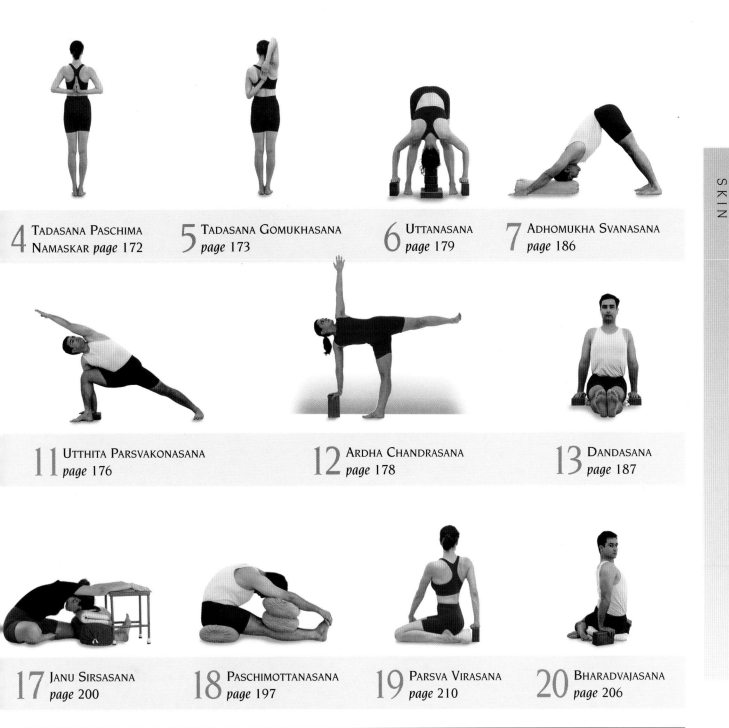

4 TADASANA PASCHIMA NAMASKAR *page* 172

5 TADASANA GOMUKHASANA *page* 173

6 UTTANASANA *page* 179

7 ADHOMUKHA SVANASANA *page* 186

11 UTTHITA PARSVAKONASANA *page* 176

12 ARDHA CHANDRASANA *page* 178

13 DANDASANA *page* 187

17 JANU SIRSASANA *page* 200

18 PASCHIMOTTANASANA *page* 197

19 PARSVA VIRASANA *page* 210

20 BHARADVAJASANA *page* 206

SKIN

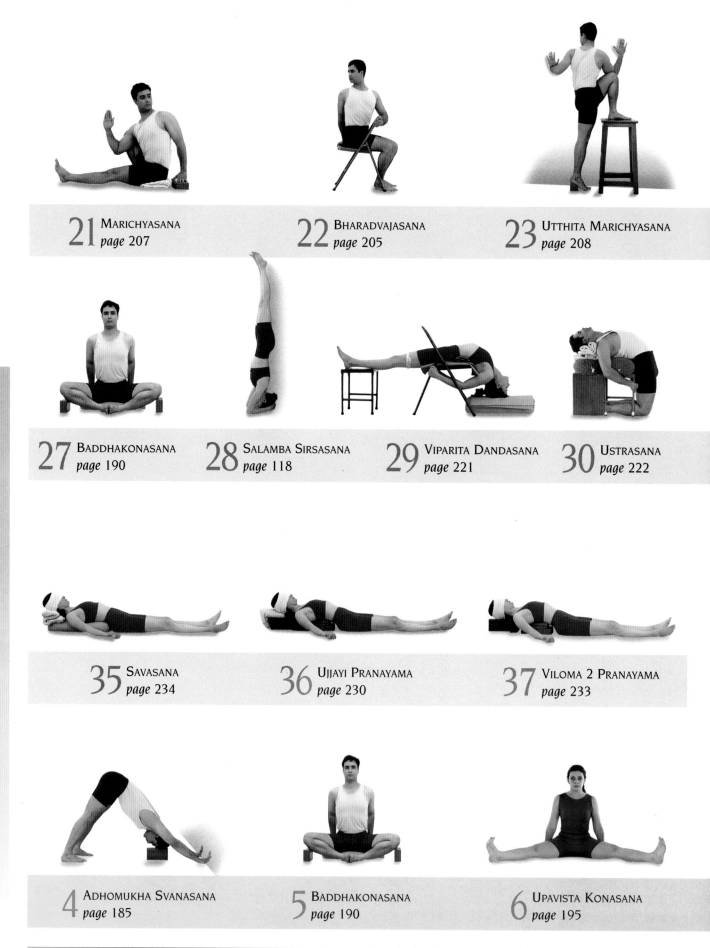

21 MARICHYASANA
page 207

22 BHARADVAJASANA
page 205

23 UTTHITA MARICHYASANA
page 208

27 BADDHAKONASANA
page 190

28 SALAMBA SIRSASANA
page 118

29 VIPARITA DANDASANA
page 221

30 USTRASANA
page 222

35 SAVASANA
page 234

36 UJJAYI PRANAYAMA
page 230

37 VILOMA 2 PRANAYAMA
page 233

4 ADHOMUKHA SVANASANA
page 185

5 BADDHAKONASANA
page 190

6 UPAVISTA KONASANA
page 195

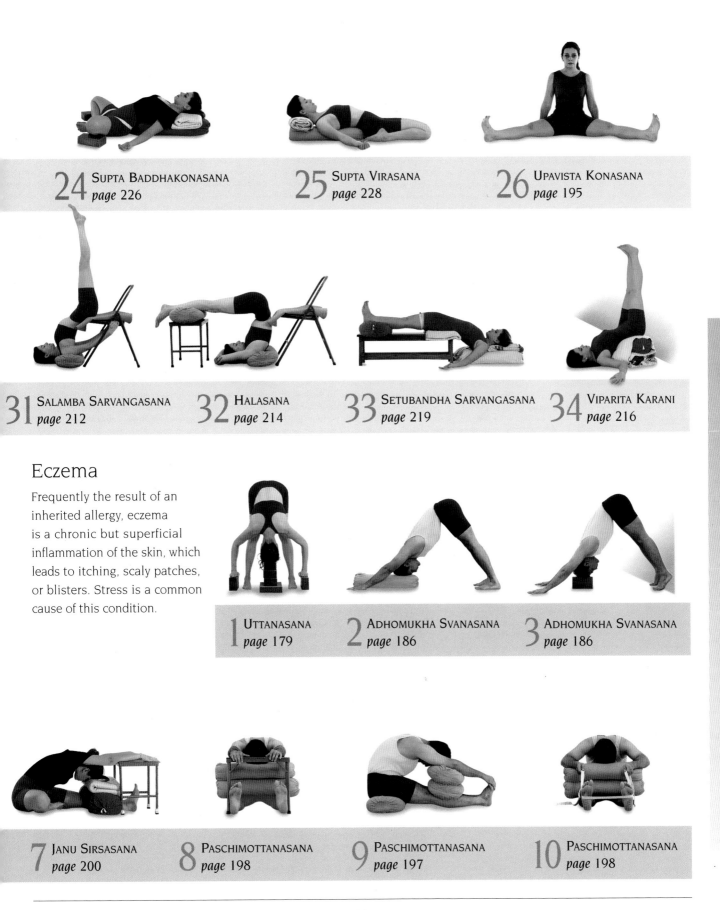

24 **SUPTA BADDHAKONASANA**
page 226

25 **SUPTA VIRASANA**
page 228

26 **UPAVISTA KONASANA**
page 195

31 **SALAMBA SARVANGASANA**
page 212

32 **HALASANA**
page 214

33 **SETUBANDHA SARVANGASANA**
page 219

34 **VIPARITA KARANI**
page 216

Eczema

Frequently the result of an inherited allergy, eczema is a chronic but superficial inflammation of the skin, which leads to itching, scaly patches, or blisters. Stress is a common cause of this condition.

1 **UTTANASANA**
page 179

2 **ADHOMUKHA SVANASANA**
page 186

3 **ADHOMUKHA SVANASANA**
page 186

7 **JANU SIRSASANA**
page 200

8 **PASCHIMOTTANASANA**
page 198

9 **PASCHIMOTTANASANA**
page 197

10 **PASCHIMOTTANASANA**
page 198

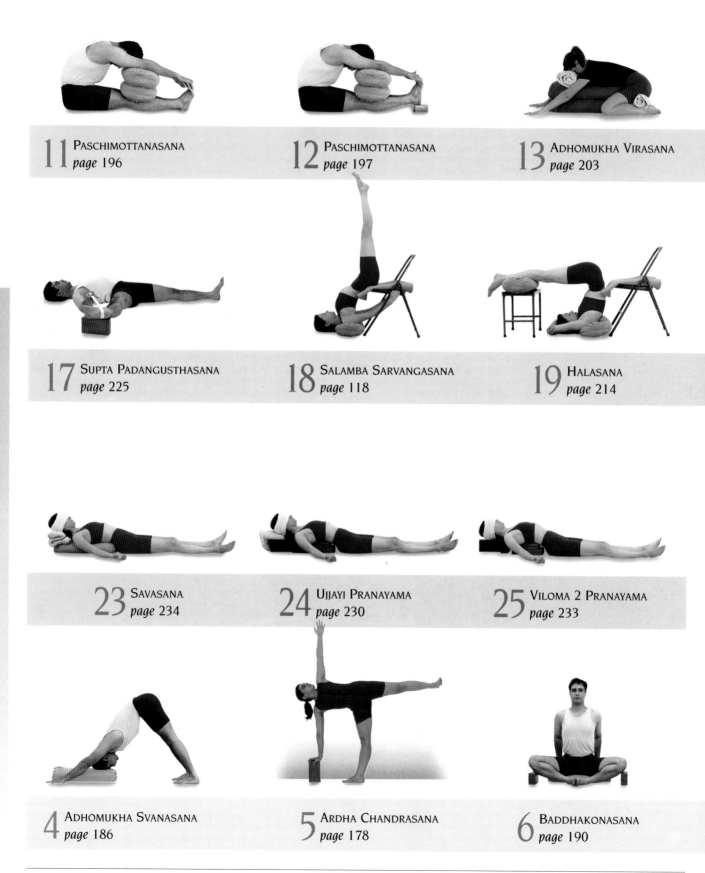

11 PASCHIMOTTANASANA
page 196

12 PASCHIMOTTANASANA
page 197

13 ADHOMUKHA VIRASANA
page 203

17 SUPTA PADANGUSTHASANA
page 225

18 SALAMBA SARVANGASANA
page 118

19 HALASANA
page 214

23 SAVASANA
page 234

24 UJJAYI PRANAYAMA
page 230

25 VILOMA 2 PRANAYAMA
page 233

4 ADHOMUKHA SVANASANA
page 186

5 ARDHA CHANDRASANA
page 178

6 BADDHAKONASANA
page 190

YOGA FOR AILMENTS

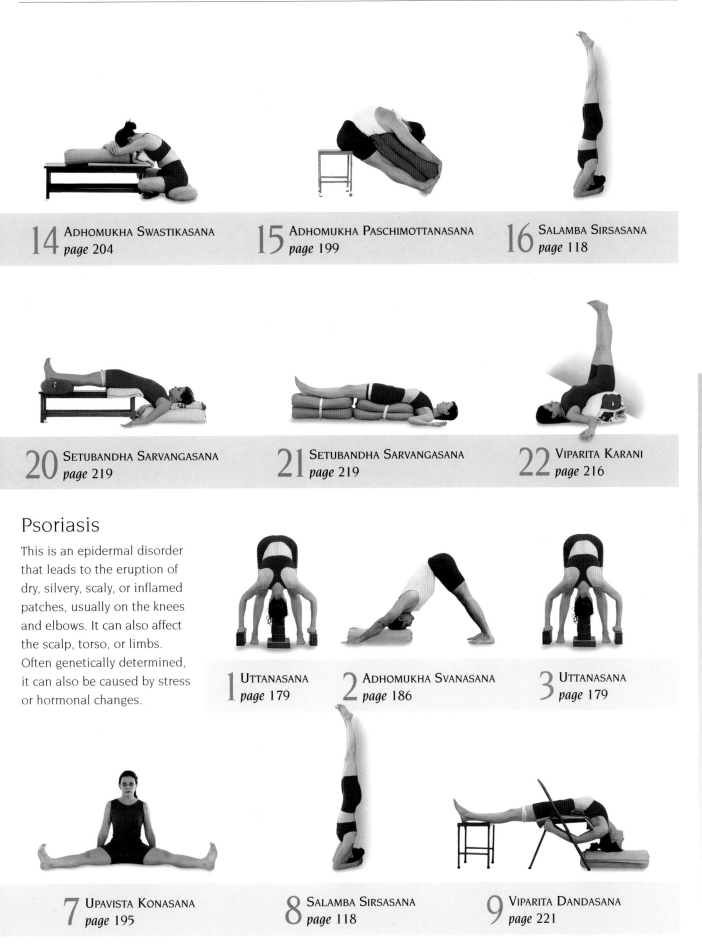

14 ADHOMUKHA SWASTIKASANA
page 204

15 ADHOMUKHA PASCHIMOTTANASANA
page 199

16 SALAMBA SIRSASANA
page 118

20 SETUBANDHA SARVANGASANA
page 219

21 SETUBANDHA SARVANGASANA
page 219

22 VIPARITA KARANI
page 216

SKIN

Psoriasis

This is an epidermal disorder that leads to the eruption of dry, silvery, scaly, or inflamed patches, usually on the knees and elbows. It can also affect the scalp, torso, or limbs. Often genetically determined, it can also be caused by stress or hormonal changes.

1 UTTANASANA
page 179

2 ADHOMUKHA SVANASANA
page 186

3 UTTANASANA
page 179

7 UPAVISTA KONASANA
page 195

8 SALAMBA SIRSASANA
page 118

9 VIPARITA DANDASANA
page 221

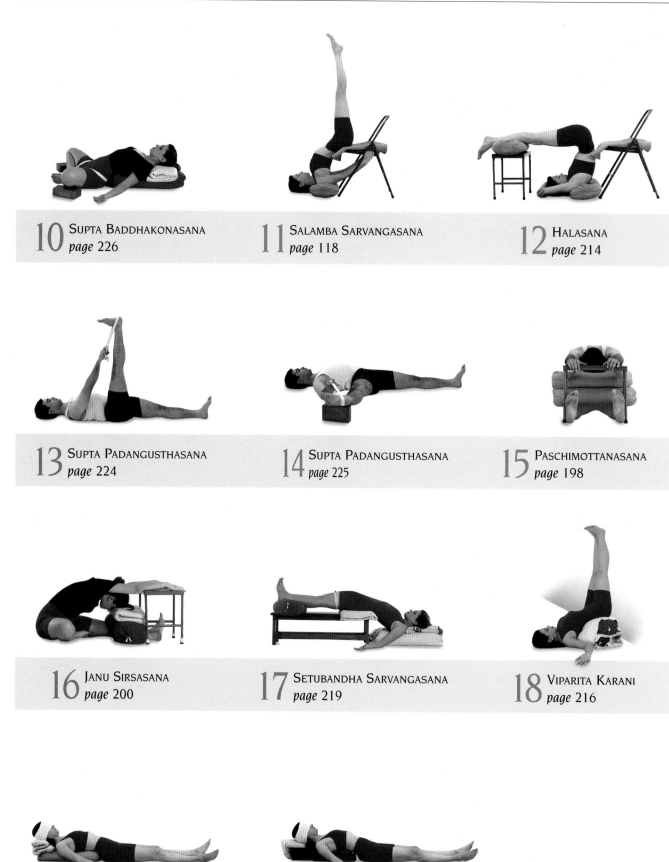

10 SUPTA BADDHAKONASANA
page 226

11 SALAMBA SARVANGASANA
page 118

12 HALASANA
page 214

13 SUPTA PADANGUSTHASANA
page 224

14 SUPTA PADANGUSTHASANA
page 225

15 PASCHIMOTTANASANA
page 198

16 JANU SIRSASANA
page 200

17 SETUBANDHA SARVANGASANA
page 219

18 VIPARITA KARANI
page 216

19 SAVASANA
page 234

20 UJJAYI PRANAYAMA
page 230

Brain & Nervous System

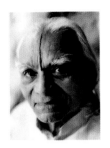

THE MAIN ENGINE OF THE NERVOUS SYSTEM is the central nervous system, composed of the brain and the spinal cord, the body's information-gathering, storage, and control center. Within this, the sympathetic and the parasympathetic nervous systems control the involuntary functions of the organs, glands, and other parts of the body. Regular practice of the recommended sequences of asanas relieves pressure on the brain and the entire nervous system.

Headache and eye strain

This is characterized by severe, piercing pain around the eyes and temples. Usually, the pain increases rapidly within 15 minutes of inception, but the attack itself can last for up to 2 hours.

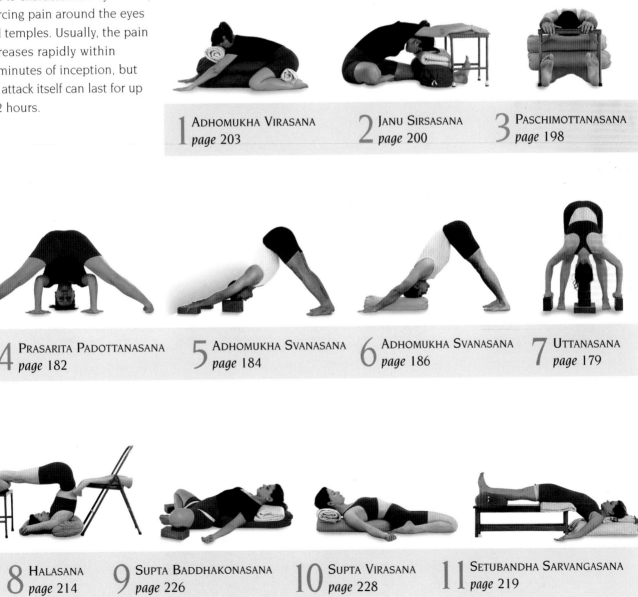

1 ADHOMUKHA VIRASANA
page 203

2 JANU SIRSASANA
page 200

3 PASCHIMOTTANASANA
page 198

4 PRASARITA PADOTTANASANA
page 182

5 ADHOMUKHA SVANASANA
page 184

6 ADHOMUKHA SVANASANA
page 186

7 UTTANASANA
page 179

8 HALASANA
page 214

9 SUPTA BADDHAKONASANA
page 226

10 SUPTA VIRASANA
page 228

11 SETUBANDHA SARVANGASANA
page 219

BRAIN & NERVOUS SYSTEM

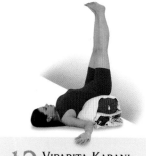

12 VIPARITA KARANI
page 216

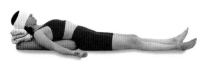

13 SAVASANA
page 234

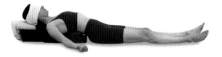

14 UJJAYI PRANAYAMA
page 230

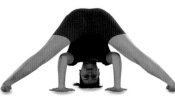

4 PRASARITA PADOTTANASANA
page 182

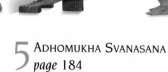

5 ADHOMUKHA SVANASANA
page 184

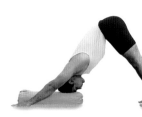

6 ADHOMUKHA SVANASANA
page 186

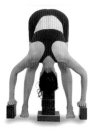

7 UTTANASANA
page 179

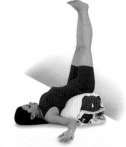

12 VIPARITA KARANI
page 216

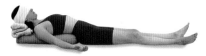

13 SAVASANA
page 234

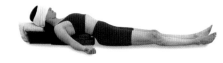

14 UJJAYI PRANAYAMA
page 230

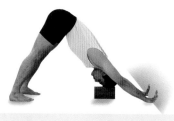

4 ADHOMUKHA SVANASANA
page 185

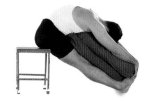

5 ADHOMUKHA PASCHIMOTTANASANA
page 199

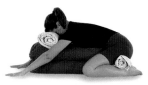

6 ADHOMUKHA VIRASANA
page 203

Stress-related headache

This condition usually takes the form of a dull ache at the back of the skull due to the tautness of the muscles of the scalp and neck. It can also occur as a dull, throbbing pain of moderate intensity, usually following a stressful event.

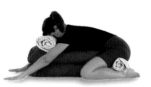

1 ADHOMUKHA VIRASANA
page 203

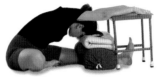

2 JANU SIRSASANA
page 200

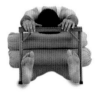

3 PASCHIMOTTANASANA
page 198

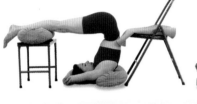

8 HALASANA
page 214

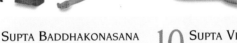

9 SUPTA BADDHAKONASANA
page 226

10 SUPTA VIRASANA
page 228

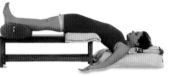

11 SETUBANDHA SARVANGASANA
page 219

Memory impairment

The ageing process is often associated with mild loss of memory. However, it is important to distinguish between this and the onset of serious progressive dementia, such as Alzheimer's disease.

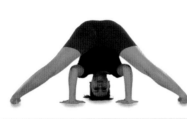

1 PRASARITA PADOTTANASANA
page 182

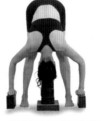

2 UTTANASANA
page 179

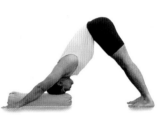

3 ADHOMUKHA SVANASANA
page 186

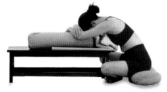

7 ADHOMUKHA SWASTIKASANA
page 204

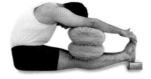

8 PASCHIMOTTANASANA
page 197

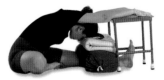

9 JANU SIRSASANA
page 200

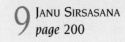

BRAIN & NERVOUS SYSTEM

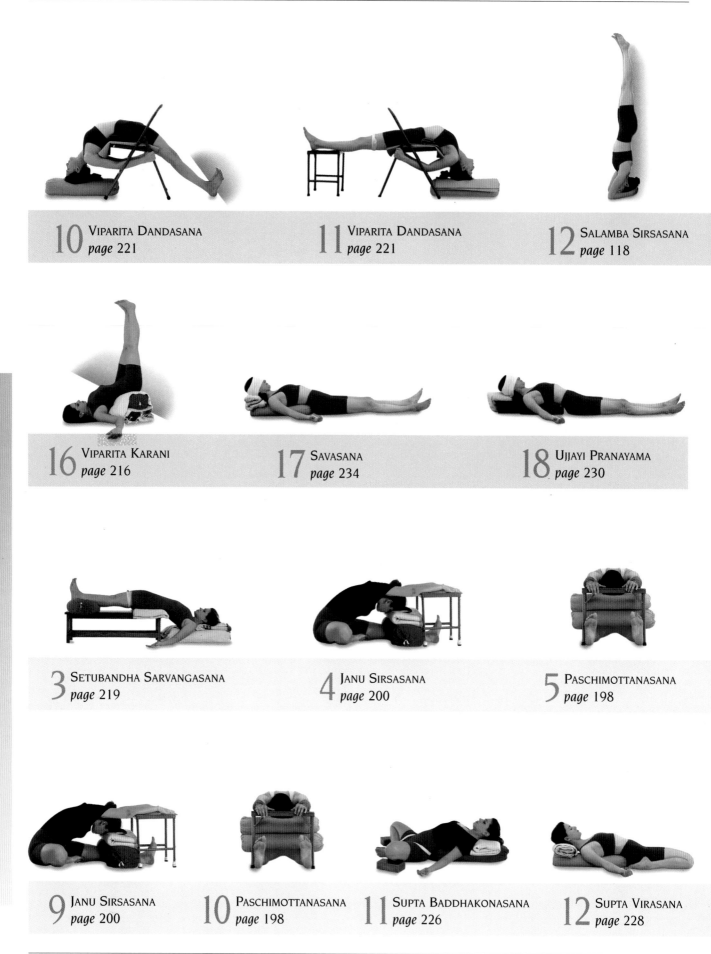

10 VIPARITA DANDASANA
page 221

11 VIPARITA DANDASANA
page 221

12 SALAMBA SIRSASANA
page 118

16 VIPARITA KARANI
page 216

17 SAVASANA
page 234

18 UJJAYI PRANAYAMA
page 230

3 SETUBANDHA SARVANGASANA
page 219

4 JANU SIRSASANA
page 200

5 PASCHIMOTTANASANA
page 198

9 JANU SIRSASANA
page 200

10 PASCHIMOTTANASANA
page 198

11 SUPTA BADDHAKONASANA
page 226

12 SUPTA VIRASANA
page 228

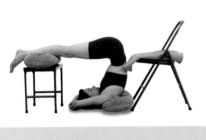

13 HALASANA
page 214

14 SALAMBA SARVANGASANA
page 212

15 SETUBANDHA SARVANGASANA
page 219

Migraine

This condition is associated with periodic, throbbing headaches, often accompanied by nausea and vomiting. The pain can be at the front, back, or sides of the skull. The attack can be preceded by sensitivity to light, partial loss of vision, and numbness in the lips.

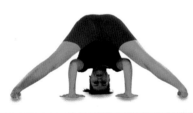

1 ADHOMUKHA VIRASANA
page 202

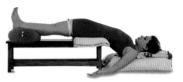

2 ADHOMUKHA SWASTIKASANA
page 204

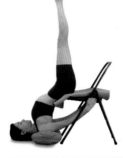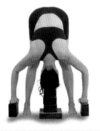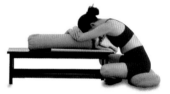

6 PRASARITA PADOTTANASANA
page 182

7 UTTANASANA
page 179

8 HALASANA
page 214

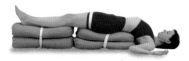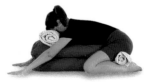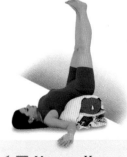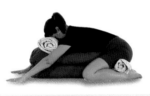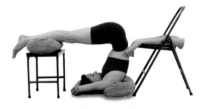

13 SETUBANDHA SARVANGASANA
page 219

14 ADHOMUKHA VIRASANA
page 203

15 VIPARITA KARANI
page 216

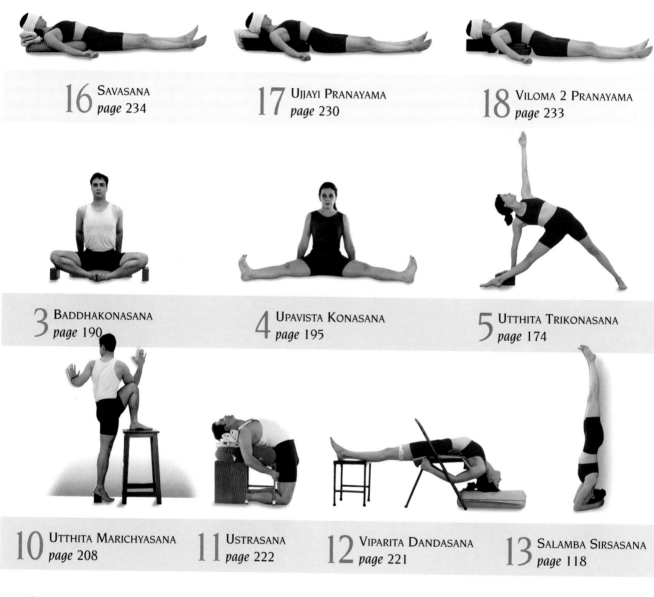

16 SAVASANA
page 234

17 UJJAYI PRANAYAMA
page 230

18 VILOMA 2 PRANAYAMA
page 233

3 BADDHAKONASANA
page 190

4 UPAVISTA KONASANA
page 195

5 UTTHITA TRIKONASANA
page 174

10 UTTHITA MARICHYASANA
page 208

11 USTRASANA
page 222

12 VIPARITA DANDASANA
page 221

13 SALAMBA SIRSASANA
page 118

Epilepsy

This condition is caused when the nerve cells of the brain emit abnormal impulses that disturb the electrical signals by which the brain controls the body. Epileptic seizures occur irregularly. The causes include head injuries, brain infections, and inherited predisposition.

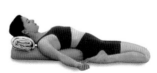

1 SUPTA VIRASANA
page 228

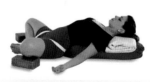

2 SUPTA BADDHAKONASANA
page 226

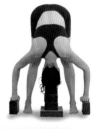

3 UTTANASANA
page 179

Sciatica

This is due to compression and inflammation of the spinal nerves. A sharp pain radiates from the lower back to the leg and foot in a pattern determined by the nerve that is affected. It feels like an electric shock, and increases with standing or walking.

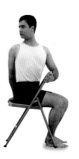

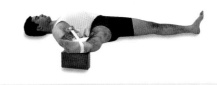

1 SUPTA PADANGUSTHASANA
page 224

2 SUPTA PADANGUSTHASANA
page 225

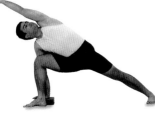

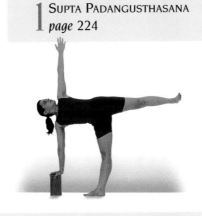

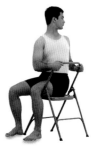

6 UTTHITA PARSVAKONASANA
page 176

7 ARDHA CHANDRASANA
page 178

8 BHARADVAJASANA
page 205

9 BHARADVAJASANA
page 205

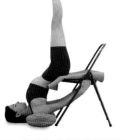

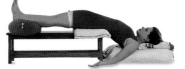

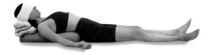

14 SALAMBA SARVANGASANA
page 212

15 SETUBANDHA SARVANGASANA
page 219

16 SAVASANA
page 234

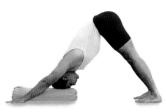

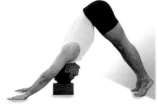

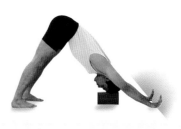

4 ADHOMUKHA SVANASANA
page 186

5 ADHOMUKHA SVANASANA
page 186

6 ADHOMUKHA SVANASANA
page 185

BRAIN & NERVOUS SYSTEM

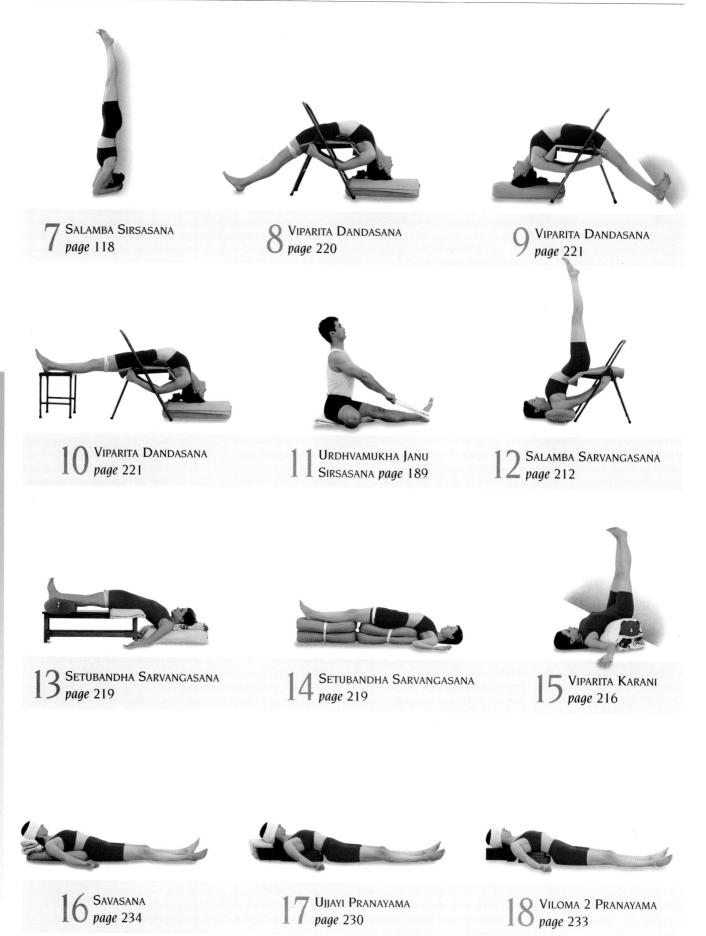

7 SALAMBA SIRSASANA
page 118

8 VIPARITA DANDASANA
page 220

9 VIPARITA DANDASANA
page 221

10 VIPARITA DANDASANA
page 221

11 URDHVAMUKHA JANU
SIRSASANA *page 189*

12 SALAMBA SARVANGASANA
page 212

13 SETUBANDHA SARVANGASANA
page 219

14 SETUBANDHA SARVANGASANA
page 219

15 VIPARITA KARANI
page 216

16 SAVASANA
page 234

17 UJJAYI PRANAYAMA
page 230

18 VILOMA 2 PRANAYAMA
page 233

Mind & Emotions

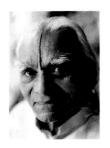

THE TENSIONS OF DAILY LIFE have an impact on our emotions. In yogic science, the secretions of the hormonal system are believed to influence the mind and the nervous system. Strong emotions are linked to hormonal imbalances which leave us vulnerable to infection and ill health. The following sequences of asanas work on the endocrine glands and the sympathetic and central nervous systems, to pacify the nerves, reduce the respiratory rate, and calm a stressed body and mind.

Irritability

Short bursts of impatience and overreaction to daily events are the result of stress factors which arise from major life changes such as divorce or bereavement, and from sleep deprivation, work-related anxieties, or allergies. These asanas help to reduce stress.

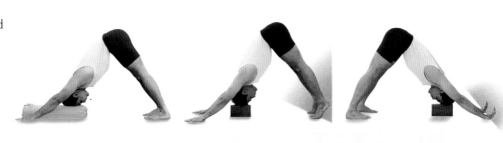

1 ADHOMUKHA SVANASANA
page 186

2 ADHOMUKHA SVANASANA
page 186

3 ADHOMUKHA SVANASANA
page 185

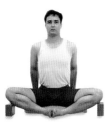

4 BADDHAKONASANA
page 190

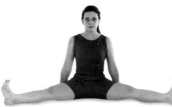

5 UPAVISTA KONASANA
page 195

6 ADHOMUKHA PASCHIMOTTANASANA
page 199

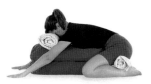

7 ADHOMUKHA VIRASANA
page 203

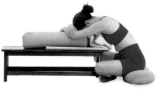

8 ADHOMUKHA SWASTIKASANA
page 204

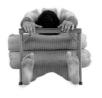

9 PASCHIMOTTANASANA
page 198

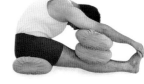

10 PASCHIMOTTANASANA
page 197

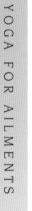

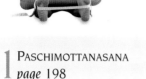

11 PASCHIMOTTANASANA
page 198

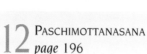

12 PASCHIMOTTANASANA
page 196

13 PASCHIMOTTANASANA
page 197

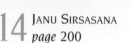

14 JANU SIRSASANA
page 200

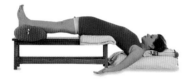

19 SETUBANDHA SARVANGASANA
page 219

20 SETUBANDHA SARVANGASANA
page 219

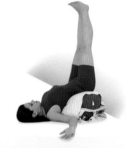

21 VIPARITA KARANI
page 216

Mental fatigue

This condition is characterized by forgetfulness, irritability, boredom, confusion, lack of concentration, and depression. Its causes include lack of sleep, emotional loss, or stress in the workplace. The potential seriousness of this condition is often underestimated.

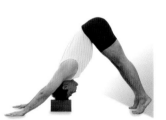

1 UTTANASANA
page 179

2 ADHOMUKHA SVANASANA
page 184

3 ADHOMUKHA SVANASANA
page 186

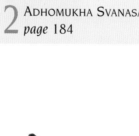

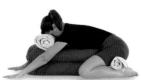

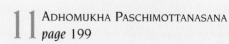

8 USTRASANA
page 222

9 SALAMBA SIRSASANA
page 118

10 ADHOMUKHA VIRASANA
page 203

11 ADHOMUKHA PASCHIMOTTANASANA
page 199

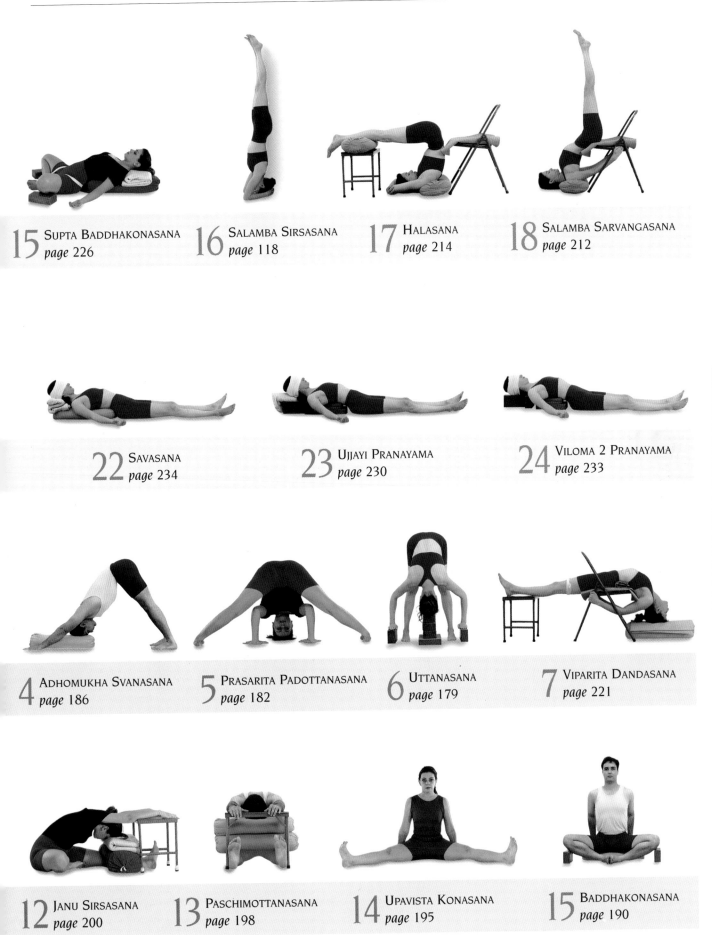

15 **SUPTA BADDHAKONASANA** *page 226*

16 **SALAMBA SIRSASANA** *page 118*

17 **HALASANA** *page 214*

18 **SALAMBA SARVANGASANA** *page 212*

22 **SAVASANA** *page 234*

23 **UJJAYI PRANAYAMA** *page 230*

24 **VILOMA 2 PRANAYAMA** *page 233*

4 **ADHOMUKHA SVANASANA** *page 186*

5 **PRASARITA PADOTTANASANA** *page 182*

6 **UTTANASANA** *page 179*

7 **VIPARITA DANDASANA** *page 221*

12 **JANU SIRSASANA** *page 200*

13 **PASCHIMOTTANASANA** *page 198*

14 **UPAVISTA KONASANA** *page 195*

15 **BADDHAKONASANA** *page 190*

MIND & EMOTIONS

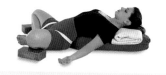

16 SUPTA BADDHAKONASANA
page 226

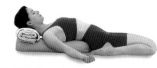

17 SUPTA VIRASANA
page 228

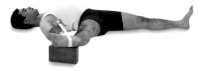

18 SUPTA PADANGUSTHASANA
page 225

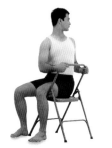

22 BHARADVAJASANA
page 205

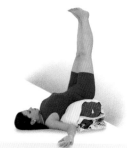

23 SETUBANDHA SARVANGASANA
page 219

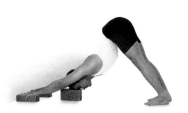

24 VIPARITA KARANI
page 216

Insomnia

Periodic wakefulness, difficulty in falling asleep, or waking up too early, are symptoms of insomnia. They can be transient and pass with life crises that cause them, or they can be chronic and associated with medical or psychiatric conditions, or medication.

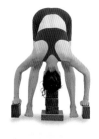

1 UTTANASANA
page 179

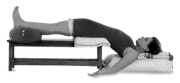

2 PRASARITA PADOTTANASANA
page 182

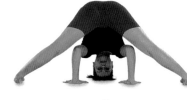

3 ADHOMUKHA SVANASANA
page 184

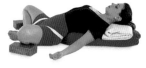

8 SUPTA BADDHAKONASANA
page 226

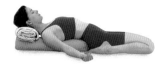

9 SUPTA VIRASANA
page 228

10 SALAMBA SIRSASANA
page 118

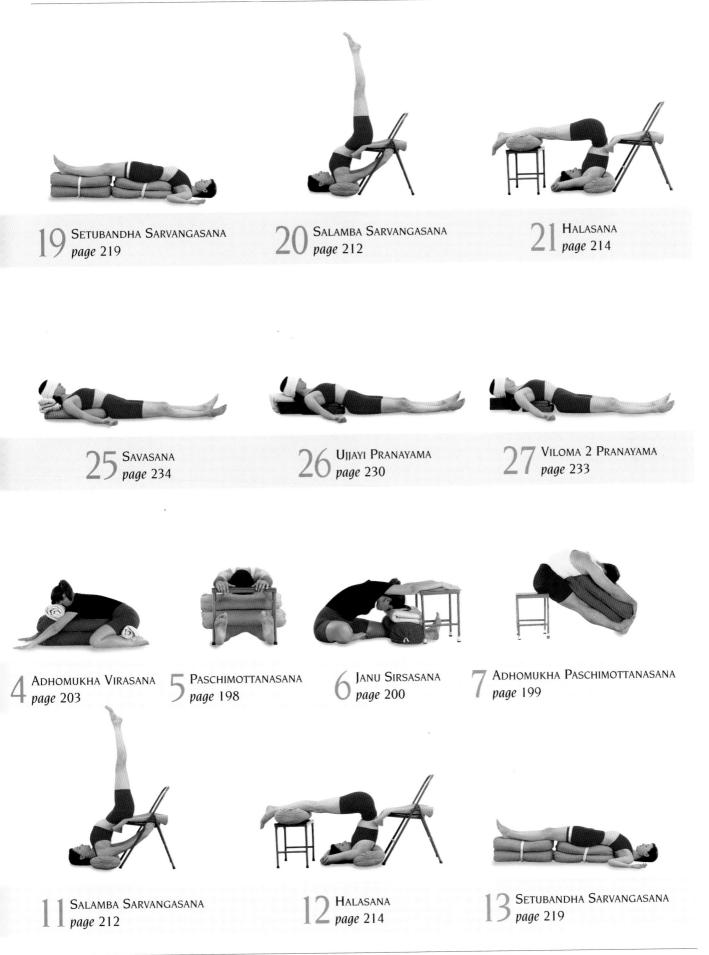

19 SETUBANDHA SARVANGASANA
page 219

20 SALAMBA SARVANGASANA
page 212

21 HALASANA
page 214

25 SAVASANA
page 234

26 UJJAYI PRANAYAMA
page 230

27 VILOMA 2 PRANAYAMA
page 233

4 ADHOMUKHA VIRASANA
page 203

5 PASCHIMOTTANASANA
page 198

6 JANU SIRSASANA
page 200

7 ADHOMUKHA PASCHIMOTTANASANA
page 199

11 SALAMBA SARVANGASANA
page 212

12 HALASANA
page 214

13 SETUBANDHA SARVANGASANA
page 219

MIND & EMOTIONS

YOGA FOR AILMENTS

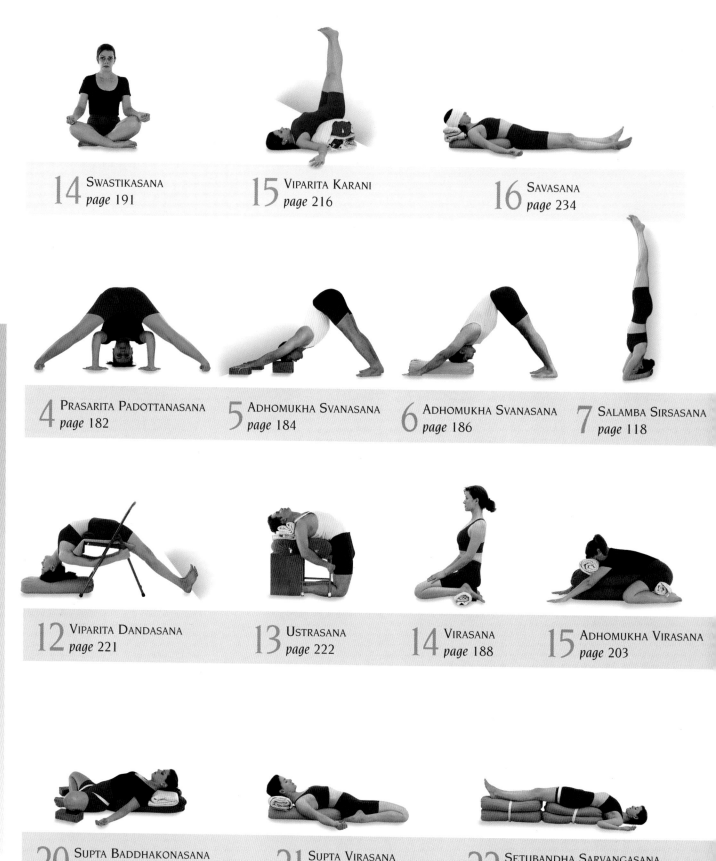

14 SWASTIKASANA
page 191

15 VIPARITA KARANI
page 216

16 SAVASANA
page 234

4 PRASARITA PADOTTANASANA
page 182

5 ADHOMUKHA SVANASANA
page 184

6 ADHOMUKHA SVANASANA
page 186

7 SALAMBA SIRSASANA
page 118

12 VIPARITA DANDASANA
page 221

13 USTRASANA
page 222

14 VIRASANA
page 188

15 ADHOMUKHA VIRASANA
page 203

20 SUPTA BADDHAKONASANA
page 226

21 SUPTA VIRASANA
page 228

22 SETUBANDHA SARVANGASANA
page 219

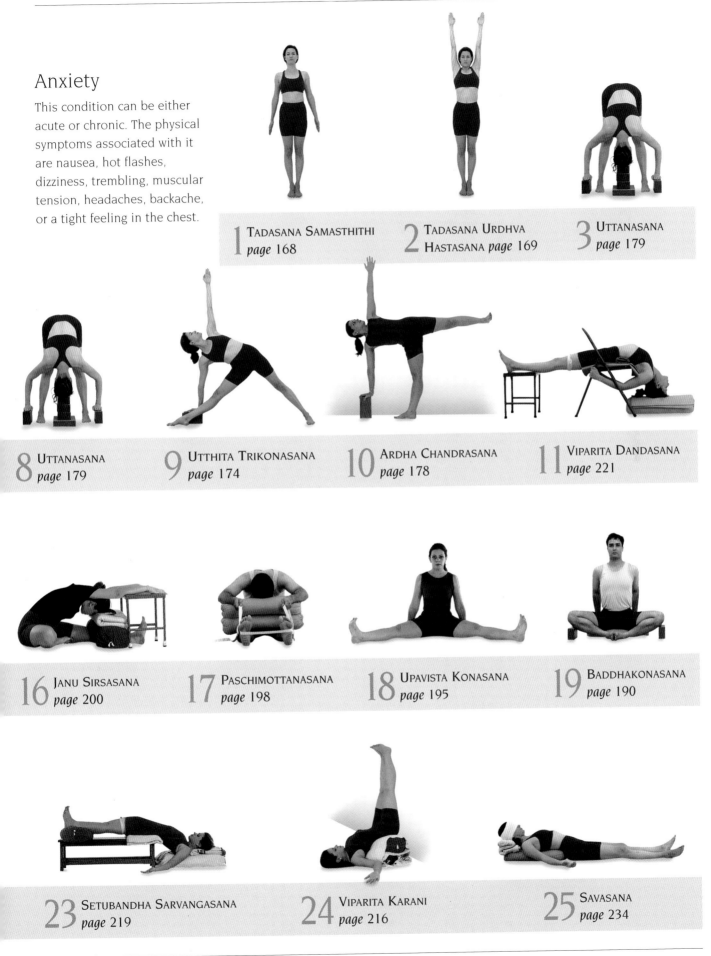

Anxiety

This condition can be either acute or chronic. The physical symptoms associated with it are nausea, hot flashes, dizziness, trembling, muscular tension, headaches, backache, or a tight feeling in the chest.

1 TADASANA SAMASTHITHI *page* 168

2 TADASANA URDHVA HASTASANA *page* 169

3 UTTANASANA *page* 179

8 UTTANASANA *page* 179

9 UTTHITA TRIKONASANA *page* 174

10 ARDHA CHANDRASANA *page* 178

11 VIPARITA DANDASANA *page* 221

16 JANU SIRSASANA *page* 200

17 PASCHIMOTTANASANA *page* 198

18 UPAVISTA KONASANA *page* 195

19 BADDHAKONASANA *page* 190

23 SETUBANDHA SARVANGASANA *page* 219

24 VIPARITA KARANI *page* 216

25 SAVASANA *page* 234

MIND & EMOTIONS

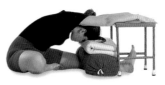

26 UJJAYI PRANAYAMA
page 230

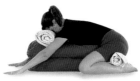

27 VILOMA 2 PRANAYAMA
page 233

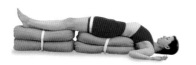

3 SETUBANDHA SARVANGASANA
page 219

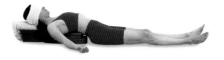

4 ADHOMUKHA VIRASANA
page 203

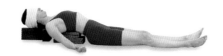

5 JANU SIRSASANA
page 200

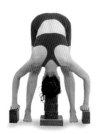

6 UTTANASANA
page 179

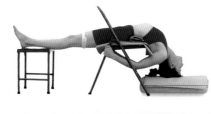

10 VIPARITA DANDASANA
page 221

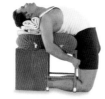

11 USTRASANA
page 222

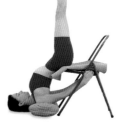

12 SALAMBA SARVANGASANA
page 212

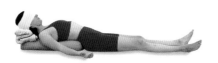

16 SAVASANA
page 234

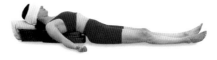

17 UJJAYI PRANAYAMA
page 230

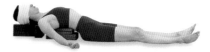

18 VILOMA 2 PRANAYAMA
page 233

Hyperventilation

This condition, triggered by stress, is associated with an increase in the rate and depth of breathing, where the body takes in much more air than what is required. If unchecked, this can lead to dizziness, tingling sensations in the fingers and toes, and chest pain.

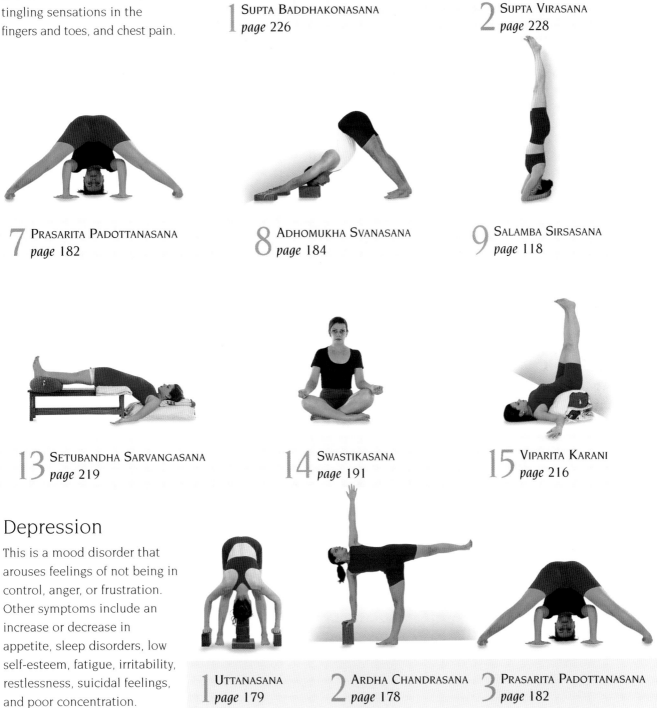

1 SUPTA BADDHAKONASANA
page 226

2 SUPTA VIRASANA
page 228

7 PRASARITA PADOTTANASANA
page 182

8 ADHOMUKHA SVANASANA
page 184

9 SALAMBA SIRSASANA
page 118

13 SETUBANDHA SARVANGASANA
page 219

14 SWASTIKASANA
page 191

15 VIPARITA KARANI
page 216

Depression

This is a mood disorder that arouses feelings of not being in control, anger, or frustration. Other symptoms include an increase or decrease in appetite, sleep disorders, low self-esteem, fatigue, irritability, restlessness, suicidal feelings, and poor concentration.

1 UTTANASANA
page 179

2 ARDHA CHANDRASANA
page 178

3 PRASARITA PADOTTANASANA
page 182

MIND & EMOTIONS

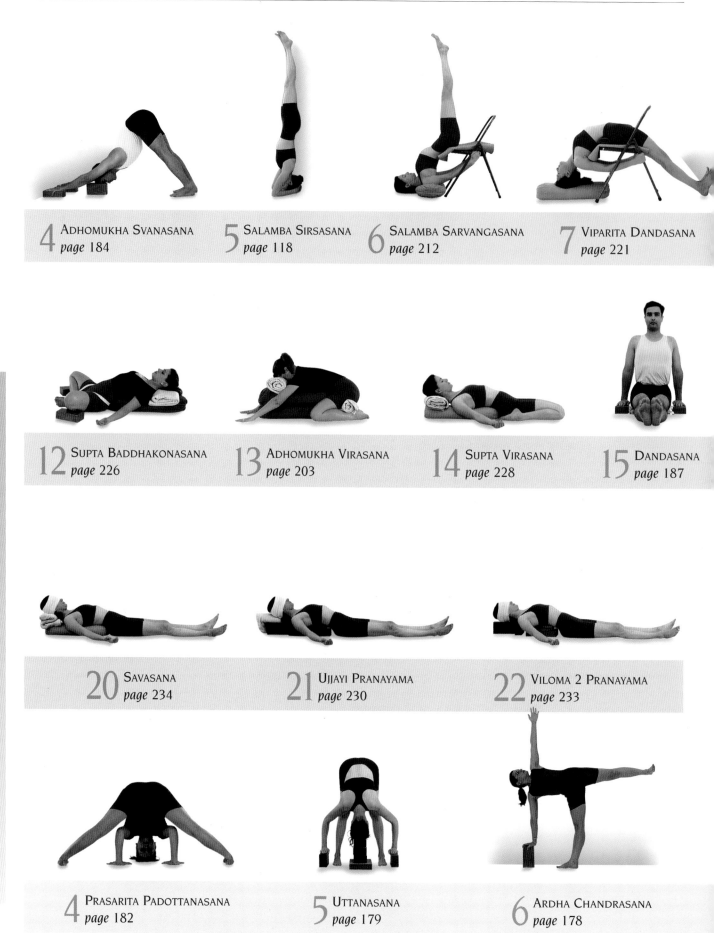

4 ADHOMUKHA SVANASANA
page 184

5 SALAMBA SIRSASANA
page 118

6 SALAMBA SARVANGASANA
page 212

7 VIPARITA DANDASANA
page 221

12 SUPTA BADDHAKONASANA
page 226

13 ADHOMUKHA VIRASANA
page 203

14 SUPTA VIRASANA
page 228

15 DANDASANA
page 187

20 SAVASANA
page 234

21 UJJAYI PRANAYAMA
page 230

22 VILOMA 2 PRANAYAMA
page 233

4 PRASARITA PADOTTANASANA
page 182

5 UTTANASANA
page 179

6 ARDHA CHANDRASANA
page 178

YOGA FOR AILMENTS

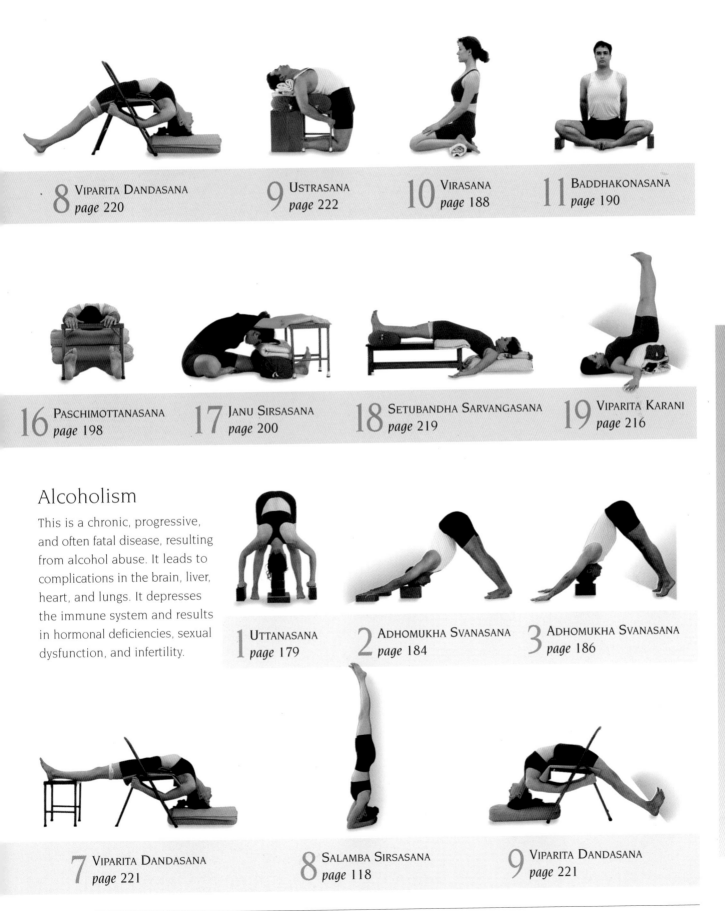

8 VIPARITA DANDASANA
page 220

9 USTRASANA
page 222

10 VIRASANA
page 188

11 BADDHAKONASANA
page 190

16 PASCHIMOTTANASANA
page 198

17 JANU SIRSASANA
page 200

18 SETUBANDHA SARVANGASANA
page 219

19 VIPARITA KARANI
page 216

Alcoholism

This is a chronic, progressive, and often fatal disease, resulting from alcohol abuse. It leads to complications in the brain, liver, heart, and lungs. It depresses the immune system and results in hormonal deficiencies, sexual dysfunction, and infertility.

1 UTTANASANA
page 179

2 ADHOMUKHA SVANASANA
page 184

3 ADHOMUKHA SVANASANA
page 186

7 VIPARITA DANDASANA
page 221

8 SALAMBA SIRSASANA
page 118

9 VIPARITA DANDASANA
page 221

MIND & EMOTIONS

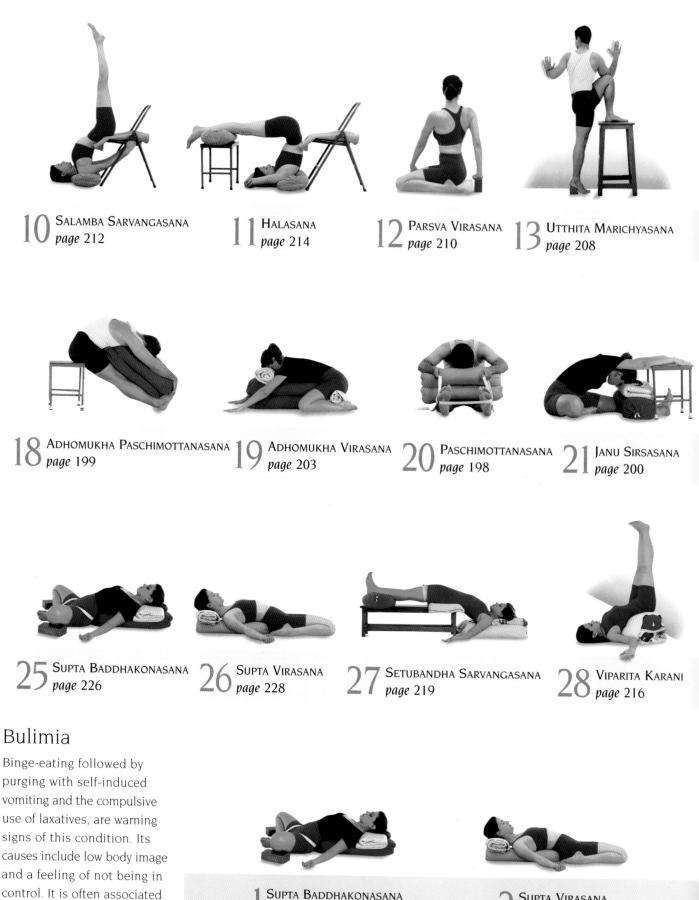

10 SALAMBA SARVANGASANA
page 212

11 HALASANA
page 214

12 PARSVA VIRASANA
page 210

13 UTTHITA MARICHYASANA
page 208

18 ADHOMUKHA PASCHIMOTTANASANA
page 199

19 ADHOMUKHA VIRASANA
page 203

20 PASCHIMOTTANASANA
page 198

21 JANU SIRSASANA
page 200

25 SUPTA BADDHAKONASANA
page 226

26 SUPTA VIRASANA
page 228

27 SETUBANDHA SARVANGASANA
page 219

28 VIPARITA KARANI
page 216

Bulimia

Binge-eating followed by purging with self-induced vomiting and the compulsive use of laxatives, are warning signs of this condition. Its causes include low body image and a feeling of not being in control. It is often associated with anorexia (see page 351).

1 SUPTA BADDHAKONASANA
page 226

2 SUPTA VIRASANA
page 228

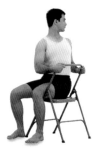
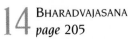

14 BHARADVAJASANA
page 205

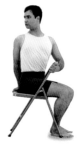
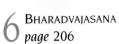

15 BHARADVAJASANA
page 205

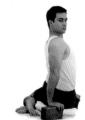
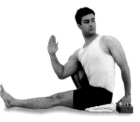

16 BHARADVAJASANA
page 206

17 MARICHYASANA
page 207

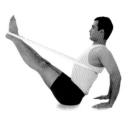
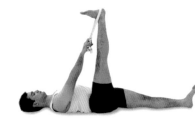
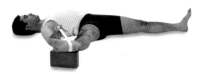

22 PARIPURNA NAVASANA
page 194

23 SUPTA PADANGUSTHASANA
page 224

24 SUPTA PADANGUSTHASANA
page 225

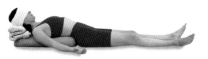
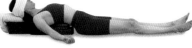
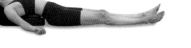
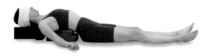

29 SAVASANA
page 234

30 UJJAYI PRANAYAMA
page 230

31 VILOMA 2 PRANAYAMA
page 233

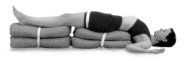
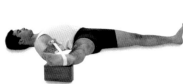
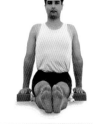
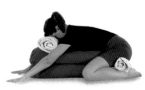

3 SETUBANDHA SARVANGASANA
page 219

4 SUPTA PADANGUSTHASANA
page 225

5 DANDASANA
page 187

6 ADHOMUKHA VIRASANA
page 203

MIND & EMOTIONS

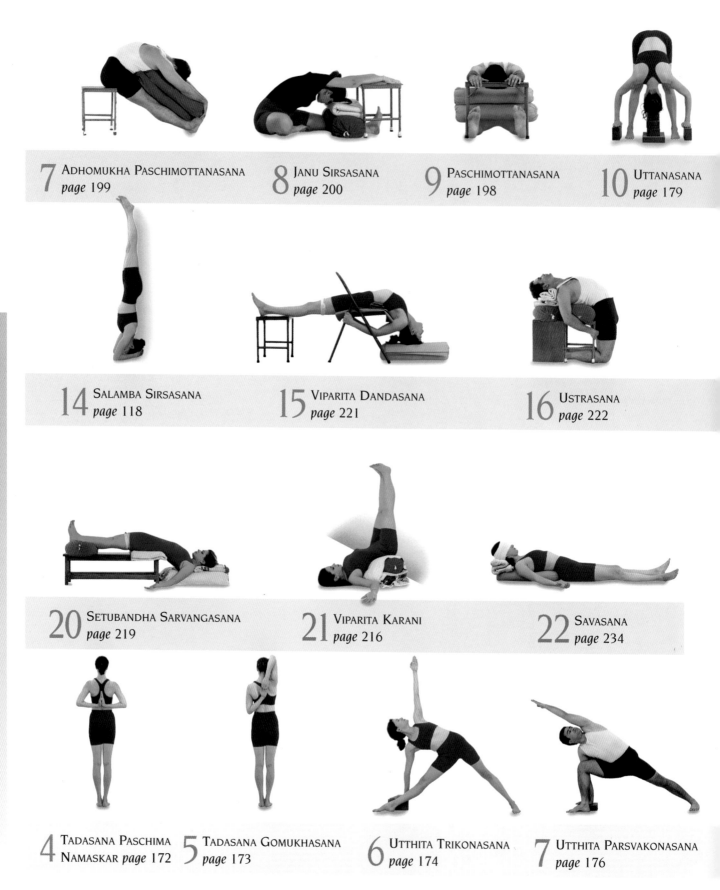

7 ADHOMUKHA PASCHIMOTTANASANA
page 199

8 JANU SIRSASANA
page 200

9 PASCHIMOTTANASANA
page 198

10 UTTANASANA
page 179

14 SALAMBA SIRSASANA
page 118

15 VIPARITA DANDASANA
page 221

16 USTRASANA
page 222

20 SETUBANDHA SARVANGASANA
page 219

21 VIPARITA KARANI
page 216

22 SAVASANA
page 234

4 TADASANA PASCHIMA
NAMASKAR *page* 172

5 TADASANA GOMUKHASANA
page 173

6 UTTHITA TRIKONASANA
page 174

7 UTTHITA PARSVAKONASANA
page 176

YOGA FOR AILMENTS

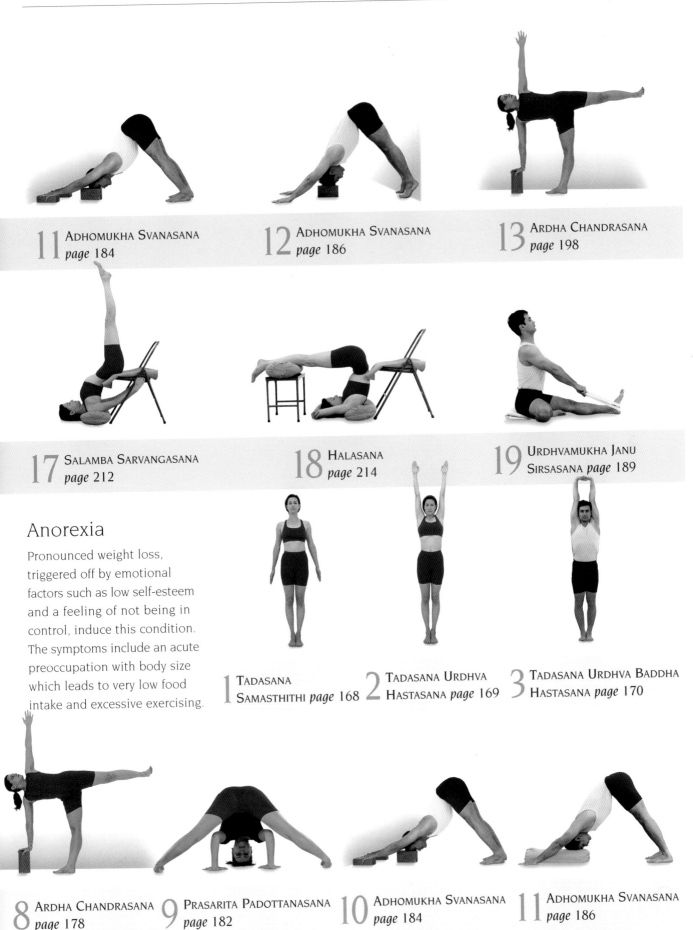

11 ADHOMUKHA SVANASANA
page 184

12 ADHOMUKHA SVANASANA
page 186

13 ARDHA CHANDRASANA
page 198

17 SALAMBA SARVANGASANA
page 212

18 HALASANA
page 214

19 URDHVAMUKHA JANU
SIRSASANA *page 189*

Anorexia

Pronounced weight loss, triggered off by emotional factors such as low self-esteem and a feeling of not being in control, induce this condition. The symptoms include an acute preoccupation with body size which leads to very low food intake and excessive exercising.

1 TADASANA
SAMASTHITHI *page 168*

2 TADASANA URDHVA
HASTASANA *page 169*

3 TADASANA URDHVA BADDHA
HASTASANA *page 170*

8 ARDHA CHANDRASANA
page 178

9 PRASARITA PADOTTANASANA
page 182

10 ADHOMUKHA SVANASANA
page 184

11 ADHOMUKHA SVANASANA
page 186

MIND & EMOTIONS

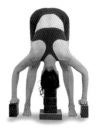
12 UTTANASANA *page* 179

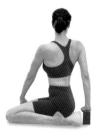
13 PARSVA VIRASANA *page* 210

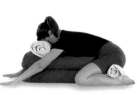
14 ADHOMUKHA VIRASANA *page* 203

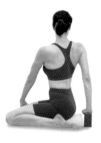
15 PARSVA VIRASANA *page* 210

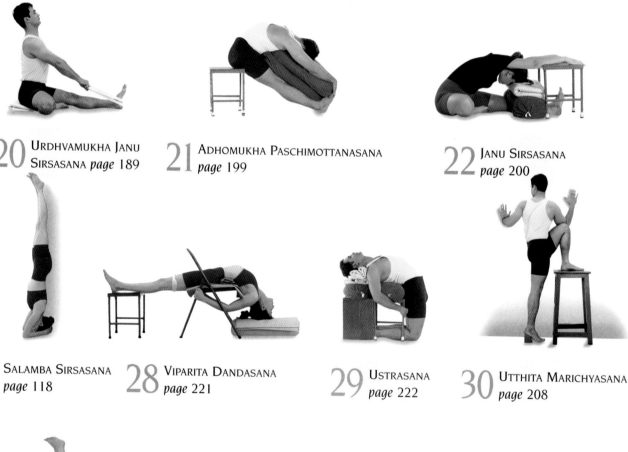

20 URDHVAMUKHA JANU SIRSASANA *page* 189

21 ADHOMUKHA PASCHIMOTTANASANA *page* 199

22 JANU SIRSASANA *page* 200

27 SALAMBA SIRSASANA *page* 118

28 VIPARITA DANDASANA *page* 221

29 USTRASANA *page* 222

30 UTTHITA MARICHYASANA *page* 208

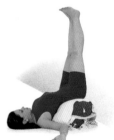
34 VIPARITA KARANI *page* 216

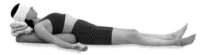
35 SAVASANA *page* 234

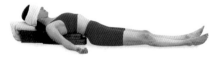
36 UJJAYI PRANAYAMA *page* 230

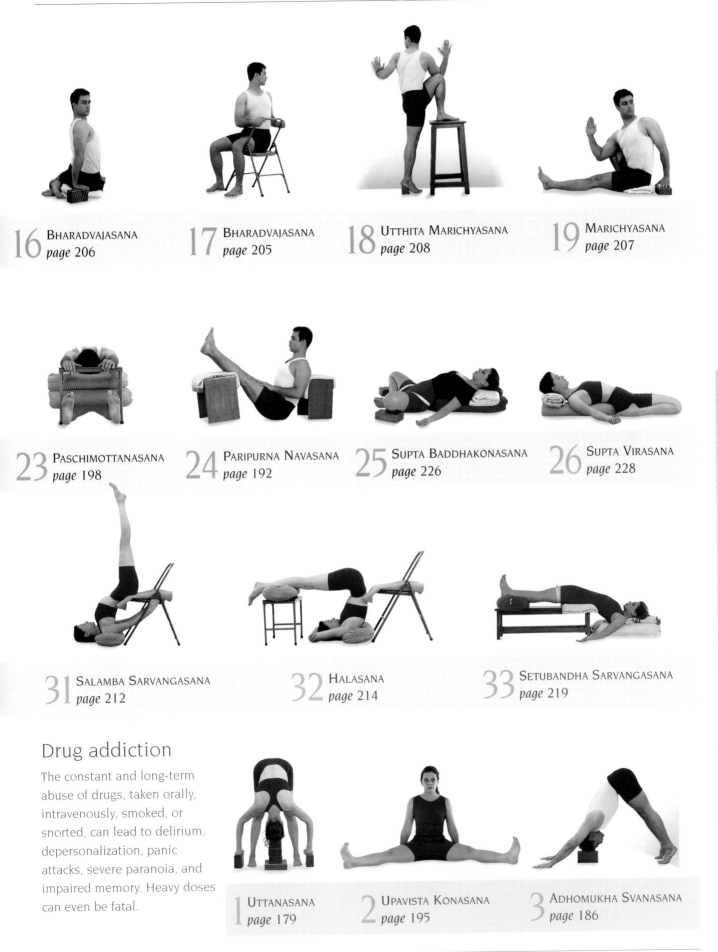

16 **BHARADVAJASANA**
page 206

17 **BHARADVAJASANA**
page 205

18 **UTTHITA MARICHYASANA**
page 208

19 **MARICHYASANA**
page 207

23 **PASCHIMOTTANASANA**
page 198

24 **PARIPURNA NAVASANA**
page 192

25 **SUPTA BADDHAKONASANA**
page 226

26 **SUPTA VIRASANA**
page 228

31 **SALAMBA SARVANGASANA**
page 212

32 **HALASANA**
page 214

33 **SETUBANDHA SARVANGASANA**
page 219

MIND & EMOTIONS

Drug addiction

The constant and long-term abuse of drugs, taken orally, intravenously, smoked, or snorted, can lead to delirium, depersonalization, panic attacks, severe paranoia, and impaired memory. Heavy doses can even be fatal.

1 **UTTANASANA**
page 179

2 **UPAVISTA KONASANA**
page 195

3 **ADHOMUKHA SVANASANA**
page 186

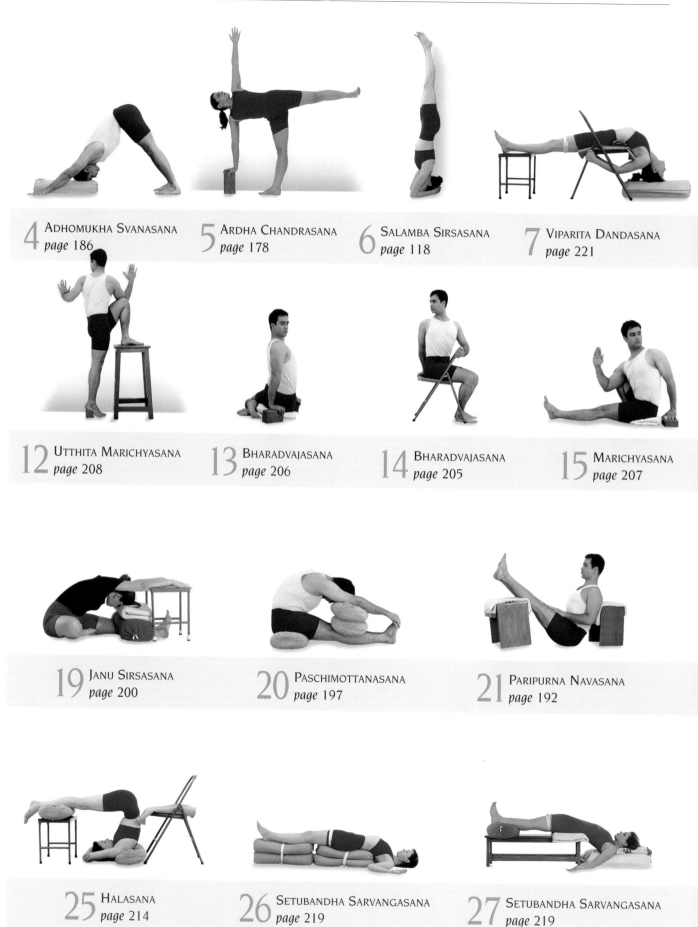

4 ADHOMUKHA SVANASANA
page 186

5 ARDHA CHANDRASANA
page 178

6 SALAMBA SIRSASANA
page 118

7 VIPARITA DANDASANA
page 221

12 UTTHITA MARICHYASANA
page 208

13 BHARADVAJASANA
page 206

14 BHARADVAJASANA
page 205

15 MARICHYASANA
page 207

19 JANU SIRSASANA
page 200

20 PASCHIMOTTANASANA
page 197

21 PARIPURNA NAVASANA
page 192

25 HALASANA
page 214

26 SETUBANDHA SARVANGASANA
page 219

27 SETUBANDHA SARVANGASANA
page 219

YOGA FOR AILMENTS

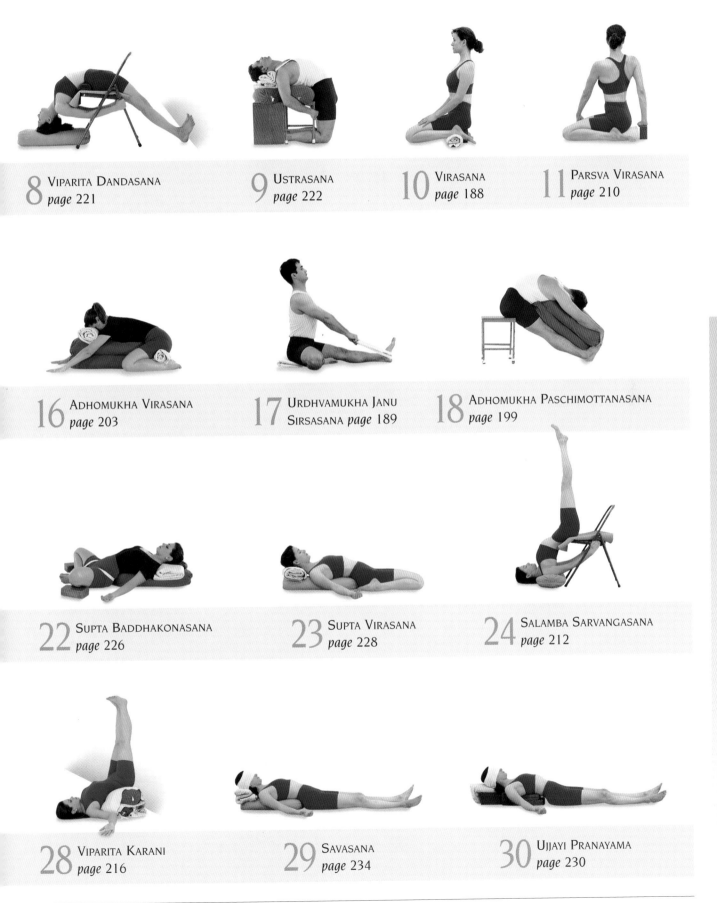

8 VIPARITA DANDASANA
page 221

9 USTRASANA
page 222

10 VIRASANA
page 188

11 PARSVA VIRASANA
page 210

16 ADHOMUKHA VIRASANA
page 203

17 URDHVAMUKHA JANU
SIRSASANA *page 189*

18 ADHOMUKHA PASCHIMOTTANASANA
page 199

22 SUPTA BADDHAKONASANA
page 226

23 SUPTA VIRASANA
page 228

24 SALAMBA SARVANGASANA
page 212

28 VIPARITA KARANI
page 216

29 SAVASANA
page 234

30 UJJAYI PRANAYAMA
page 230

MIND & EMOTIONS

Women's Health

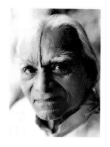

Pᴿᴬᶜᵀᴵᶜᴵᴺᴳ ʸᴼᴳᴬ ᶜᴬᴺ ᴴᴱᴸᴾ prevent or reduce the severity of many ailments that specifically affect women by providing a form of treatment directed at the basic causes. For instance, yoga can help correct gynaecological factors that lead to hypertension, diabetes, indigestion, degeneration in the bones and joints, hernia, and varicose veins. Yoga also helps to regulate menstrual disorders, thyroid imbalance, the effects of osteoporosis, and the side effects of menopause.

Menstruation

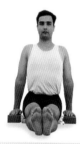

Menstruation is not an ailment, but it can sometimes cause discomfort. When menstruating avoid inversions and standing postures, but practice forward bends, since they control the flow of blood and check excess discharge. The following sequence tones your system.

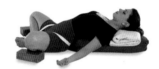

1 **SUPTA BADDHAKONASANA** *page 226*

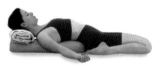

2 **SUPTA VIRASANA** *page 228*

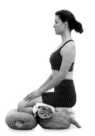

6 **DANDASANA** *page 187*

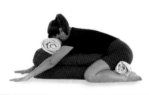

7 **ADHOMUKHA VIRASANA** *page 203*

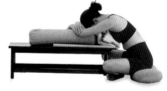

8 **ADHOMUKHA SWASTIKASANA** *page 204*

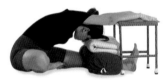

9 **JANU SIRSASANA** *page 200*

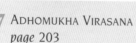

13 **VIRASANA** *page 188*

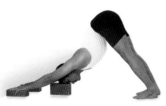

14 **ADHOMUKHA SVANASANA** *page 184*

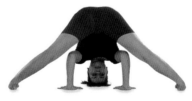

15 **PRASARITA PADOTTANASANA** *page 182*

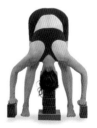

16 **UTTANASANA** *page 179*

"Spiritual yoga uses the intellect of the heart as well as the head."

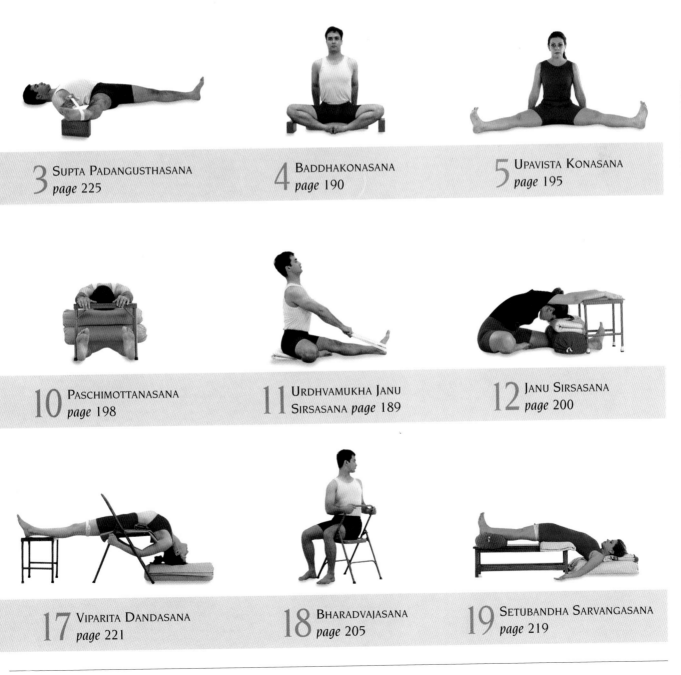

3 SUPTA PADANGUSTHASANA
page 225

4 BADDHAKONASANA
page 190

5 UPAVISTA KONASANA
page 195

10 PASCHIMOTTANASANA
page 198

11 URDHVAMUKHA JANU
SIRSASANA *page* 189

12 JANU SIRSASANA
page 200

17 VIPARITA DANDASANA
page 221

18 BHARADVAJASANA
page 205

19 SETUBANDHA SARVANGASANA
page 219

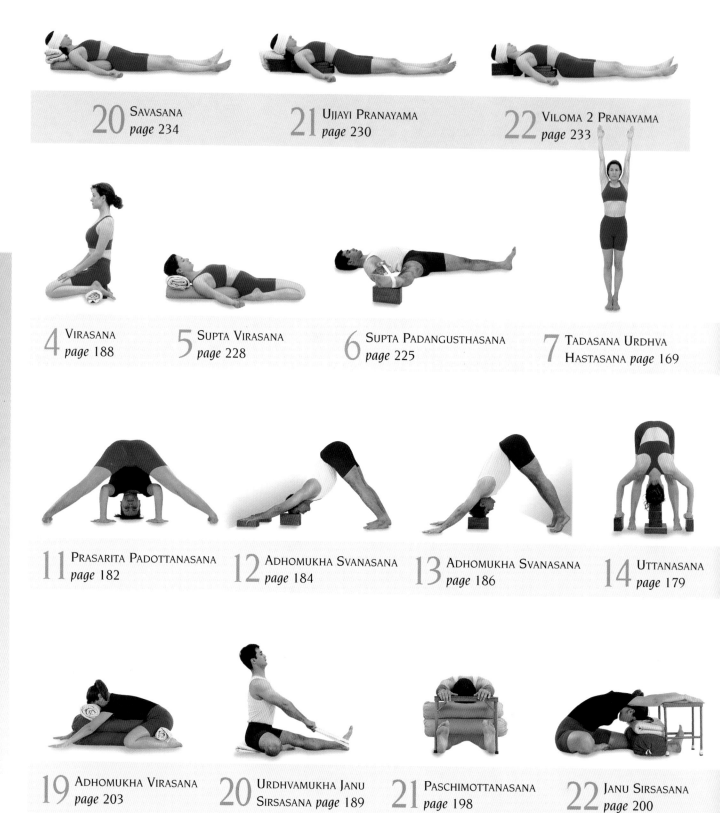

20 SAVASANA
page 234

21 UJJAYI PRANAYAMA
page 230

22 VILOMA 2 PRANAYAMA
page 233

4 VIRASANA
page 188

5 SUPTA VIRASANA
page 228

6 SUPTA PADANGUSTHASANA
page 225

7 TADASANA URDHVA
HASTASANA page 169

11 PRASARITA PADOTTANASANA
page 182

12 ADHOMUKHA SVANASANA
page 184

13 ADHOMUKHA SVANASANA
page 186

14 UTTANASANA
page 179

19 ADHOMUKHA VIRASANA
page 203

20 URDHVAMUKHA JANU
SIRSASANA page 189

21 PASCHIMOTTANASANA
page 198

22 JANU SIRSASANA
page 200

Menstrual pain

Cramps in the pelvic region, just before or during menstruation, are caused by contractions of the uterus while it sheds its lining. Nausea, headaches, and frequent bowel movements, often accompany these cramps.

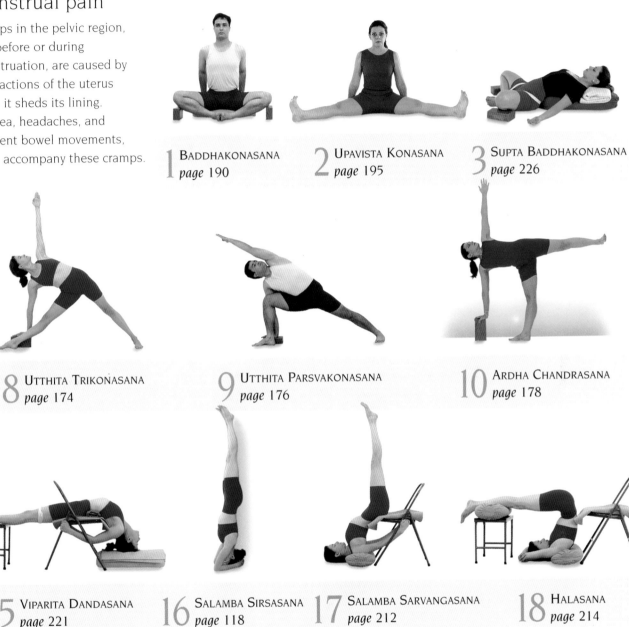

1 BADDHAKONASANA
page 190

2 UPAVISTA KONASANA
page 195

3 SUPTA BADDHAKONASANA
page 226

8 UTTHITA TRIKONASANA
page 174

9 UTTHITA PARSVAKONASANA
page 176

10 ARDHA CHANDRASANA
page 178

15 VIPARITA DANDASANA
page 221

16 SALAMBA SIRSASANA
page 118

17 SALAMBA SARVANGASANA
page 212

18 HALASANA
page 214

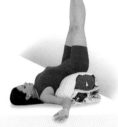

23 SETUBANDHA SARVANGASANA
page 219

24 VIPARITA KARANI
page 216

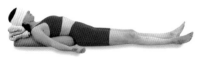

25 SAVASANA
page 234

Premenstrual syndrome

This is a condition that occurs 3-4 days before menstruation, and is relieved by its onset. The symptoms include mood swings, abdominal cramps, lower backache, and aching legs.

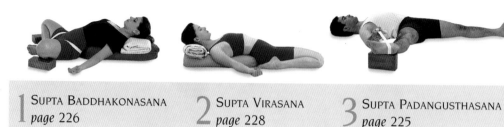

1 SUPTA BADDHAKONASANA
page 226

2 SUPTA VIRASANA
page 228

3 SUPTA PADANGUSTHASANA
page 225

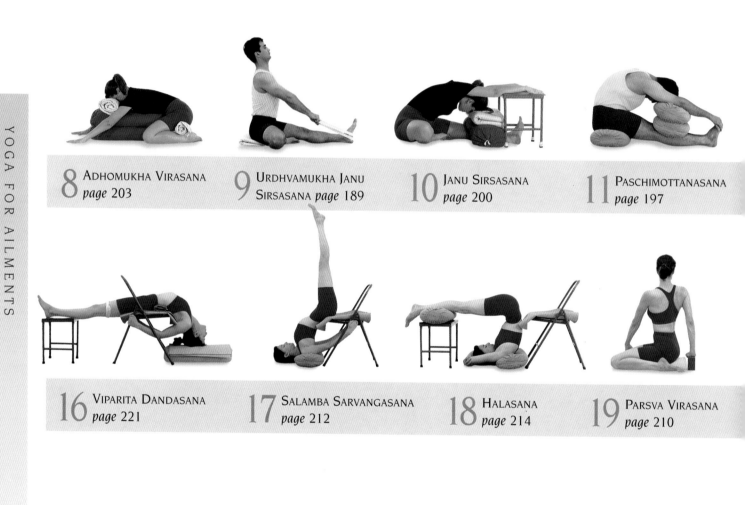

8 ADHOMUKHA VIRASANA
page 203

9 URDHVAMUKHA JANU
SIRSASANA *page 189*

10 JANU SIRSASANA
page 200

11 PASCHIMOTTANASANA
page 197

16 VIPARITA DANDASANA
page 221

17 SALAMBA SARVANGASANA
page 212

18 HALASANA
page 214

19 PARSVA VIRASANA
page 210

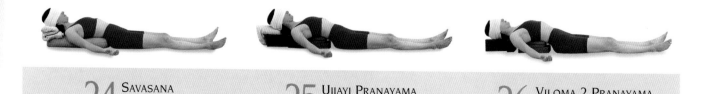

24 SAVASANA
page 234

25 UJJAYI PRANAYAMA
page 230

26 VILOMA 2 PRANAYAMA
page 233

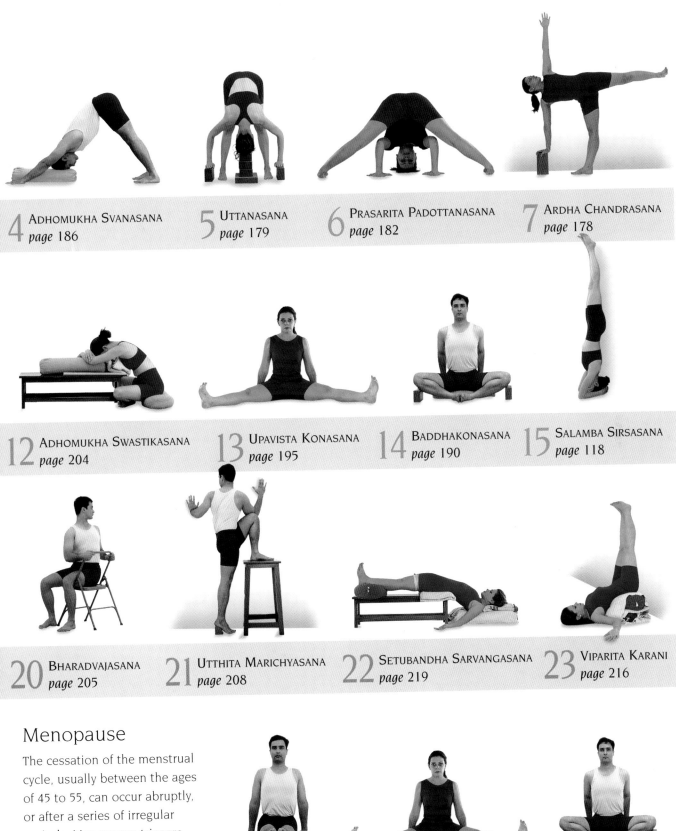

4 ADHOMUKHA SVANASANA
page 186

5 UTTANASANA
page 179

6 PRASARITA PADOTTANASANA
page 182

7 ARDHA CHANDRASANA
page 178

12 ADHOMUKHA SWASTIKASANA
page 204

13 UPAVISTA KONASANA
page 195

14 BADDHAKONASANA
page 190

15 SALAMBA SIRSASANA
page 118

20 BHARADVAJASANA
page 205

21 UTTHITA MARICHYASANA
page 208

22 SETUBANDHA SARVANGASANA
page 219

23 VIPARITA KARANI
page 216

WOMEN'S HEALTH

Menopause

The cessation of the menstrual cycle, usually between the ages of 45 to 55, can occur abruptly, or after a series of irregular periods. Menopause triggers hormonal changes and may cause sweating, hot flashes, depression, insomnia, and mood swings.

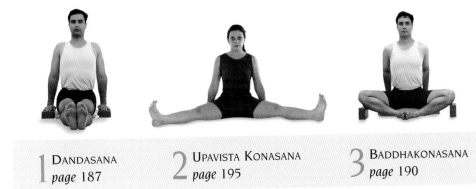

1 DANDASANA
page 187

2 UPAVISTA KONASANA
page 195

3 BADDHAKONASANA
page 190

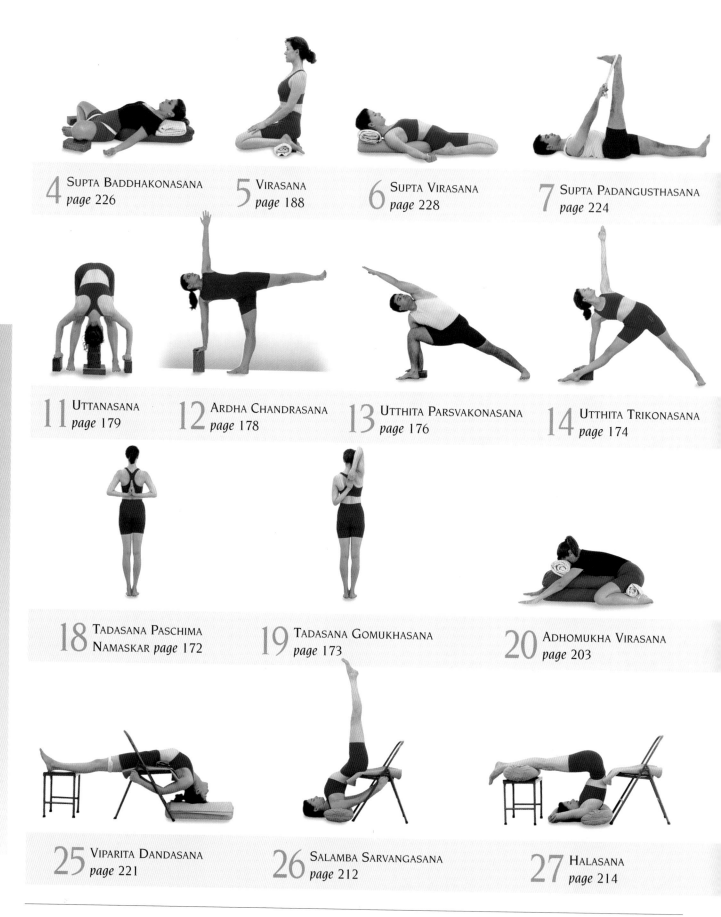

4 SUPTA BADDHAKONASANA
page 226

5 VIRASANA
page 188

6 SUPTA VIRASANA
page 228

7 SUPTA PADANGUSTHASANA
page 224

11 UTTANASANA
page 179

12 ARDHA CHANDRASANA
page 178

13 UTTHITA PARSVAKONASANA
page 176

14 UTTHITA TRIKONASANA
page 174

18 TADASANA PASCHIMA
NAMASKAR *page* 172

19 TADASANA GOMUKHASANA
page 173

20 ADHOMUKHA VIRASANA
page 203

25 VIPARITA DANDASANA
page 221

26 SALAMBA SARVANGASANA
page 212

27 HALASANA
page 214

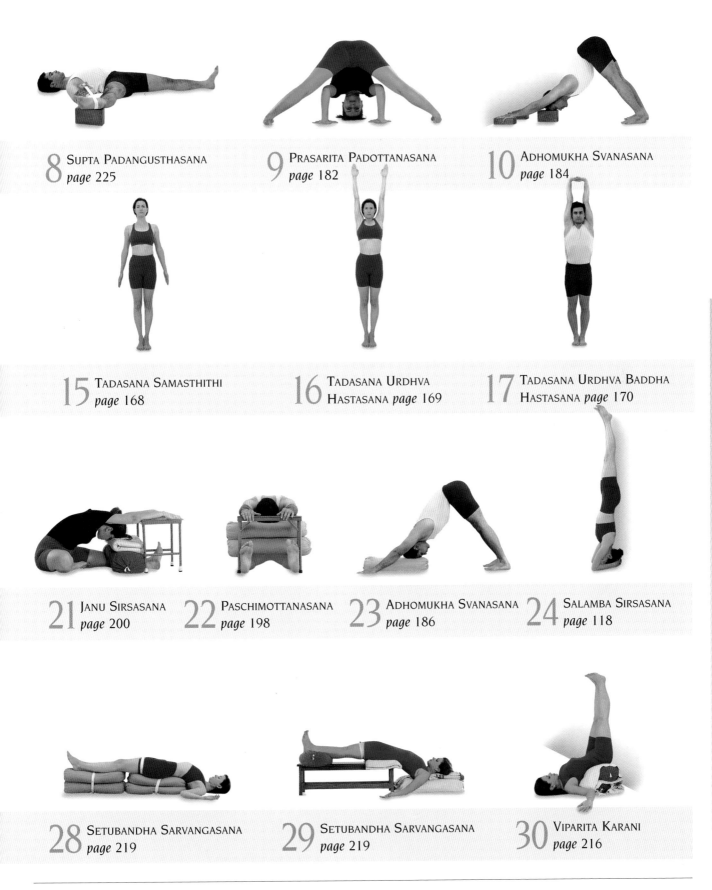

8 SUPTA PADANGUSTHASANA
page 225

9 PRASARITA PADOTTANASANA
page 182

10 ADHOMUKHA SVANASANA
page 184

15 TADASANA SAMASTHITHI
page 168

16 TADASANA URDHVA
HASTASANA *page 169*

17 TADASANA URDHVA BADDHA
HASTASANA *page 170*

21 JANU SIRSASANA
page 200

22 PASCHIMOTTANASANA
page 198

23 ADHOMUKHA SVANASANA
page 186

24 SALAMBA SIRSASANA
page 118

28 SETUBANDHA SARVANGASANA
page 219

29 SETUBANDHA SARVANGASANA
page 219

30 VIPARITA KARANI
page 216

WOMEN'S HEALTH

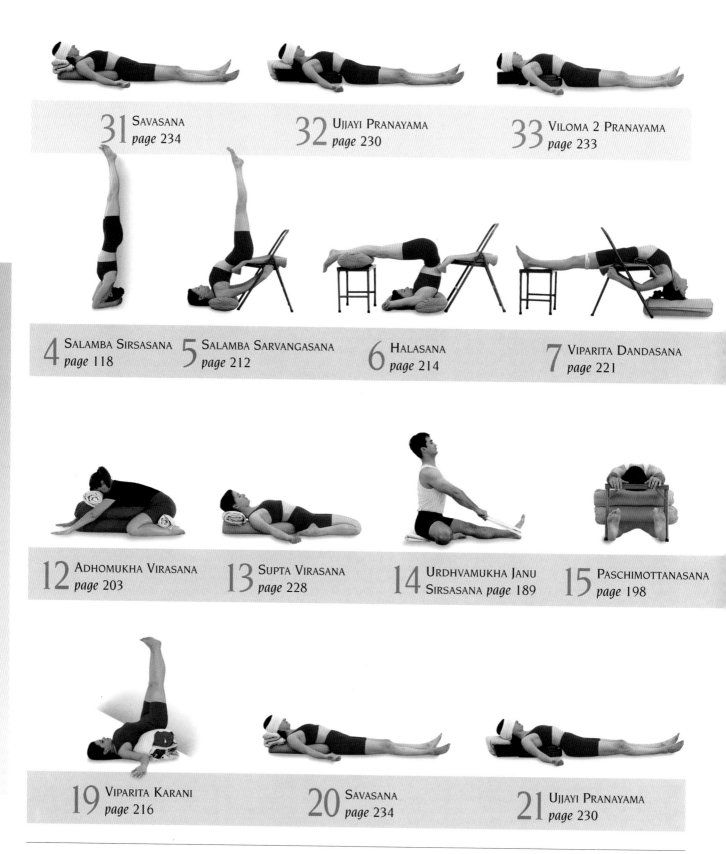

31 SAVASANA
page 234

32 UJJAYI PRANAYAMA
page 230

33 VILOMA 2 PRANAYAMA
page 233

4 SALAMBA SIRSASANA
page 118

5 SALAMBA SARVANGASANA
page 212

6 HALASANA
page 214

7 VIPARITA DANDASANA
page 221

12 ADHOMUKHA VIRASANA
page 203

13 SUPTA VIRASANA
page 228

14 URDHVAMUKHA JANU
SIRSASANA page 189

15 PASCHIMOTTANASANA
page 198

19 VIPARITA KARANI
page 216

20 SAVASANA
page 234

21 UJJAYI PRANAYAMA
page 230

Metrorrhagia

This condition is characterized by irregular and heavy bleeding between menstrual periods. The causes include uterine cysts and fibroids, miscarriage, uterine inflammation, or displacement of the uterus.

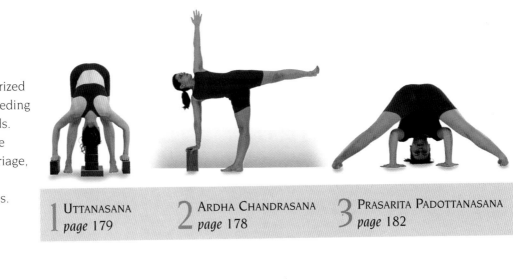

1 **UTTANASANA**
page 179

2 **ARDHA CHANDRASANA**
page 178

3 **PRASARITA PADOTTANASANA**
page 182

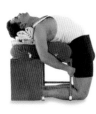

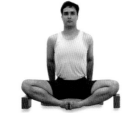

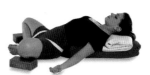

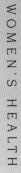

8 **USTRASANA**
page 222

9 **UPAVISTA KONASANA**
page 195

10 **BADDHAKONASANA**
page 190

11 **SUPTA BADDHAKONASANA**
page 226

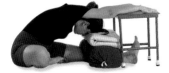

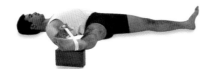

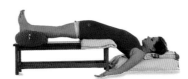

16 **JANU SIRSASANA**
page 200

17 **SUPTA PADANGUSTHASANA**
page 225

18 **SETUBANDHA SARVANGASANA**
page 219

Leukorrhea

Excess white discharge from the vagina can cause acute discomfort and embarrassment. It is usually caused by stress, the presence of a foreign body in the vagina, or an infection.

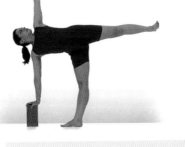

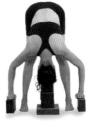

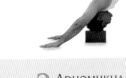

1 **ARDHA CHANDRASANA**
page 178

2 **UTTANASANA**
page 179

3 **ADHOMUKHA SVANASANA**
page 186

WOMEN'S HEALTH

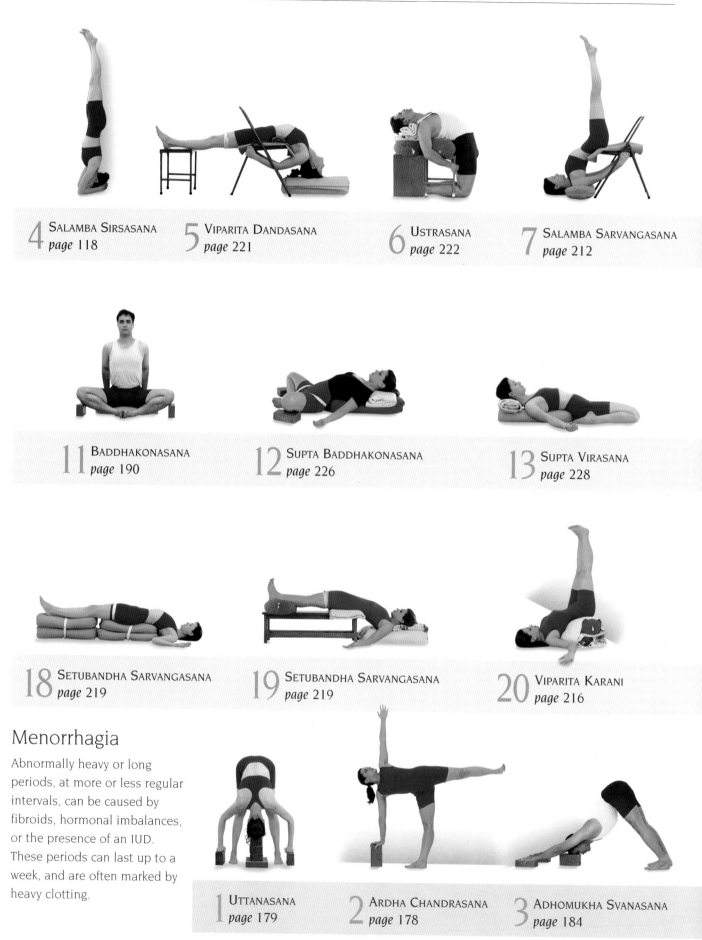

4 SALAMBA SIRSASANA
page 118

5 VIPARITA DANDASANA
page 221

6 USTRASANA
page 222

7 SALAMBA SARVANGASANA
page 212

11 BADDHAKONASANA
page 190

12 SUPTA BADDHAKONASANA
page 226

13 SUPTA VIRASANA
page 228

18 SETUBANDHA SARVANGASANA
page 219

19 SETUBANDHA SARVANGASANA
page 219

20 VIPARITA KARANI
page 216

Menorrhagia

Abnormally heavy or long periods, at more or less regular intervals, can be caused by fibroids, hormonal imbalances, or the presence of an IUD. These periods can last up to a week, and are often marked by heavy clotting.

1 UTTANASANA
page 179

2 ARDHA CHANDRASANA
page 178

3 ADHOMUKHA SVANASANA
page 184

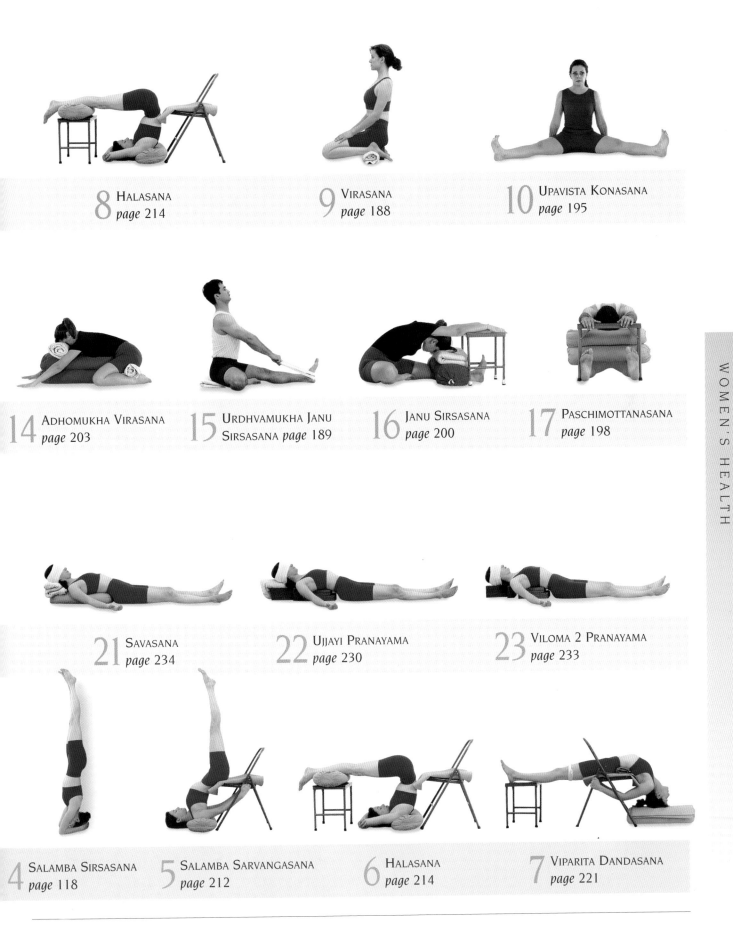

8 HALASANA
page 214

9 VIRASANA
page 188

10 UPAVISTA KONASANA
page 195

14 ADHOMUKHA VIRASANA
page 203

15 URDHVAMUKHA JANU
SIRSASANA *page* 189

16 JANU SIRSASANA
page 200

17 PASCHIMOTTANASANA
page 198

WOMEN'S HEALTH

21 SAVASANA
page 234

22 UJJAYI PRANAYAMA
page 230

23 VILOMA 2 PRANAYAMA
page 233

4 SALAMBA SIRSASANA
page 118

5 SALAMBA SARVANGASANA
page 212

6 HALASANA
page 214

7 VIPARITA DANDASANA
page 221

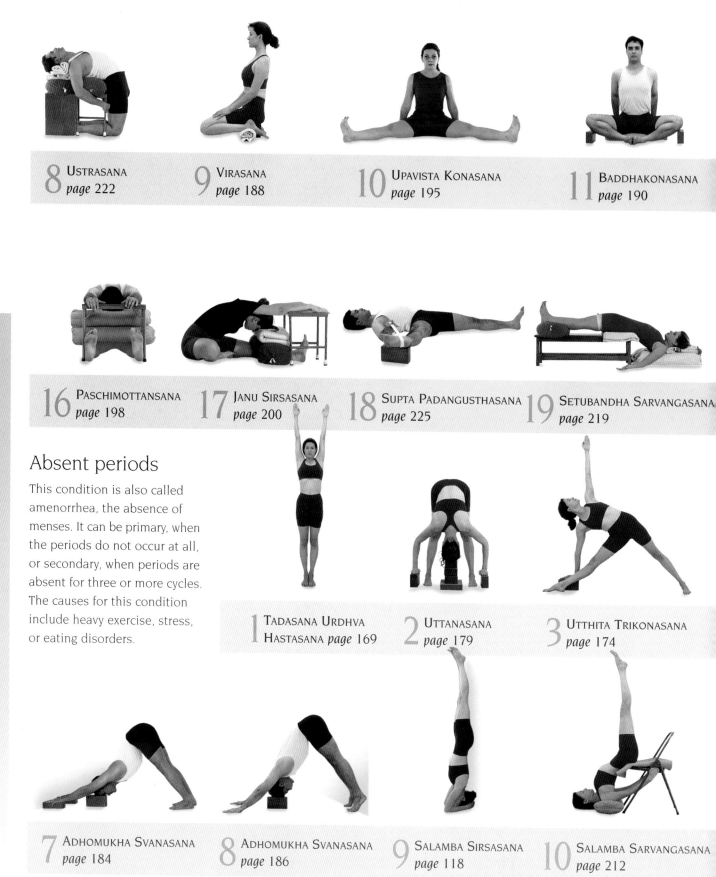

8 USTRASANA
page 222

9 VIRASANA
page 188

10 UPAVISTA KONASANA
page 195

11 BADDHAKONASANA
page 190

16 PASCHIMOTTANSANA
page 198

17 JANU SIRSASANA
page 200

18 SUPTA PADANGUSTHASANA
page 225

19 SETUBANDHA SARVANGASANA
page 219

Absent periods

This condition is also called amenorrhea, the absence of menses. It can be primary, when the periods do not occur at all, or secondary, when periods are absent for three or more cycles. The causes for this condition include heavy exercise, stress, or eating disorders.

1 TADASANA URDHVA
HASTASANA page 169

2 UTTANASANA
page 179

3 UTTHITA TRIKONASANA
page 174

7 ADHOMUKHA SVANASANA
page 184

8 ADHOMUKHA SVANASANA
page 186

9 SALAMBA SIRSASANA
page 118

10 SALAMBA SARVANGASANA
page 212

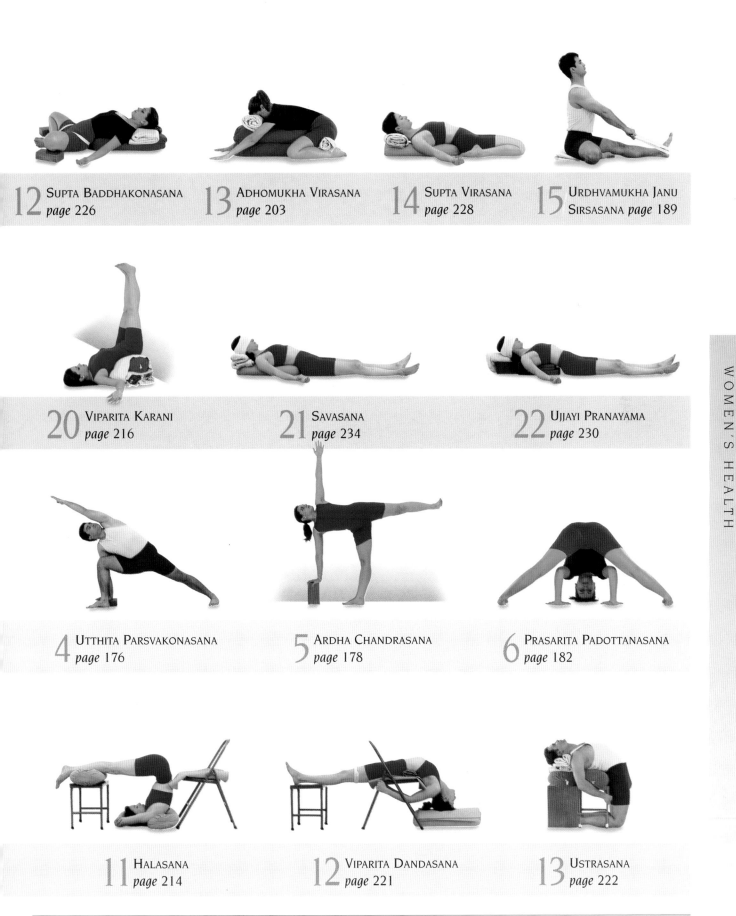

12 SUPTA BADDHAKONASANA *page* 226

13 ADHOMUKHA VIRASANA *page* 203

14 SUPTA VIRASANA *page* 228

15 URDHVAMUKHA JANU SIRSASANA *page* 189

20 VIPARITA KARANI *page* 216

21 SAVASANA *page* 234

22 UJJAYI PRANAYAMA *page* 230

4 UTTHITA PARSVAKONASANA *page* 176

5 ARDHA CHANDRASANA *page* 178

6 PRASARITA PADOTTANASANA *page* 182

11 HALASANA *page* 214

12 VIPARITA DANDASANA *page* 221

13 USTRASANA *page* 222

WOMEN'S HEALTH

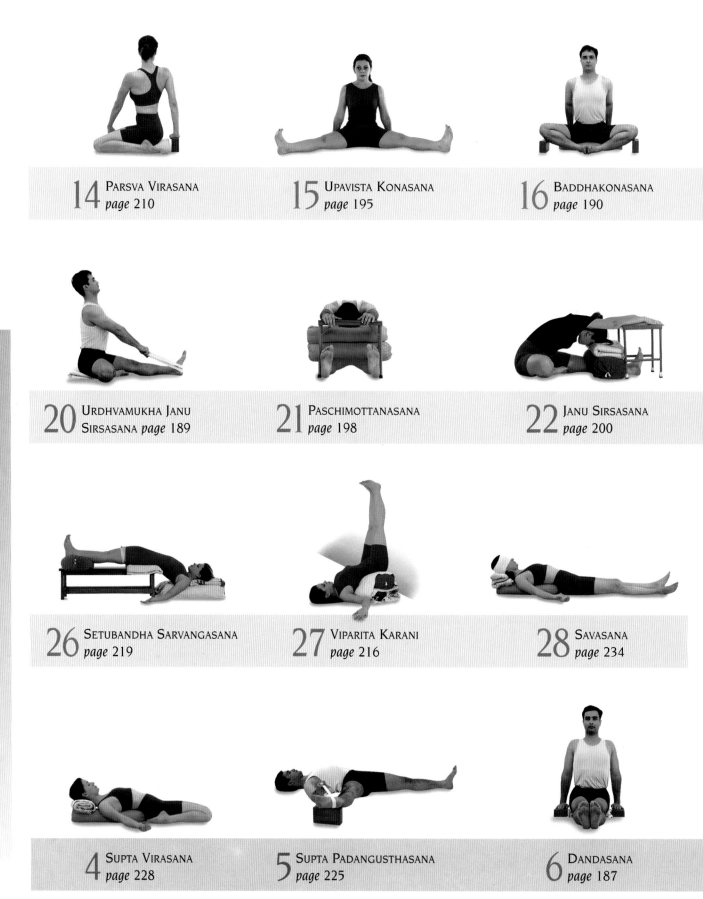

14 PARSVA VIRASANA
page 210

15 UPAVISTA KONASANA
page 195

16 BADDHAKONASANA
page 190

20 URDHVAMUKHA JANU
SIRSASANA *page* 189

21 PASCHIMOTTANASANA
page 198

22 JANU SIRSASANA
page 200

26 SETUBANDHA SARVANGASANA
page 219

27 VIPARITA KARANI
page 216

28 SAVASANA
page 234

4 SUPTA VIRASANA
page 228

5 SUPTA PADANGUSTHASANA
page 225

6 DANDASANA
page 187

YOGA FOR AILMENTS

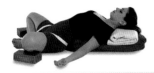

17 SUPTA BADDHAKONASANA
page 226

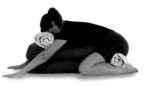

18 ADHOMUKHA VIRASANA
page 203

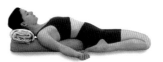

19 SUPTA VIRASANA
page 228

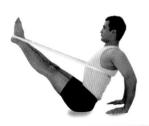

23 PARIPURNA NAVASANA
page 194

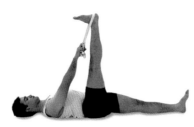

24 SUPTA PADANGUSTHASANA
page 224

25 SUPTA PADANGUSTHASANA
page 225

Prolapsed uterus

This condition occurs when the muscles and ligaments of the pelvis become weak and slack, and results in the uterus slipping out of position. It can be caused by age, obesity, or frequent childbirth.

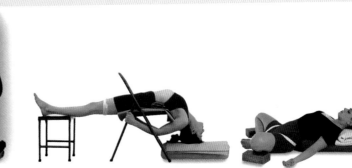

1 SALAMBA SIRSASANA
page 118

2 VIPARITA DANDASANA
page 221

3 SUPTA BADDHAKONASANA
page 226

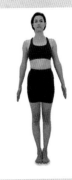

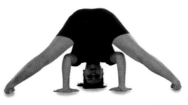

7 URDHVAMUKHA JANU
SIRSASANA *page 189*

8 PRASARITA PADOTTANASANA
page 182

9 TADASANA
SAMASTHITHI *page 168*

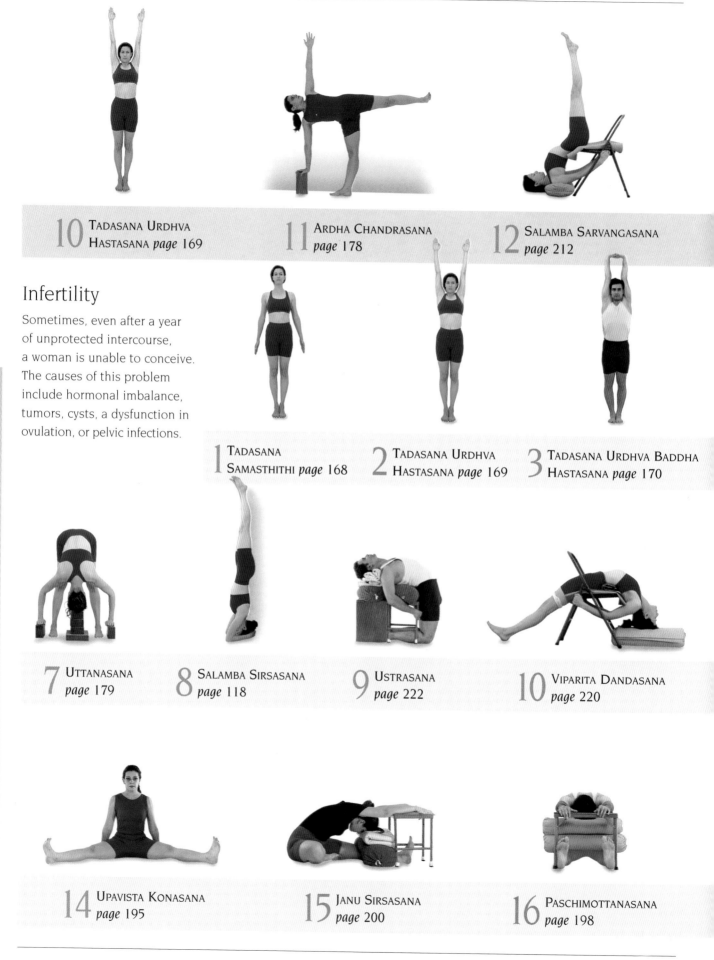

10 TADASANA URDHVA HASTASANA *page* 169

11 ARDHA CHANDRASANA *page* 178

12 SALAMBA SARVANGASANA *page* 212

Infertility

Sometimes, even after a year of unprotected intercourse, a woman is unable to conceive. The causes of this problem include hormonal imbalance, tumors, cysts, a dysfunction in ovulation, or pelvic infections.

1 TADASANA SAMASTHITHI *page* 168

2 TADASANA URDHVA HASTASANA *page* 169

3 TADASANA URDHVA BADDHA HASTASANA *page* 170

7 UTTANASANA *page* 179

8 SALAMBA SIRSASANA *page* 118

9 USTRASANA *page* 222

10 VIPARITA DANDASANA *page* 220

14 UPAVISTA KONASANA *page* 195

15 JANU SIRSASANA *page* 200

16 PASCHIMOTTANASANA *page* 198

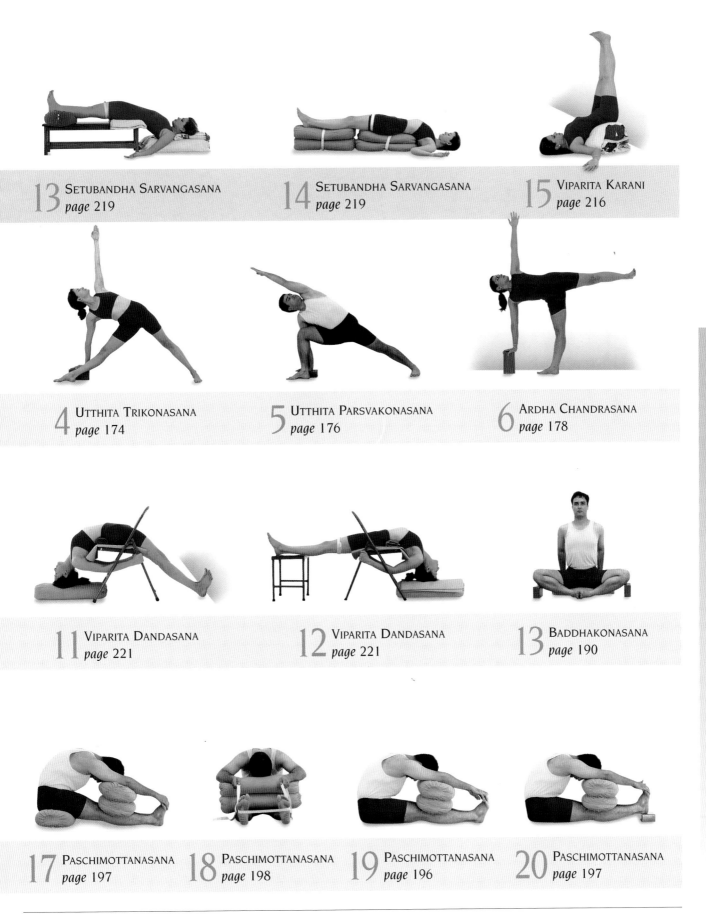

13 SETUBANDHA SARVANGASANA
page 219

14 SETUBANDHA SARVANGASANA
page 219

15 VIPARITA KARANI
page 216

4 UTTHITA TRIKONASANA
page 174

5 UTTHITA PARSVAKONASANA
page 176

6 ARDHA CHANDRASANA
page 178

11 VIPARITA DANDASANA
page 221

12 VIPARITA DANDASANA
page 221

13 BADDHAKONASANA
page 190

17 PASCHIMOTTANASANA
page 197

18 PASCHIMOTTANASANA
page 198

19 PASCHIMOTTANASANA
page 196

20 PASCHIMOTTANASANA
page 197

WOMEN'S HEALTH

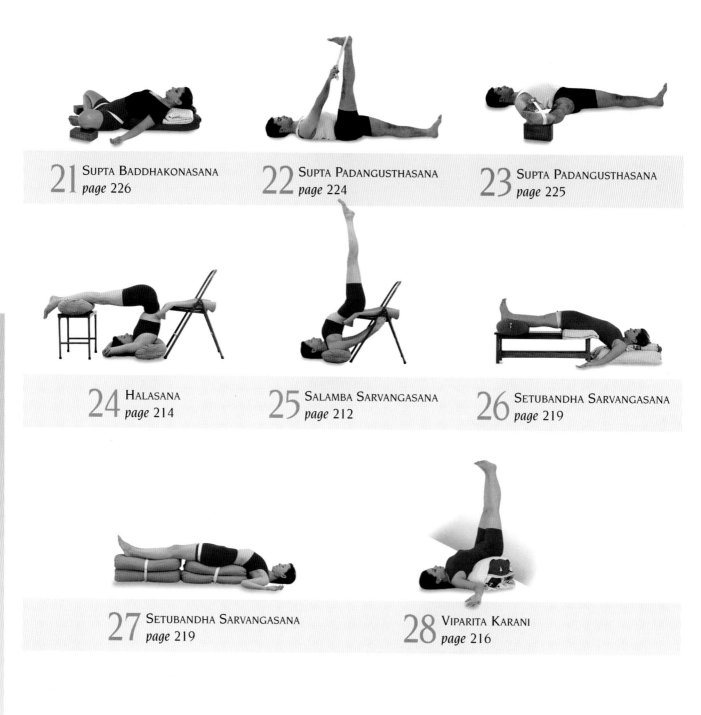

21 **SUPTA BADDHAKONASANA**
page 226

22 **SUPTA PADANGUSTHASANA**
page 224

23 **SUPTA PADANGUSTHASANA**
page 225

24 **HALASANA**
page 214

25 **SALAMBA SARVANGASANA**
page 212

26 **SETUBANDHA SARVANGASANA**
page 219

27 **SETUBANDHA SARVANGASANA**
page 219

28 **VIPARITA KARANI**
page 216

"Do not stop trying just because perfection eludes you."

Men's Health

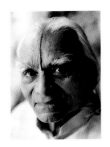

NEARLY HALF OF ALL ADULT MEN face some form of impotence at some time in their lives. The treatment of this and many other disorders that relate to the male reproductive organs and glands is helped by regular practice of the prescribed sequences of asanas. The enlargement of the prostate gland and various forms of hernia are common problems that affect men above the age of 50. These ailments respond to the practice of yoga.

Impotence

This is the inability, often temporary, to achieve or maintain an erection. The causes can be structural, hormonal, neurological, or psychological. It can also be caused by the side effects of medicines or substance abuse.

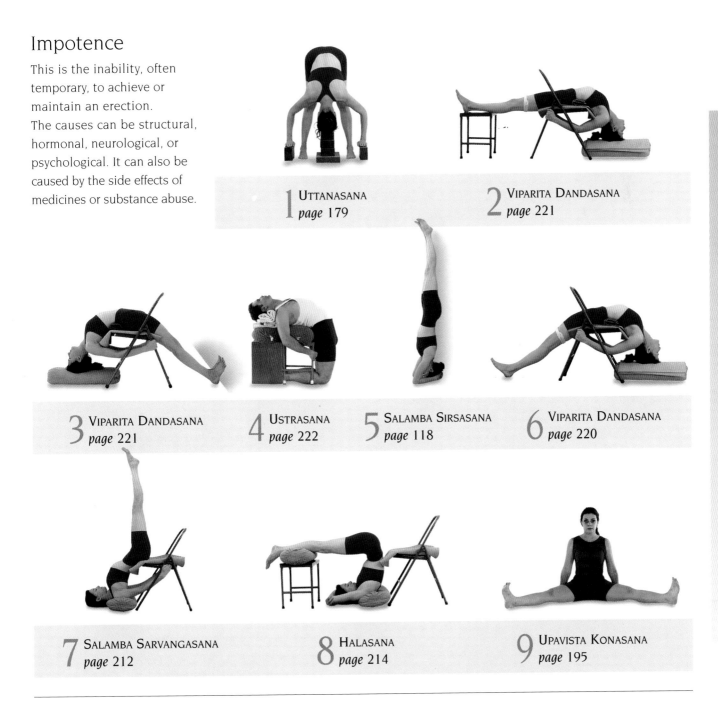

1 UTTANASANA
page 179

2 VIPARITA DANDASANA
page 221

3 VIPARITA DANDASANA
page 221

4 USTRASANA
page 222

5 SALAMBA SIRSASANA
page 118

6 VIPARITA DANDASANA
page 220

7 SALAMBA SARVANGASANA
page 212

8 HALASANA
page 214

9 UPAVISTA KONASANA
page 195

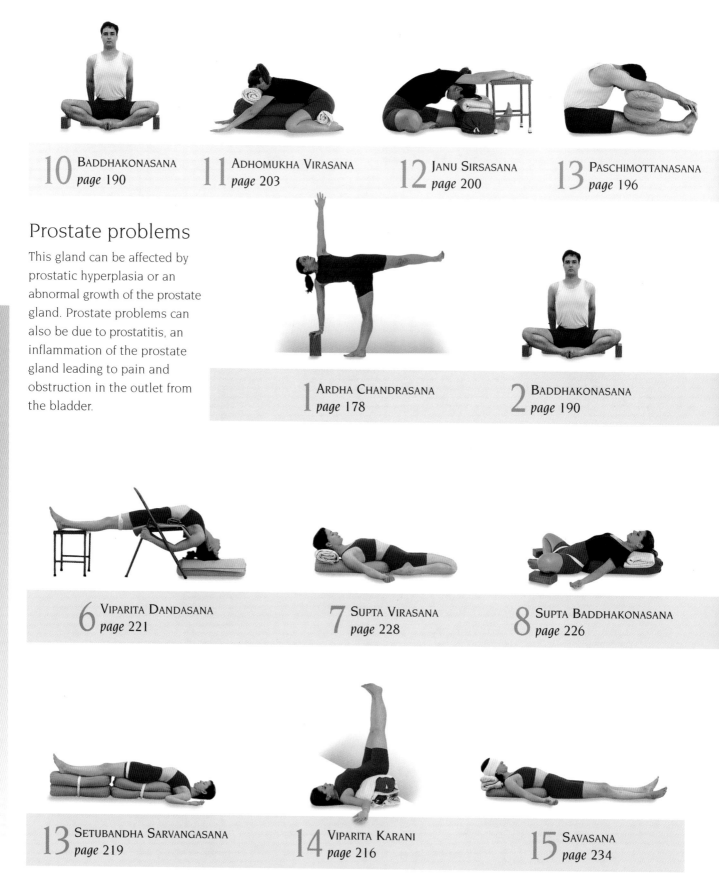

10 **BADDHAKONASANA**
page 190

11 **ADHOMUKHA VIRASANA**
page 203

12 **JANU SIRSASANA**
page 200

13 **PASCHIMOTTANASANA**
page 196

Prostate problems

This gland can be affected by prostatic hyperplasia or an abnormal growth of the prostate gland. Prostate problems can also be due to prostatitis, an inflammation of the prostate gland leading to pain and obstruction in the outlet from the bladder.

1 **ARDHA CHANDRASANA**
page 178

2 **BADDHAKONASANA**
page 190

6 **VIPARITA DANDASANA**
page 221

7 **SUPTA VIRASANA**
page 228

8 **SUPTA BADDHAKONASANA**
page 226

13 **SETUBANDHA SARVANGASANA**
page 219

14 **VIPARITA KARANI**
page 216

15 **SAVASANA**
page 234

YOGA FOR AILMENTS

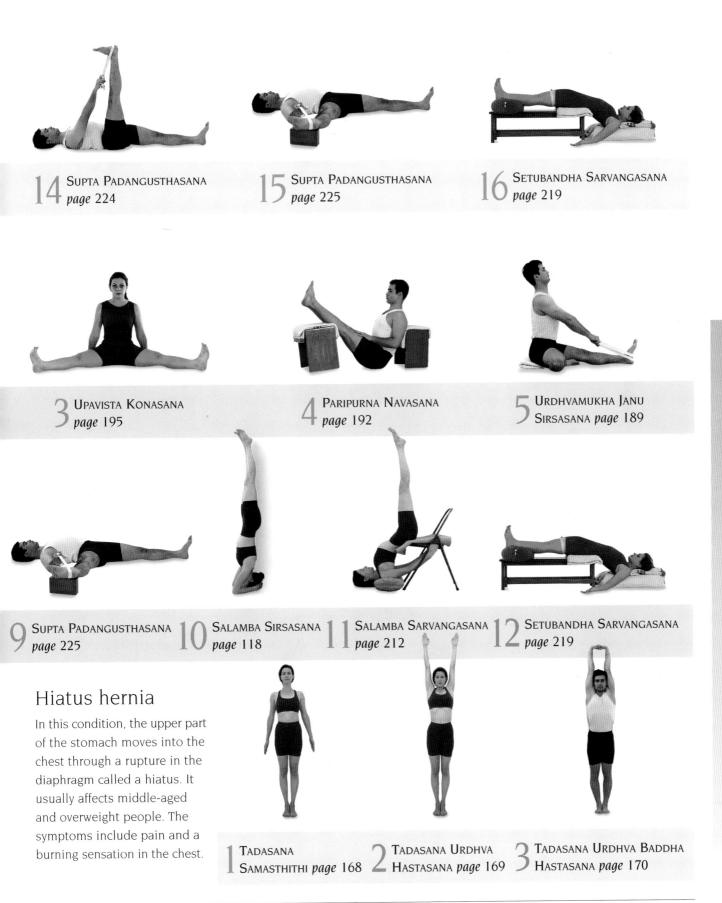

14 SUPTA PADANGUSTHASANA *page 224*

15 SUPTA PADANGUSTHASANA *page 225*

16 SETUBANDHA SARVANGASANA *page 219*

3 UPAVISTA KONASANA *page 195*

4 PARIPURNA NAVASANA *page 192*

5 URDHVAMUKHA JANU SIRSASANA *page 189*

9 SUPTA PADANGUSTHASANA *page 225*

10 SALAMBA SIRSASANA *page 118*

11 SALAMBA SARVANGASANA *page 212*

12 SETUBANDHA SARVANGASANA *page 219*

Hiatus hernia

In this condition, the upper part of the stomach moves into the chest through a rupture in the diaphragm called a hiatus. It usually affects middle-aged and overweight people. The symptoms include pain and a burning sensation in the chest.

1 TADASANA SAMASTHITHI *page 168*

2 TADASANA URDHVA HASTASANA *page 169*

3 TADASANA URDHVA BADDHA HASTASANA *page 170*

MEN'S HEALTH

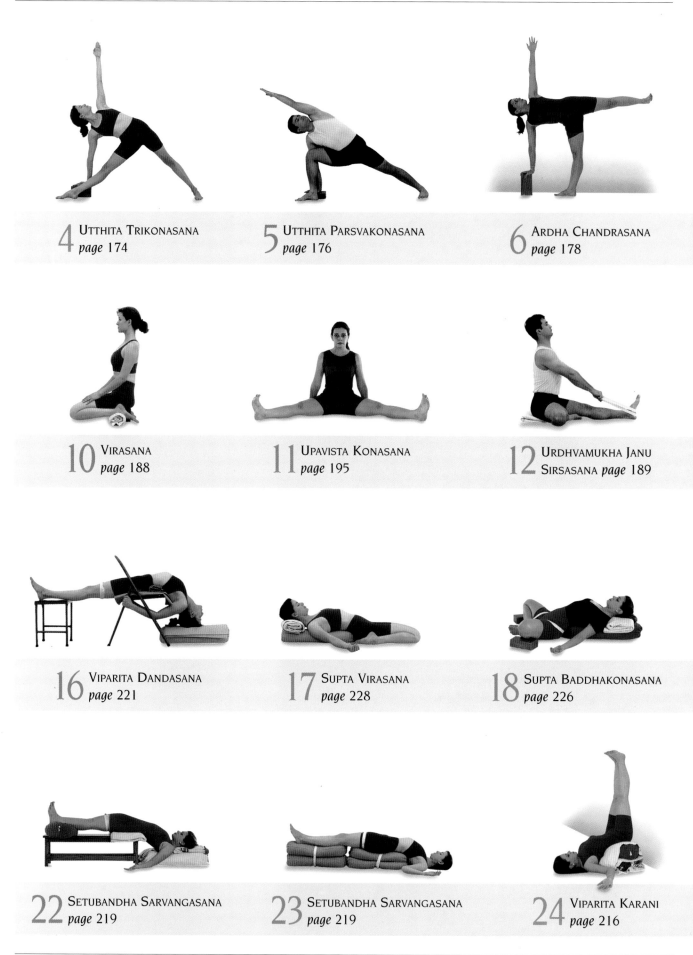

4 **UTTHITA TRIKONASANA** *page* 174

5 **UTTHITA PARSVAKONASANA** *page* 176

6 **ARDHA CHANDRASANA** *page* 178

10 **VIRASANA** *page* 188

11 **UPAVISTA KONASANA** *page* 195

12 **URDHVAMUKHA JANU SIRSASANA** *page* 189

16 **VIPARITA DANDASANA** *page* 221

17 **SUPTA VIRASANA** *page* 228

18 **SUPTA BADDHAKONASANA** *page* 226

22 **SETUBANDHA SARVANGASANA** *page* 219

23 **SETUBANDHA SARVANGASANA** *page* 219

24 **VIPARITA KARANI** *page* 216

YOGA FOR AILMENTS

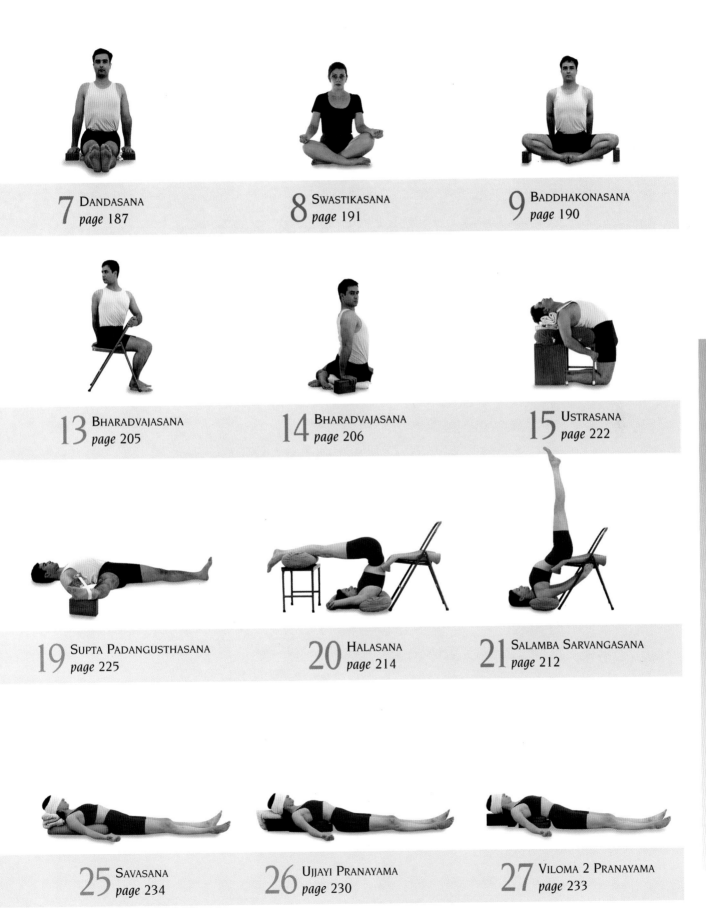

7 DANDASANA
page 187

8 SWASTIKASANA
page 191

9 BADDHAKONASANA
page 190

13 BHARADVAJASANA
page 205

14 BHARADVAJASANA
page 206

15 USTRASANA
page 222

19 SUPTA PADANGUSTHASANA
page 225

20 HALASANA
page 214

21 SALAMBA SARVANGASANA
page 212

25 SAVASANA
page 234

26 UJJAYI PRANAYAMA
page 230

27 VILOMA 2 PRANAYAMA
page 233

MEN'S HEALTH

Inguinal hernia

This occurs when the intestine protrudes through a weak point or tear in the lower layers of the abdominal wall. A direct inguinal hernia creates a bulge in the groin area while an indirect inguinal hernia descends into the scrotum.

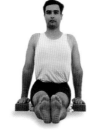

1 DANDASANA
page 187

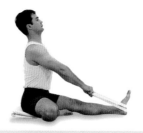

2 URDHVAMUKHA JANU
SIRSASANA page 189

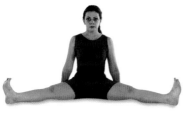

6 UPAVISTA KONASANA
page 195

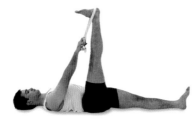

7 SUPTA PADANGUSTHASANA
page 224

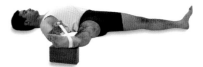

8 SUPTA PADANGUSTHASANA
page 225

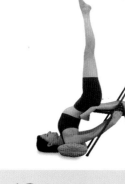

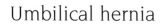

12 SALAMBA SARVANGASANA
page 212

13 SETUBANDHA SARVANGASANA
page 219

14 SETUBANDHA SARVANGASANA
page 219

Umbilical hernia

This condition sometimes affects infants, and occurs in the region of the umbilicus. It usually corrects itself naturally. It also occurs in adults when the intestine protrudes through the abdominal wall at the navel.

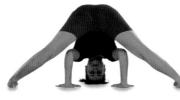

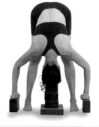

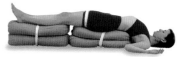

1 PRASARITA PADOTTANASANA
page 182

2 UTTANASANA
page 179

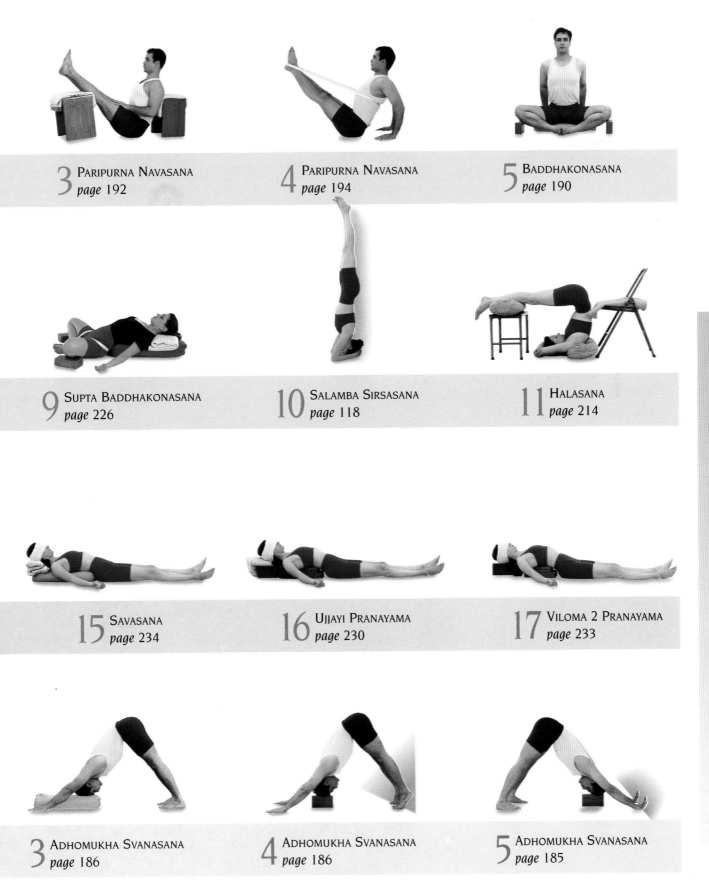

3 PARIPURNA NAVASANA
page 192

4 PARIPURNA NAVASANA
page 194

5 BADDHAKONASANA
page 190

9 SUPTA BADDHAKONASANA
page 226

10 SALAMBA SIRSASANA
page 118

11 HALASANA
page 214

15 SAVASANA
page 234

16 UJJAYI PRANAYAMA
page 230

17 VILOMA 2 PRANAYAMA
page 233

3 ADHOMUKHA SVANASANA
page 186

4 ADHOMUKHA SVANASANA
page 186

5 ADHOMUKHA SVANASANA
page 185

MEN'S HEALTH

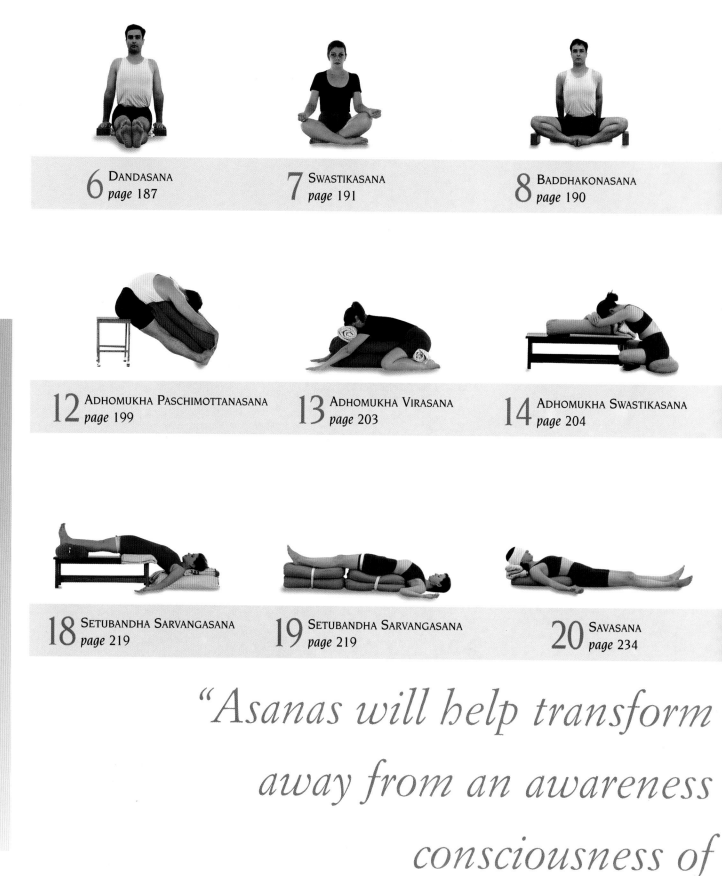

6 DANDASANA
page 187

7 SWASTIKASANA
page 191

8 BADDHAKONASANA
page 190

12 ADHOMUKHA PASCHIMOTTANASANA
page 199

13 ADHOMUKHA VIRASANA
page 203

14 ADHOMUKHA SWASTIKASANA
page 204

18 SETUBANDHA SARVANGASANA
page 219

19 SETUBANDHA SARVANGASANA
page 219

20 SAVASANA
page 234

"Asanas will help transform
away from an awareness
consciousness of

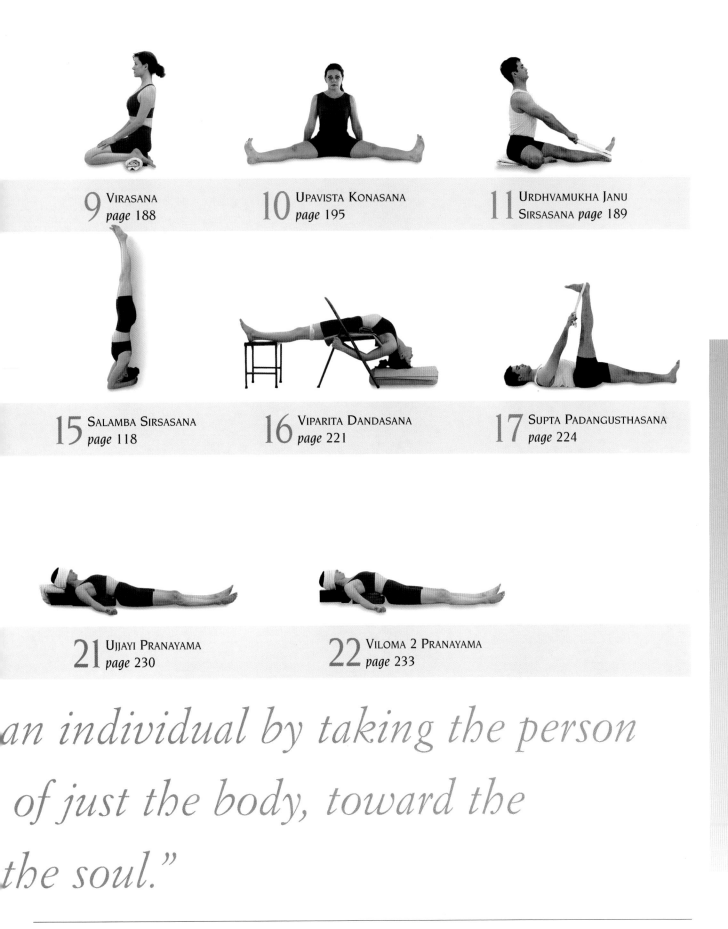

9 VIRASANA
page 188

10 UPAVISTA KONASANA
page 195

11 URDHVAMUKHA JANU
SIRSASANA *page* 189

15 SALAMBA SIRSASANA
page 118

16 VIPARITA DANDASANA
page 221

17 SUPTA PADANGUSTHASANA
page 224

21 UJJAYI PRANAYAMA
page 230

22 VILOMA 2 PRANAYAMA
page 233

MEN'S HEALTH

an individual by taking the person

of just the body, toward the

the soul."

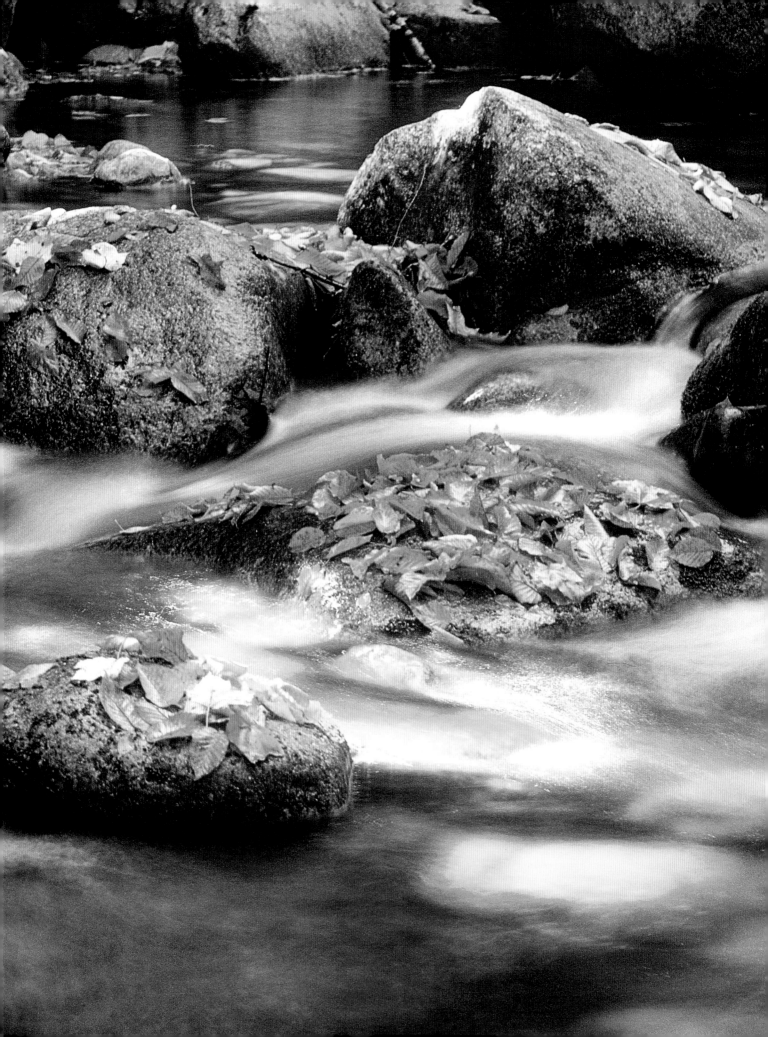

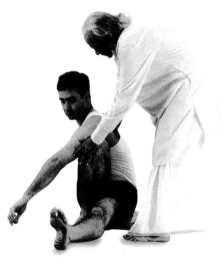

CHAPTER 6

"Our body is the bow and the asanas are the arrows to hit the target – the soul."

Iyengar Yoga Course

Learning a new subject requires dedication and perseverance. In yoga, the physical body, the sense organs, the emotions, mind, and consciousness are trained slowly and gradually. A beginner starts with simple asanas and progresses to more complex ones by building strength and concentration. Advanced students of yoga, too, should practice asanas in a logical sequence that allows them to experience the full effectiveness of each asana. Understanding sequencing is a gradual process. Just as a car cannot pick up speed in first gear, we cannot understand the subtleties and technical requirements of asanas.without time and patience.

Guide to your Yoga Practice

This course takes you from simple to complex asanas. Follow the sequence listed for each week, since this not only makes your practice more effective, but also minimizes the possibility of injury or strain.

People start yoga with many preconceptions. Some expect instant cures to ailments, and others assume that the simplest asanas will be difficult to achieve. These are usually people whose muscles are stiff, and whose posture is often faulty. Even the physically fit may not possess the stability of body or mind needed to practice correctly. A beginner must, therefore, practice asanas at a very basic level at first, and then continue practicing regularly, until the intelligence penetrates all the sheaths of his or her body (*see page* 24).

ADVICE FOR BEGINNERS

Initially, practice as many asanas of the sequence as you feel comfortable with. Do not exhaust your strength or stamina. Begin with small expectations. Restructuring muscles, bones, tissues, posture, and internal organs takes time. In Iyengar yoga, basic movements, like turning out the right foot or interlocking the fingers, are called "motions." More subtle movements like lifting the kneecap, tightening the groin, and drawing in the kidneys, are regarded as "actions." Motions get you into a posture, and actions refine it. Understand the motions first. Learn *how* to observe, rather than *what* you must observe. Grasping the essence of the asana is more important than getting the movements right. Some instructions may seem absurd or even impossible to beginners. Gradually, however, you will become aware of the complexity and subtlety of the body's movements in each increasingly simple maneuver, not

as an abstraction, but as a necessity. Eventually, understanding the actions of an asana will establish the rhythm and pace of your practice.

The yoga course begins with simple asanas which prepare the body to perform the more complicated asanas with ease. You will learn to access levels of yourself that you were unaware existed. The asana connects you to the inner world within you.

SCHEDULING YOUR PRACTICE

Practice asanas when you feel fresh and energetic. Early in the morning, if your muscles are not stiff, or in the early evenings, when the muscles are supple and free, is advisable. Do not practice after a heavy meal. The duration of your practice is flexible. Learn to know when to stop.

Make your yoga sessions a daily practice. If you are tired or a part of your body is aching, practicing asanas will relieve your body of tension and strain. Just keep the cautions at the beginning of each asana in mind.

GENERAL GUIDELINES

If you do not get a particular asana right, practice one with similar movements. The physical body, sense organs, emotions, mind, and consciousness are trained gradually in yoga. If you stop practicing a particular asana, the body loses a part of its intelligence. Practice different types of asanas.

If your legs ache, for instance, do not avoid your yoga session. Locate the discomfort, think about its cause, and understand how to remove it. Through your

HOLDING THE POSTURE
Concentrate completely when you are in the final posture

intelligence, introduce a soothing sensation into that area. Delve deep into your consciousness and extend a feeling of calm to the part of your body that needs it most.

YOUR ENVIRONMENT

Coordinate your practice with the state of your body and mind. Hot summer days can make you feel exhausted or dehydrated. Practice with props to relax. For example, perform Salamba Sarvangasana with the help of a chair and a bolster. Reclining asanas, inversions, and resting asanas are also suitable since they slow down the metabolism, calm all parts of the body and mind, and conserve energy. In winter, standing asanas, back bends, and inversions help combat colds, arthritis, and seasonal depression. Twists, forward bends, and inversions help counter the effects of damp conditions.

SEQUENCE

Practicing asanas in the prescribed order enhances their effectiveness as well as your experience of each asana. Understanding the significance of sequencing takes time. Grasp the subtleties and movements of each asana and its impact on your body before attempting to formulate an order which suits your personal needs. Follow the 20-Week Yoga Course until you feel confident enough to develop your own sequence. Those suffering from specific ailments, however, should follow the asana sequences appropriate to their condition, given in Chapter 5 (*see pages* 238-283).

TIMING

For as long as possible, hold the final posture for the recommended time to maximize the benefits and build strength. However, timing also depends on attention. The intelligence of the brain rises and drops very fast, but the body's intelligence cannot be awakened at the same speed. You have to bring awareness to all parts of the body for the whole time you are in the posture.

Ultimately, use your discrimination to decide the sequence, timing, and nature of the asanas you want

to practice, according to your age and physical condition. Keep your progress in developing an awareness and understanding of the asanas in mind. First, stretch and awaken your body and mind to the logic behind a series of asanas. Do not begin your session with a back bend, for instance. For those in perfect physical condition, cycles of asanas can be worked out fairly easily. If your condition is less than perfect, evolve a sequence which suits your body's requirements. There should be a physical, physiological, psychological, and spiritual rhythm in your practice of yoga.

BALANCE AND HARMONY
Yogacharya Iyengar in a variation of Bharadvajasana

FORMULATING YOUR OWN PRACTICE

All the asanas listed in the 20-Week Yoga Course are simple postures, made even easier with props. Practice Virabhadrasana 1 and 2 (*see pages 76 and 56*), against a wall for the first few weeks. Once you feel comfortable in the posture, practice without the support of the wall. Similarly, after about 6 months (although this can vary from person to person) of practicing Utthita Trikonasana, place your hand on the floor, instead of on the block. Attempt Halasana, Salamba Sarvangasana, and Urdhva Dhanurasana without props after 6 months. It might take up to 8 months to achieve Salamba Sirsasana without the support of the wall. Attempt Trianga Mukhaikapada Paschimottanasana after 6 months, sequencing it after Janu Sirsasana and Paschimottanasana. As your muscles and joints become supple, props will become a hindrance, and you will progress smoothly to the classic postures without them.

20-Week Yoga Course

Week 1

Asanas	Page
1. Tadasana Samasthithi *against a wall*	168
2. Tadasana Urdhva Hastasana *against a wall*	169
3. Tadasana Urdhva Baddha Hastasana *against a wall*	170
4. Uttanasana 1 *foam block & 5 wooden blocks*	179
5. Adhomukha Svanasana *3 blocks**	184
6. Dandasana *1 blanket & 2 blocks*	187
7. Virasana *2 blankets & 2 bolsters*	188
8. Adhomukha Virasana *2 blankets & 2 bolsters*	203
9. Paschimottanasana *1 stool & 2 bolsters (legs apart)*	198
10. Bharadvajasana *1 blanket & 2 blocks*	206
11. Setubandha Sarvangasana *4 bolsters*	219
12. Savasana	150

*blocks are wooden unless otherwise specified

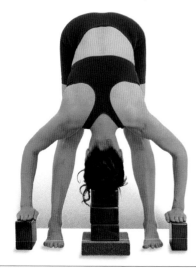

Week 2

Asanas	Page
1. Tadasana Samasthithi *against a wall*	168
2. Tadasana Urdhva Hastasana *against a wall*	169
3. Tadasana Urdhva Baddha Hastasana *against a wall*	170
4. Tadasana Paschima Baddha Namaskar	171
5. Utthita Trikonasana *1 block*	174
6. Uttanasana 1 *foam block & 5 wooden blocks*	179
7. Adhomukha Svanasana *3 blocks*	184
8. Dandasana *1 blanket & 2 blocks*	187
9. Virasana *2 blankets & 2 bolsters*	188
10. Urdhvamukha Janu Sirsasana *1 belt*	189
11. Baddhakonasana *2 blocks & 1 bolster (parallel to the hips)*	190
12. Adhomukha Virasana *2 blankets & 2 bolsters*	203
13. Paschimottanasana *2 bolsters & 1 belt (legs apart)*	198
14. Bharadvajasana *1 chair (sitting sideways)*	205
15. Supta Baddhakonasana *1 blanket, 1 bolster, 2 blocks & 1 belt*	226
16. Setubandha Sarvangasana *4 bolsters*	219
17. Savasana	150

Week 3

Asanas	Page
1. Tadasana Samasthithi *against a wall*	168
2. Tadasana Urdhva Hastasana *against a wall*	169
3. Tadasana Urdhva Baddha Hastasana *against a wall*	170
4. Tadasana Paschima Baddha Namaskar	171
5. Utthita Trikonasana *1 block*	174
6. Uttanasana 1 *foam block & 5 wooden blocks*	179
7. Adhomukha Svanasana *1 block (heels against a wall)*	186
8. Dandasana *1 blanket & 2 blocks*	187
9. Virasana *2 blankets & 2 bolsters*	188
10. Urdhvamukha Janu Sirsasana *1 belt*	189
11. Baddhakonasana *2 blocks & 1 bolster (parallel to the hips)*	190
12. Adhomukha Virasana *2 blankets & 2 bolsters*	203
13. Paschimottanasana *2 bolsters & 1 belt (legs apart)*	198
14. Bharadvajasana *1 chair (sitting sideways)*	205
15. Utthita Marichyasana *1 stool, 1 rounded block & a wall*	208
16. Supta Baddhakonasana *1 blanket, 1 bolster, 2 blocks & 1 belt*	226
17. Setubandha Sarvangasana *4 bolsters*	219
18. Savasana	150

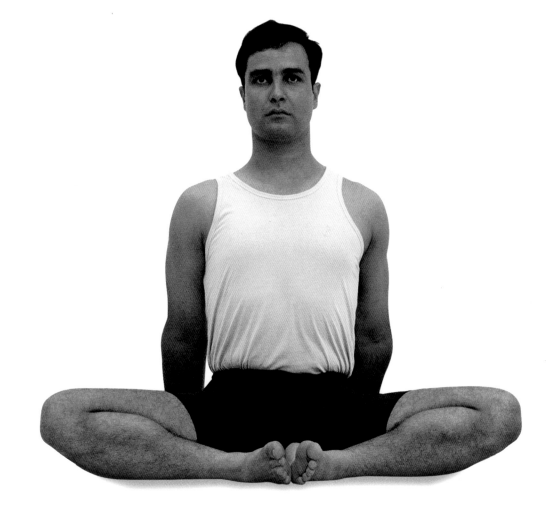

Week 4

Asanas	Page
1. Tadasana Samasthithi *against a wall*	168
2. Tadasana Urdhva Hastasana *against a wall*	169
3. Tadasana Urdhva Baddha Hastasana *against a wall*	170
4. Tadasana Paschima Baddha Namaskar	171
5. Tadasana Gomukhasana	173
6. Utthita Trikonasana *1 block*	174
7. Utthita Parsvakonasana *1 block*	176
8. Uttanasana *1 foam block & 5 wooden blocks*	179
9. Adhomukha Svanasana *1 block (heels against a wall)*	186

Asanas	Page
10. Dandasana *1 blanket & 2 blocks*	187
11. Virasana *1 rolled blanket & 1 block*	188
12. Urdhvamukha Janu Sirsasana *1 belt*	189
13. Swastikasana	191
14. Baddhakonasana *2 blocks & 1 bolster (parallel to the hips)*	190
15. Upavista Konasana	195
16. Adhomukha Virasana *2 blankets & 2 bolsters*	203
17. Paschimottanasana *2 bolsters & 1 belt (legs apart)*	198
18. Janu Sirsasana *1 stool, 1 blanket & 1 bolster*	200

Asanas	Page
19. Paschimottanasana *3 bolsters*	197
20. Bharadvajasana *1 chair (sitting sideways)*	205
21. Bharadvajasana *1 chair (legs through a chair back)*	205
22. Utthita Marichyasana *1 stool, 1 rounded block & a wall*	208
23. Parsva Virasana *1 rolled blanket & 2 blocks*	210
24. Supta Baddhakonasana *1 blanket, 1 bolster, 2 blocks & 1 belt*	226
25. Supta Padangusthasana *1 belt*	224
26. Setubandha Sarvangasana *4 bolsters*	219
27. Savasana	150

Week 5

Asanas	Page
1. Tadasana Samasthithi *against a wall*	168
2. Tadasana Urdhva Hastasana *against a wall*	169
3. Tadasana Urdhva Baddha Hastasana *against a wall*	170
4. Tadasana Paschima Baddha Namaskar	171
5. Tadasana Gomukhasana	173
6. Utthita Trikonasana *1 block*	174
7. Utthita Parsvakonasana *1 block*	176
8. Virabhadrasana 1	76
9. Virabhadrasana 2	56
10. Adhomukha Svanasana *1 block (heels against a wall)*	186
11. Prasarita Padottanasana *1 block or 1 bolster*	183
12. Uttanasana *1 foam block & 5 wooden blocks*	179
13. Dandasana *1 blanket & 2 blocks*	187
14. Virasana *1 rolled blanket & 1 block*	188
15. Urdhvamukha Janu Sirsasana *1 belt*	189
16. Swastikasana	191
17. Baddhakonasana 2 *blocks & 1 bolster (parallel to the hips)*	190
18. Upavista Konasana	195
19. Adhomukha Virasana *2 blankets & 2 bolsters*	203
20. Adhomukha Swastikasana *1 bench, 1 blanket & 2 bolsters*	204
21. Paschimottanasana *3 bolsters*	197
22. Janu Sirsasana *1 stool, 1 blanket & 1 bolster*	200

Asanas	Page
23. Paschimottanasana *1 stool & 2 bolsters*	198
24. Bharadvajasana *1 chair (sitting sideways)*	205
25. Bharadvajasana 1 *chair (legs through a chair back)*	205
26. Bharadvajasana *1 blanket & 2 blocks*	206
27. Utthita Marichyasana *1 stool, 1 rounded block & a wall*	208
28. Parsva Virasana *1 rolled blanket & 2 blocks*	211
29. Supta Baddhakonasana *1 blanket, 1 bolster, 2 blocks & 1 belt*	226
30. Supta Padangusthasana *1 belt*	224
31. Supta Padangusthasana *1 block & 1 belt*	225
32. Setubandha Sarvangasana *1 bench, 1 blanket & 2 bolsters*	219
33. Savasana	150

Week 6

Asanas	Page
1. Tadasana Samasthithi *against a wall*	168
2. Tadasana Urdhva Hastasana *against a wall*	169
3. Tadasana Urdhva Baddha Hastasana *against a wall*	170
4. Tadasana Paschima Namaskar	172
5. Tadasana Gomukhasana	173
6. Utthita Trikonasana *1 block*	174
7. Utthita Parsvakonasana *1 block*	176
8. Virabhadrasana 1	76
9. Virabhadrasana 2	56
10. Ardha Chandrasana *1 block*	178
11. Adhomukha Svanasana *1 bolster*	186
12. Prasarita Padottanasana *1 block or 1 bolster*	183
13. Uttanasana *1 foam block & 5 wooden blocks*	179
14. Adhomukha Paschimottanasana *1 stool & 2 bolsters*	199
15. Dandasana *1 blanket & 2 blocks*	187
16. Virasana *2 blankets & 2 bolsters*	188
17. Urdhvamukha Janu Sirsasana *1 belt*	189
18. Swastikasana	191
19. Baddhakonasana *2 blocks & 1 bolster*	190
20. Upavista Konasana	195
21. Paripurna Navasana *2 stools & 3 mats*	192
22. Adhomukha Virasana *2 blankets & 2 bolsters*	203

Week 7

WEEKS 5-7

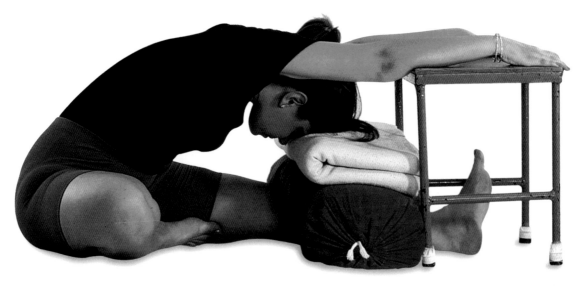

Week 8

Week 9

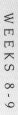

Week 10

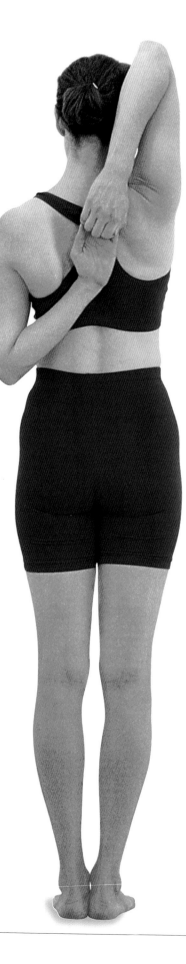

Week 11

Asanas	Page
1. Tadasana Samasthithi *against a wall*	168
2. Tadasana Urdhva Hastasana *against a wall*	169
3. Tadasana Urdhva Baddha Hastasana *against a wall*	170
4. Tadasana Paschima Namaskar	172
5. Tadasana Gomukhasana	173
6. Utthita Trikonasana *1 block*	174
7. Utthita Parsvakonasana *1 block*	176
8. Virabhadrasana 1	76
9. Virabhadrasana 2	56
10. Ardha Chandrasana *1 block*	178
11. Parsvottanasana	64
12. Adhomukha Svanasana *1 bolster*	186
13. Prasarita Padottanasana *1 block or 1 bolster*	183
14. Uttanasana *1 foam block & 5 wooden blocks*	179
15. Adhomukha Paschimottanasana *1 stool & 2 bolsters*	199
16. Dandasana *1 blanket & 2 blocks*	187
17. Virasana *2 blankets & 2 bolsters*	188

Asanas	Page
18. Urdhvamukha Janu Sirsasana *1 belt*	189
19. Swastikasana	191
20. Baddhakonasana *2 blocks & 1 bolster*	190
21. Upavista Konasana	195
22. Paripurna Navasana *2 belts*	194
23. Adhomukha Virasana *2 blankets & 1 bolster*	202
24. Adhomukha Swastikasana *1 bench, 1 blanket & 1 bolster*	204
25. Paschimottanasana *1 stool & 2 bolsters (legs together)*	198
26. Janu Sirsasana *1 stool, 1 blanket & 1 bolster*	200
27. Paschimottanasana *2 bolsters*	196
28. Bharadvajasana *1 chair (sitting sideways)*	205
29. Bharadvajasana *1 chair (legs through a chair back)*	205
30. Bharadvajasana *1 blanket & 2 blocks*	206
31. Marichyasana *1 blanket & 1 block*	207

Asanas	Page
32. Utthita Marichyasana *1 stool, 1 rounded block & a wall*	208
33. Parsva Virasana *1 blanket & 1 block*	210
34. Supta Baddhakonasana *1 blanket, 1 bolster, 2 blocks & 1 belt*	226
35. Supta Virasana *1 blanket & 1 bolster*	228
36. Supta Padangusthasana *1 belt*	224
37. Supta Padangusthasana *1 belt & 1 block*	225
38. Salamba Sarvangasana *1 chair, 1 blanket & 2 bolsters*	212
39. Halasana *1 chair, 1 stool, 1 blanket & 1 bolster*	214
40. Setubandha Sarvangasana *1 bench, 3 blankets & 1 bolster*	218
41. Viparita Karani *1 blanket, 1 block & 2 bolsters*	216
42. Savasana *1 blanket, 1 bolster & 1 bandage*	234

WEEKS 10-11

Week 12

Week 13

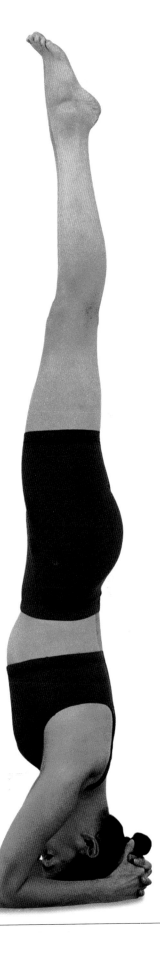

Week 14

Asanas	Page
1. Tadasana Samasthithi *against a wall*	168
2. Tadasana Urdhva Hastasana *against a wall*	169
3. Tadasana Urdhva Baddha Hastasana *against a wall*	170
4. Tadasana Paschima Namaskar	172
5. Tadasana Gomukhasana	173
6. Utthita Trikonasana 1 *block*	174
7. Utthita Parsvakonasana 1 *block*	176
8. Virabhadrasana 1	76
9. Virabhadrasana 2	56
10. Ardha Chandrasana 1 *block*	178
11. Parsvottanasana	64
12. Adhomukha Svanasana 1 *bolster*	186
13. Prasarita Padottanasana 1 *block or 1 bolster*	183
14. Uttanasana 1 *foam block & 5 wooden blocks*	179
15. Adhomukha Paschimottanasana 1 *stool & 2 bolsters*	199
16. Dandasana 1 *blanket & 2 blocks*	187
17. Virasana 2 *blankets & 2 bolsters*	188
18. Urdhvamukha Janu Sirsasana 1 *belt*	189
19. Swastikasana	191
20. Baddhakonasana 2 *blocks & 1 bolster*	190
21. Upavista Konasana	195
22. Paripurna Navasana 2 *belts*	194
23. Adhomukha Virasana 2 *blankets & 1 bolster*	202

Asanas	Page
24. Adhomukha Swastikasana 1 *bench, 1 blanket & 1 bolster*	204
25. Paschimottanasana 1 *stool & 2 bolsters (legs together)*	198
26. Janu Sirsasana 1 *stool, 1 blanket & 1 bolster*	200
27. Paschimottanasana 2 *bolsters*	196
28. Bharadvajasana 1 *chair (sitting sideways)*	205
29. Bharadvajasana *(legs through a chair back)*	205
30. Bharadvajasana 1 *chair 1 blanket & 2 blocks*	206
31. Marichyasana 1 *blanket & 1 block*	207
32. Utthita Marichyasana 1 *stool, 1 rounded block & a wall*	208
33. Parsva Virasana 1 *blanket & 1 block*	210
34. Supta Baddhakonasana 1 *blanket, 1 bolster, 2 blocks & 1 belt*	226
35. Supta Virasana 1 *blanket & 1 bolster*	228
36. Supta Padangusthasana 1 *belt*	224
37. Supta Padangusthasana 1 *belt & 1 block*	225
38. Salamba Sirsasana *against a wall*	118
39. Salamba Sarvangasana 1 *chair, 1 blanket & 1 bolster*	212
40. Halasana 1 *chair, 1 stool, 1 blanket & 2 bolsters*	214
41. Setubandha Sarvangasana 1 *bench, 3 blankets & 1 bolster*	218
42. Viparita Karani 1 *blanket, 1 block & 2 bolsters*	216
43. Savasana 1 *blanket, 1 bolster & 1 bandage*	234

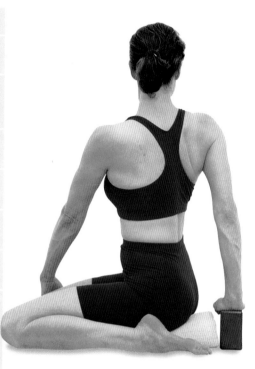

Week 15

Asanas	Page
1. Tadasana Samasthithi *against a wall*	168
2. Tadasana Urdhva Hastasana *against a wall*	169
3. Tadasana Urdhva Baddha Hastasana *against a wall*	170
4. Tadasana Paschima Namaskar	172
5. Tadasana Gomukhasana	173
6. Utthita Trikonasana 1 *block*	174
7. Utthita Parsvakonasana 1 *block*	176
8. Virabhadrasana 1	76
9. Virabhadrasana 2	56
10. Ardha Chandrasana 1 *block*	178
11. Parsvottanasana	64
12. Adhomukha Svanasana 1 *bolster*	186
13. Prasarita Padottanasana 1 *block or 1 bolster*	183

Week 16

Week 17

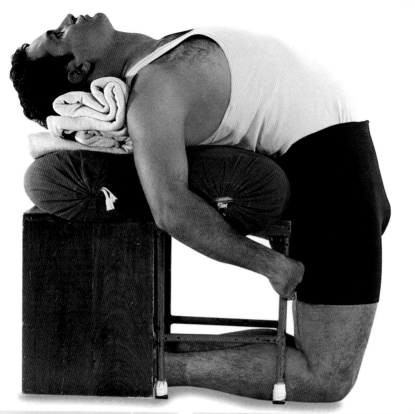

Asanas	Page
1. Tadasana Samasthithi *against a wall*	168
2. Tadasana Urdhva Hastasana *against a wall*	169
3. Tadasana Urdhva Baddha Hastasana *against a wall*	170
4. Tadasana Paschima Namaskar	172
5. Tadasana Gomukhasana	173
6. Utthita Trikonasana 1 *block*	174
7. Utthita Parsvakonasana 1 *block*	176
8. Virabhadrasana 1	76
9. Virabhadrasana 2	56
10. Ardha Chandrasana 1 *block*	178
11. Parsvottanasana	64
12. Adhomukha Svanasana 1 *bolster*	186
13. Prasarita Padottanasana 1 *block or 1 bolster*	183
14. Uttanasana 1 *foam block & 5 wooden blocks*	179
15. Adhomukha Paschimottanasana 1 *stool & 2 bolsters*	199
16. Dandasana 1 *blanket & 2 blocks*	187
17. Virasana 2 *blankets & 2 bolsters*	188
18. Urdhvamukha Janu Sirsasana 1 *belt*	189
19. Swastikasana	191
20. Baddhakonasana 2 *blocks & 1 bolster*	190
21. Upavista Konasana	195
22. Paripurna Navasana 2 *belts*	194
23. Adhomukha Virasana 2 *blankets & 1 bolster*	202
24. Adhomukha Swastikasana 1 *bench, 1 blanket & 1 bolster*	204

Asanas	Page
24. Adhomukha Swastikasana 1 *bench, 1 blanket & 1 bolster*	204
25. Paschimottanasana 1 *stool & 2 bolsters (legs together)*	198
26. Janu Sirsasana 1 *stool, 1 blanket & 1 bolster*	200
27. Paschimottanasana 2 *bolsters*	196
28. Bharadvajasana 1 *chair (sitting sideways)*	205
29. Bharadvajasana 1 *chair (legs through a chair back)*	205
30. Bharadvajasana 1 *blanket & 2 blocks*	206
31. Marichyasana 1 *blanket & 1 block*	207
32. Utthita Marichyasana 1 *stool, 1 rounded block & a wall*	208
33. Parsva Virasana 1 *blanket & 1 block*	210
34. Viparita Dandasana 1 *chair, 1 stool, 2 blankets 1 bolster & 1 belt*	221
35. Ustrasana 2 *stools, 1 blanket & 2 bolsters*	222

Asanas	Page
36. Supta Baddhakonasana 1 *blanket, 1 bolster, 2 blocks & 1 belt*	226
37. Supta Virasana 1 *blanket & 1 bolster*	228
38. Supta Padangusthasana 1 *belt*	224
39. Supta Padangusthasana 1 *belt & 1 block*	225
40. Salamba Sirsasana *against a wall*	118
41. Salamba Sarvangasana 1 *chair, 1 blanket & 1 bolster*	212
42. Halasana 1 *chair, 1 stool, 1 blanket & 2 bolsters*	214
43. Setubandha Sarvangasana 1 *bench, 3 blankets & 1 bolster*	218
44. Viparita Karani 1 *blanket, 1 block & 2 bolsters*	216
45. Savasana 1 *blanket, 1 bolster & 1 bandage*	234
46. Ujjayi Pranayama 2 *blankets, 2 foam blocks, 2 wooden blocks & 1 bandage*	230

Week 18

Asanas	Page
25. Paschimottanasana 1 *stool & 2 bolsters (legs together)*	198
26. Janu Sirsasana 1 *stool, 1 blanket & 1 bolster*	200
27. Paschimottanasana 2 *bolsters*	196
28. Bharadvajasana 1 *chair (sitting sideways)*	205
29. Bharadvajasana 1 *chair* *(legs through a chair back)*	205
30. Bharadvajasana 1 *blanket & 2 blocks*	206
31. Marichyasana 1 *blanket & 1 block*	207
32. Utthita Marichyasana 1 *stool, 1 rounded block & a wall*	208
33. Parsva Virasana 1 *blanket & 1 block*	210
34. Viparita Dandasana 1 *chair, 2 blankets & 1 bolster* *(feet against a wall)*	221
35. Ustrasana 2 *stools, 1 blanket & 2 bolsters*	222
36. Supta Baddhakonasana 1 *blanket, 1 bolster, 2 blocks & 1 belt*	226
37. Supta Virasana 1 *blanket & 1 bolster*	228
38. Supta Padangusthasana 1 *belt*	224
39. Supta Padangusthasana 1 *belt & 1 block*	225
40. Salamba Sirsasana *against a wall*	118
41. Salamba Sarvangasana 1 *chair, 1 blanket & 1 bolster*	212
42. Halasana 1 *chair, 1 stool,* 1 *blanket & 2 bolsters*	214
43. Setubandha Sarvangasana 1 *bench, 3 blankets & 1 bolster*	218
44. Viparita Karani 1 *blanket, 1 block & 2 bolsters*	216
45. Savasana 1 *blanket, 1 bolster & 1 bandage*	234
46. Ujjayi Pranayama 2 *blankets, 2 foam blocks* 2 *wooden blocks & 1 bandage*	230

Asanas	Page
1. Tadasana Samasthithi *against a wall*	168
2. Tadasana Urdhva Hastasana *against a wall*	169
3. Tadasana Urdhva Baddha Hastasana *against a wall*	170
4. Tadasana Paschima Namaskar	172
5. Tadasana Gomukhasana	173
6. Utthita Trikonasana 1 *block*	174
7. Utthita Parsvakonasana 1 *block*	176
8. Virabhadrasana 1	76
9. Virabhadrasana 2	56
10. Ardha Chandrasana 1 *block*	178
11. Parsvottanasana	64
12. Adhomukha Svanasana 1 *bolster*	186
13. Prasarita Padottanasana 1 *block or 1 bolster*	183
14. Uttanasana 1 *foam block* & 5 *wooden blocks*	179
15. Adhomukha Paschimottanasana 1 *stool & 2 bolsters*	199
16. Dandasana 1 *blanket & 2 blocks*	187
17. Virasana 2 *blankets & 2 bolsters*	188
18. Urdhvamukha Janu Sirsasana 1 *belt*	189
19. Swastikasana	191
20. Baddhakonasana 2 *blocks & 1 bolster*	190
21. Upavista Konasana	195
22. Paripurna Navasana 2 *belts*	194
23. Adhomukha Virasana 2 *blankets & 1 bolster*	202
24. Adhomukha Swastikasana 1 *bench, 1 blanket & 1 bolster*	204
25. Paschimottanasana 1 *stool & 2 bolsters (legs together)*	198

Asanas	Page
26. Janu Sirsasana 1 *stool, 1 blanket & 1 bolster*	200
27. Paschimottanasana 2 *bolsters*	196
28. Bharadvajasana 1 *chair (sitting sideways)*	205
29. Bharadvajasana 1 *chair* *(legs through a chair back)*	205
30. Bharadvajasana 1 *blanket & 2 blocks*	206
31. Marichyasana 1 *blanket & 1 block*	207
32. Utthita Marichyasana 1 *stool, 1 rounded block & a wall*	208
33. Parsva Virasana 1 *blanket & 1 block*	210
34. Viparita Dandasana 1 *chair, 2 blankets & 1 bolster* *(feet against a wall)*	221
35. Ustrasana 2 *stools, 1 blanket & 2 bolsters*	222
36. Supta Baddhakonasana 1 *blanket, 1 bolster, 2 blocks* & 1 *belt*	226
37. Supta Virasana 1 *blanket & 1 bolster*	228
38. Supta Padangusthasana 1 *belt*	224
39. Supta Padangusthasana 1 *belt & 1 block*	225
40. Salamba Sirsasana *against a wall*	118
41. Salamba Sarvangasana 1 *chair, 1 blanket & 1 bolster*	212
42. Halasana 1 *chair, 1 stool,* 1 *blanket & 2 bolsters*	214
43. Setubandha Sarvangasana 1 *bench, 3 blankets & 1 bolster*	218
44. Viparita Karani 1 *blanket, 1 block & 2 bolsters*	216
45. Savasana 1 *blanket, 1 bolster & 1 bandage*	234
46. Ujjayi Pranayama 2 *blankets, 2 foam blocks* 2 *wooden blocks & 1 bandage*	230

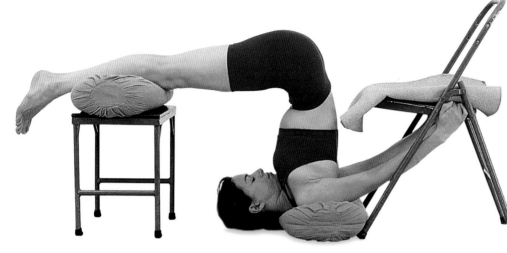

Week 19

20-WEEK YOGA COURSE

Week 20

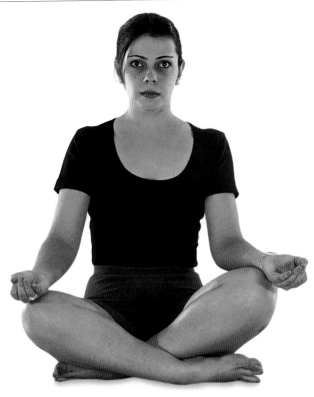

WEEKS 19-20

Internal Organs

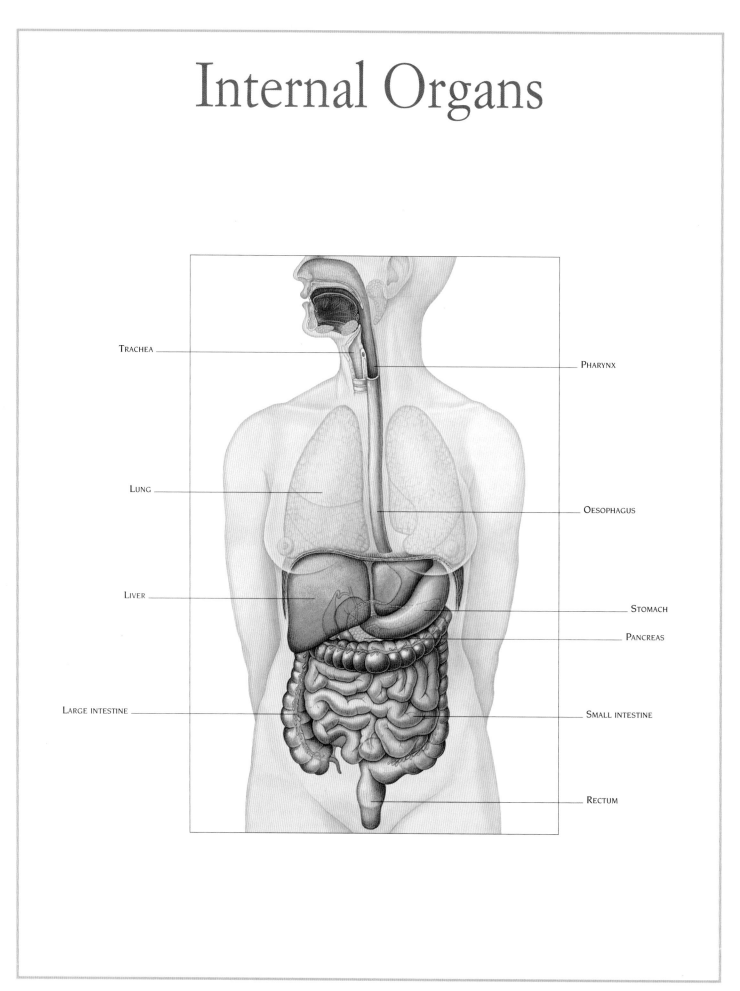

TRACHEA

PHARYNX

LUNG

OESOPHAGUS

LIVER

STOMACH

PANCREAS

LARGE INTESTINE

SMALL INTESTINE

RECTUM

Skeletal System

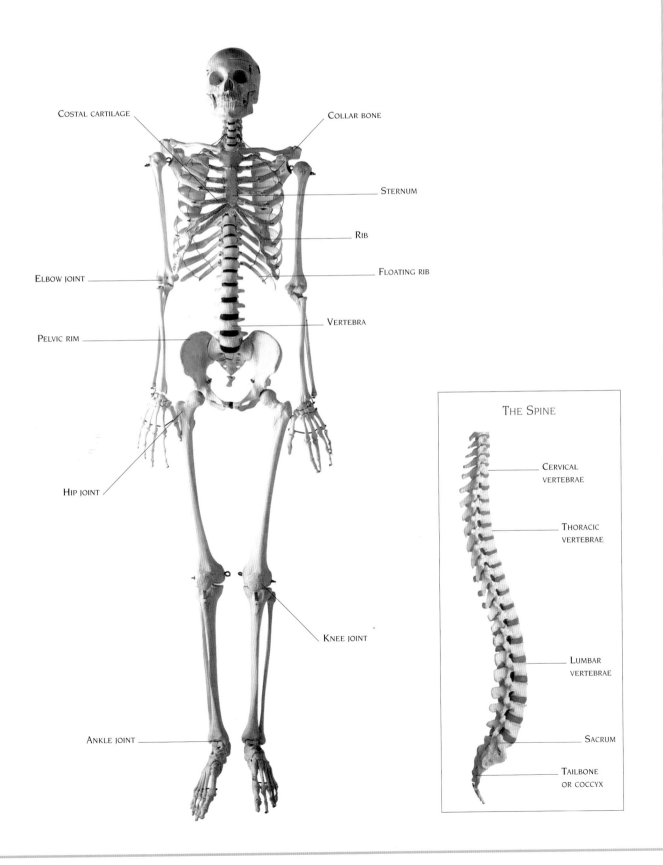

COSTAL CARTILAGE

COLLAR BONE

STERNUM

RIB

FLOATING RIB

ELBOW JOINT

VERTEBRA

PELVIC RIM

HIP JOINT

KNEE JOINT

ANKLE JOINT

THE SPINE

CERVICAL
VERTEBRAE

THORACIC
VERTEBRAE

LUMBAR
VERTEBRAE

SACRUM

TAILBONE
OR COCCYX

Muscular System

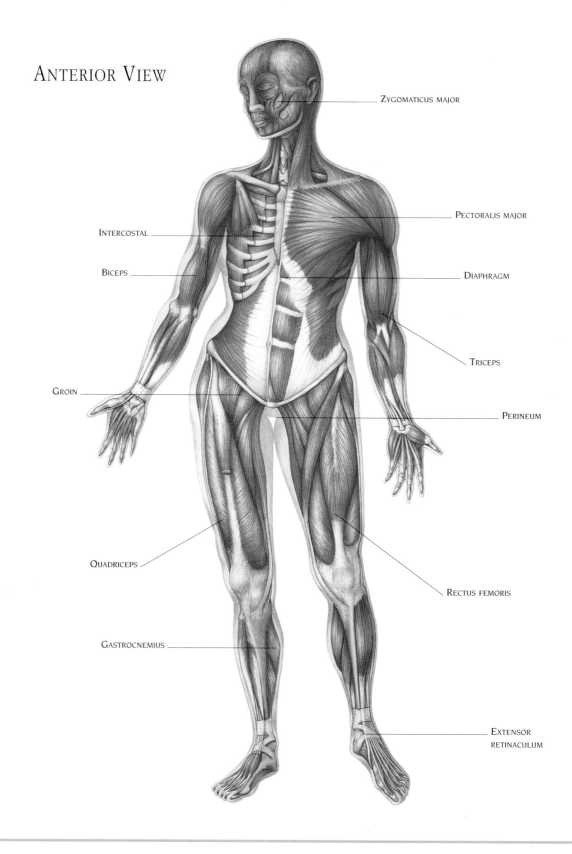

ANTERIOR VIEW

ZYGOMATICUS MAJOR

PECTORALIS MAJOR

INTERCOSTAL

DIAPHRAGM

BICEPS

TRICEPS

GROIN

PERINEUM

QUADRICEPS

RECTUS FEMORIS

GASTROCNEMIUS

EXTENSOR
RETINACULUM

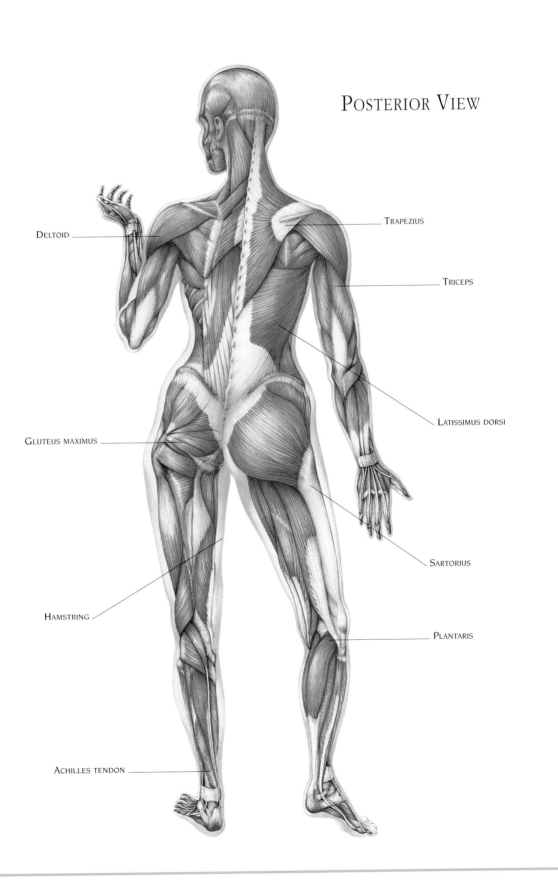

POSTERIOR VIEW

DELTOID

TRAPEZIUS

TRICEPS

LATISSIMUS DORSI

GLUTEUS MAXIMUS

SARTORIUS

HAMSTRING

PLANTARIS

ACHILLES TENDON

Glossary

Abhyantara inhalation

Ahankara false pride

Ahimsa creed of nonviolence

Ajna chakra energy or command chakra

Alabdha bhumikatva indisposition

Alasya laziness

Anahata chakra spiritual heart chakra

Anandamaya kosha the sheath of bliss, the most important of the 5 sheaths of the body, reached by the practice of yoga

Angamejaytatva unsteadiness in the body

Annamaya kosha anatomical sheath, one of 5 sheaths of the body

Antara-kumbhaka suspension of breath with empty lungs

Antaranga-sadhana emotional and mental discipline gained through following the 8 limbs or steps of yoga

Antaratma-sadhana quest for the soul gained through following the 8 limbs or steps of yoga

Anusaswami discipline

Aparigraha freedom from desire

Arambhavastha beginners' stage of yoga, practiced at the level of the physical body alone

Asmita egoism

Astanga yoga eight limbs: the steps to self-realization through the practice of yoga

Asteya freedom from avarice

Atman the self or soul

Avirati desire for sensual satisfaction

Ayama expansion or distribution of energy

Bahya exhalation

Bahya-kumbhaka suspension of breath with full lungs

Bahiranga-sadhana one of 3 yogic disciplines, comprising the practice of ethics

Bhakti marg path of love and devotion

Bharadvaja a sage, the father of the warrior Dronacharya

Bharanti darshana false knowledge

Brahmacharya chastity

Buddhi intelligence

Chitta the restraint of consciousness

Chittavritti an imbalance in the mental state

Chakras critical junctions in the body, notionally located along the spine, which, when activated by asanas and pranayama, transform cosmic energy into spiritual energy

Dharana concentration, the sixth limb or step of Astanga yoga

Dhyana freedom from attachments, the seventh stage of the 8 limbs or steps of Astanga yoga

Dronacharya son of the sage Bharadvaja and a major character in the epic, *Mahabharata*

Dorsal region the upper part of the body, relating especially to the back

Dukha misery or pain

Ekagra a focused state of mind

Floating ribs the last 2 pairs of ribs which are not attached to the sternum

Ghatavastha intermediate stage of yoga, when the mind and body learn to move together

Gheranda Samhita text on yoga, written by the sage Gheranda in the 15th century

Guru teacher; one who hands down a system of knowledge to a disciple

Guru-sishya parampara the tradition of teaching, dating back centuries, of teacher and student

Hatha yoga sighting the soul through the restraint of energy

Hathayoga Pradipika treatise on yoga compiled in the 15th century by the sage Svatmarama

Isvara pranidhana devotion to God

Jivatma the individual self

Jnana marg path of knowledge whereby the seeker learns to discriminate between the real and the unreal

Kaivalya freedom of emancipation

Karma marg path of selfless service without thought of reward

Karana sharira causal body, one of the 3 layers of the body

Karya sharira gross body, one of the 3 layers of the body

Kathopanishad ancient text circa 300-400 BC

Klesha sorrow caused by egoism, desire, ignorance and hatred

Ksipta a distracted mind

Kundalini divine, cosmic energy which is latent in every human being

Kumbhaka retention of energy

Leukorrhea excessive white vaginal discharge

Manas the mind

Manava (manusya) an intelligent and conscious being

Mahabharata the most ancient of the Indian epics, dating to the first millennium BC

Manipuraka chakra site of the sense of fear and apprehension

Manomaya kosha psychological sheath, one of the 5 sheaths of the body

Marichi a sage, son of Brahma, the creator of the universe

Menorrhagia abnormally heavy or long periods

Metrorrhagia bleeding in-between periods

Mudha a dull, inert mind

Muladhara chakra controls sexual energy

Nadi notional channels which distribute energy from the chakras through the body

Nirbija seedless

Niruddha a controlled and restrained mind

Nispattyavastha ultimate stage of yoga practice, the state of perfection

Niyama self-restraint

Parmatama the universal self

Parichayavastha third stage of yoga practice, when the intelligence and the body become one

Parigraha possessiveness

Patanjali, a sage, the founder of yoga; believed to have lived sometime between 300 BC-AD 300

Patanjali Yoga Darshana corpus of aphorisms on yoga, compiled between 300 BC-AD 300 and usually attributed to the sage Patanjali

Perineum the area between the thighs, behind the genital organs and in front of the anus

Pramada indifference

Prakriti shakti energy of nature

Prana vital energy or life-force

Pranamaya kosha life-force sheath, one of the 5 sheaths of the body

Pranayama control of energy through breathing

Pratyahara mental detachment from the external world

Psoriasis an ailment leading to dry and scaly patches on the skin

Purusha shakti energy of the soul

Raja yoga sighting the soul through the restraint of consciousness

Rajasic spicy, pungent foods that overstimulate the body and mind

Sahasrara chakra the most important chakra which, when uncoiled, brings the seeker to freedom

Samadhi self-realization

Samsahya doubt

Samayama integration of the body, breath, mind, intellect, and self

Santosha contentment

Sarvaanga sadhana holistic practice which integrates the body, mind and the self

Sattvic natural, organic vegetarian food

Satya truth

Saucha cleanliness

Scoliosis a curved spine

Shakti vital energy and the sense of self, which determine a person's emotions, will power and discrimination

Shvasa-prashvasa uneven respiration or unsteadiness

Styana reluctance to work

Suksma sharira the subtle body, one of the 3 layers of the body

Svadhyaya to study one's body, mind, intellect, and ego

Svatmarama sage, author of *Hathayoga Pradipika*

Swadhishtana chakra site of worldly desires

Tamasic food containing meat or alcohol

Tapas austerity gained through the committed practice of yoga

Vijnamaya kosha intellectual sheath, one of the 5 sheaths of the body

Viksipta a scattered, fearful mind

Virabhadra a legendary warrior

Vishuddhi chakra seat of intellectual awareness

Vyadhi physical ailments

Yama ethical codes for daily life

Yoga the path which integrates the body, senses, mind, and the intelligence, with the self

Yogacharya a teacher and a master of yogic traditions

Yoga-agni the fire of yoga which, when lit, ignites the kundalini

Yogabhrastha falling from the grace of yoga

Yoga marg penultimate stage of the journey to self-realization, when the mind and its actions are brought under control

Yoga Sutras a collection of aphorisms on the practice of yoga, attributed to the sage Patanjali

Yogi a student, a seeker of truth

Names of Asanas

NAME	TRANSLATION
Adhomukha Paschimottanasana	Downward-facing intense west stretch
Adhomukha Svanasana	Downward-facing dog posture
Adhomukha Swastikasana	Downward-facing cross-legged posture
Adhomukha Virasana	Downward-facing hero posture
Ardha Chandrasana	Half moon posture
Baddhakonasana	Bound angle posture
Bharadvajasana	Torso stretch
Bharadvajasana on a chair	Torso twist
Dandasana	Staff posture
Halasana	Plough posture
Janu Sirsasana	Head on knee posture
Marichyasana	Spinal twist
Paripurna Navasana	Full boat posture
Parsva Virasana	Spinal twist in hero posture
Parsvottanasana	Intense chest stretch
Paschimottanasana	Intense west stretch posture
Prasarita Padottanasana	Expanded leg intense stretch
Salamba Sarvangasana	Shoulderstand
Salamba Sirsasana	Headstand
Savasana	Corpse posture
Setubandha Sarvangasana	Full bridge posture
Supta Baddhakonasana	Reclining bound angle posture
Supta Padangusthasana	Reclining big toe posture
Supta Virasana	Reclining hero posture
Swastikasana	Cross-legged posture
Tadasana	Mountain posture
Tadasana Samasthithi	Steady and firm mountain posture
Tadasana Gomukhasana	Mountain posture with hands held in the shape of a cow's face
Tadasana Paschima Baddha Namaskar	Mountain posture with bound arms
Tadasana Paschima Namaskar	Mountain posture with hands in prayer position
Tadasana Urdhva Baddha Hastasana	Mountain posture with bound hands
Tadasana Urdhva Hastasana	Mountain posture with arms stretched up
Trianga Mukhaikapada Paschimottanasana	Three limbs intense west stretch posture
Ujjayi Pranayama	Expanding conquest of life-force energy
Upavista Konasana	Seated wide-angle posture
Urdhva Dhanurasana	Upward-facing bow posture
Urdhvamukha Janu Sirsasana	Upward-facing single leg forward bent knee posture
Ustrasana	Camel posture
Uttanasana	Intense forward stretch posture
Utthita Marichyasana	Standing spinal twist
Utthita Parsvakonasana	Extended side angle stretch
Utthita Trikonasana	Extended triangle posture
Viloma 2 Pranayama	Interrupted breathing cycle
Viparita Dandasana	Inverted staff posture
Viparita Karani	Inverted lake posture
Virabhadrasana 1	Warrior posture 1
Virabhadrasana 2	Warrior posture 2
Virasana	Hero posture

Index

Acknowledgments

AUTHOR'S ACKNOWLEDGMENTS
B.K.S. Iyengar would like to thank
Dr Geeta S. Iyengar for her expert advice as
a consultant on this project; Parth Amin,
producer of the CDs *Yoga for You* and *Yoga for
Stress*; Prof R.N. Kulhali, for his help on the
text; Zarina Kolah, yoga consultant, for her
help in compiling the text and liaising with the
DK editorial team. The author also wishes to
thank the photographer, Harminder Singh, and
the models, Roshen Amin, Leslie Peters,
Ali Dashti, and Jawahar Bangera.

PUBLISHER'S ACKNOWLEDGMENTS
Dorling Kindersley would like to thank the
Ramayani Memorial Yoga Institute, Pune for
their permission to use photographs of
B.K.S. Iyengar from their archives; Sudha Malik,
the yoga consultant for the project; Amit
Kharsani for the Sanskrit calligraphy; and
R.C. Sharma for indexing. The publishers would
also like to thank Clare Sheddon and Salima
Hirani for their help and advice during the
early stages of the project; and Abhijeet
Mukherjee for production support.

PICTURE CREDITS
Dorling Kindersley would like to thank the
following for their kind permission to
reproduce their photographs: National
Museum, New Delhi p10, p21 bl, p25 t, p33 t,
& b, p35 b, p37; American Institute of Indian
Studies, New Delhi p11 tl, p12,p24, p28 t, p39;
Max Alexander p22; Akhil Bakshi p13 b, p36;
Subhash Bhargava p31; Joe Cornish p29; Andy
Crawford p11 tr & b; Antonia Deutch p19 b;
Ashok Dilwali p8 , p161; Ashim Ghosh p40;
Steve Gorton p11 tr; Alistair Hughes p26;
Madan Mohan Jain p13 t (2 photographs
superimposed), p34 t; Subir Kumedan p384;
Ashok Nath p21; Stephen Parker p6; Janet
Peckam p15; Kim Sayer p158; Hashmat Singh
p154; Arvind Teki p157; Pankaj Usrani p28 b;
Amar Talwar p236; Colin Walton p159 tc.
DK Copyright pages (shot by Harminder Singh)
48-49, 56-59, 76-79, 177 b, 178, 182, 183 t
184-185, 186 tr, 191-195, 199-203, 216-218,
219 t, 222-223, 226-227.
Every effort has been made to trace the
copyright holders of photographs. The
publisher apologizes for any omissions and
will amend further editions.

KEY: t=top; r=right; l=left; c=center; b=bottom

Useful Addresses

B.K.S. Iyengar website: **www.bksiyengar.com**

USA

Iyengar Yoga Institute of Greater New York,
27 W. 24th Street, NY 10010 USA

BKS Iyengar Yoga Center of Philadelphia
125 No. 23rd St., Philadephia,
PA 19103 USA

Iyengar Yoga Institute of Los Angeles,
8233 West 3rd Street, LA, CA 90048 USA

Iyengar Yoga Institute of San Francisco,
2404 27th Ave, SF, CA 94116, USA

Full Circle Yoga Institute
3910 El Cajon Blvd.
San Diego, California 92105 USA

Intermountain BKS Iyengar Yoga Association.
c/o Craig Kurtz
154 W. Bayaud Ave
Denver, Colorado 80223-1824 USA

Yoga Institute of Miami
9350 So. Dadeland Blvd.
Miami, Florida 33143 USA

Big Island Yoga Center
P.O. Box 2233
Kealakekua, Hawaii 96750 USA

Boise Yoga Center
3541 Ticonderoga
Boise, Idaho 83706 USA

BKS Iyengar Yoga Association of Massachusetts
c/o Tina Goldsmith 144 Pearl St. #3,
Cambridge, Massachusetts 02139 USA

Yoga Circle
c/o Gabriel Halpern 401 W Ontario,
Chicago, IL 60610 USA
TheMeiste@yogacircle.com

Yoyoga, Inc
c/o Joan Budilovsky P.O. Box 5013
Oak Brook, IL 60522 USA
www.yoyoga.com

BKS Iyengar Yoga Association of the Midwest Bioregions
P.O. Box 8051,Ann Arbor,
Michigan 48103 USA

Winona Yoga Center
686 W. 5th St.,Winona,
Minnesota 55987 USA

Iyengar Yoga School of Northern New Jersey
10 Franklin Turnpike Waldwick
New Jersey 07463 USA

CANADA

Yoga Center Toronto
2428 Yonge Street, Toronto, ON M4P 2H4,
Canada

Center de Yoga Iyengar de Montréal
919 Mont-Royal Est
Montréal, Québec Canada H2J 1X3

Ottawa Iyengar Yoga Teachers
10 Henderson Avenue, Suite 105
Ottawa, Ontario, Canada K1N 7P1